Social Work in Health Settings

Practice in Context

Fourth edition

Judith L. M. McCoyd, Toba Schwaber Kerson, and Associates

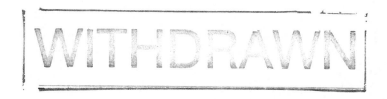

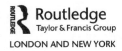

Routledge
Taylor & Francis Group

LONDON AND NEW YORK

First edition published 1989 (revised) by Haworth Press Inc
Second edition published 1997 by Haworth Press Inc
Third edition published 2010 by Routledge

This edition published 2016
by Routledge
2 Park Square, Milton Park, Abingdon, Oxon OX14 4RN

and by Routledge
711 Third Avenue, New York, NY 10017

Routledge is an imprint of the Taylor & Francis Group, an informa business

British Library Cataloguing-in-Publication Data
A catalogue record for this book is available from the British Library.

Library of Congress Cataloging in Publication Data
A catalog record for this book has been requested.

ISBN: 978-1-138-92435-2 (hbk)
ISBN: 978-1-138-92436-9 (pbk)
ISBN: 978-1-315-68442-0 (ebk)

Typeset in Times New Roman
by Swales & Willis Ltd, Exeter, Devon, UK

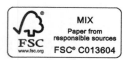

Printed and bound by CPI Group (UK) Ltd, Croydon, CR0 4YY

Social Work in Health Settings

Social Work in Health Settings: Practice in Context maintains its use of the Practice in Context (PiC) decision-making framework to explore a wide range of social work services in health care settings. The PiC framework is used to cover a broad range of social work practice sites, settings, and populations over 30 case chapters.

Fully updated to reflect the landscape of health care provision in the United States since the Affordable Care Act was passed, the cases are grounded by "primer" chapters to illustrate the necessary decisional and foundational skills for best practices in social work in health settings. The cases cover working with both individuals and groups of clients across the life course and the PiC framework helps maintain focus on each of the practice decisions a social worker must make when working with a variety of clients from military veterans to HIV-positive children.

The ideal textbook for social work in health care and clinical social work classes, this thought-provoking volume thoroughly integrates social work theory and practice, and provides an excellent opportunity for understanding particular techniques and interventions.

Judith L. M. McCoyd is Associate Professor of Social Work at Rutgers University, The State University of New Jersey, School of Social Work, USA, with focus on clinical practice, loss and grief, and interprofessional education.

Toba Schwaber Kerson is Mary Hale Chase Professor Emeritus in Social Science at the Graduate School of Social Work and Social Research, Bryn Mawr College, Bryn Mawr, Pennsylvania, USA, and a Fulbright Specialist.

"The new edition of this classic text offers the most comprehensive and insightful analysis of social work practice in health care found in any textbook. The cases are new and discuss cutting-edge issues including transgender health, genetic testing and counseling, immigrant health, and international public health. Of particular value are the discussions of each case that identify new learning and that model reflective practice skills. Because it presents contemporary issues influencing the context for, and the process of, social work decision-making in the accessible form of case studies, *Social Work in Health Settings* is strongly recommended as a textbook for students as well as advanced practitioners."

Goldie Kadushin, University of Wisconsin-Milwaukee, USA

"The fourth edition of McCoyd and Kerson's *Social Work in Health Settings* makes a strong case for its impact and utility for social workers in health care. This well-written and consistently edited book allows each contributor to speak in her own voice. The range of settings and social work roles presented expands our understanding of social work in health care while the casebook format helps the reader to see reflective social workers in action. Social work educators will also find the book useful for teaching generalist social work practice."

Julie S. Abramson, University at Albany, SUNY, USA

Contents

Figures

Tables

Contributors

Senayish Addis, M.S.S., has been a social worker at the Hospital of the University of Pennsylvania, USA, for the past 9 years and a Liver Transplant Social Worker for the past 7 years.

Annick Barker, M.S.S., L.C.S.W., is a mental health therapist at Health Care for the Homeless, a Federally Qualified Health Center in Baltimore, MD, USA.

Juli E. Birmingham, M.Ed., is a counselor at the Special Immunology Family Care Center at the Children's Hospital of Philadelphia, USA.

Laura Boyd, M.S.W., is a Team Lead in the EPSDT Department at Health Partners Plans in Philadelphia. She was formerly a social worker in the Center for Children with Special Health Care Needs at St. Christopher's Hospital for Children, also in Philadelphia, USA.

Michelle K. Brooks, M.S.S., L.C.S.W., is the Director of Psychosocial Services for Penn Homecare and Hospice, an entity of the University of Pennsylvania Health System. Ms. Brooks' social work practice focus has been working with patients and families at the end of life and in bereavement.

Laudy Burgos, M.S.W., L.C.S.W., is a social worker at Mount Sinai Hospital in New York City, USA, where she works in the OB/GYN unit. She is also faculty for Icahn School of Medicine at Mt. Sinai Hospital.

Deborah Calvert, M.S.W., L.S.W., is a social worker at the Special Immunology Family Care Center at the Children's Hospital of Philadelphia, USA.

Helaine Ciporen, M.S.W., M.Ed., L.C.S.W., is a social worker at Mount Sinai Hospital in New York City, USA. She works in the Pediatric Endocrinology and Diabetes department.

Rachel E. Condon, B.A., is a graduate student in social work at Boston University, USA.

Reneé C. Cunningham, M.S.S., is the Associate Director at Center in the Park, USA, where she is responsible for general operations, strategic planning, and evaluation, as well as supervising key staff and managing contractual obligations for major contracts.

Judith A. DeBonis, Ph.D., L.C.S.W., is an assistant professor at the California State University, Northridge, USA, and is the Principal Investigator for the Garrett Lee Smith Suicide Prevention Campus Grant. As part of the CSWE Social Work and Integrated Behavioral Healthcare Project, she is working to infuse integrated behavioral health and primary care into master's level social work education.

Helen Dombalis, M.S.W., M.P.H., is the Director of Programs for the National Farm to School Network in Washington, DC, USA.

Emily Duffy, L.C.S.W., served as the Camp Achieve coordinator from 2005 to 2007 and has continued to work with children and families as a pediatric behavioral health consultant, and most recently as a school social worker.

Kathleen "Casey" Durkin, M.S.S.A., L.I.S.W.-S., is a clinical social worker with over 30 years' experience, and has a private practice serving individuals aged 3–93: groups, couples, and families.

Jennifer L. Fenstermacher, M.S.S., L.C.S.W., is a social worker at the Nemours/A. I. duPont Hospital for Children in Wilmington, DE, USA, where she works on the general pediatrics short stay unit.

Patricia A. Findley, Dr.P.H., M.S.W., L.C.S.W., is Associate Professor of Social Work at the Rutgers University School of Social Work, USA, the Special Assistant to the Dean for Interprofessional Health Initiatives, and the Newark MSW Campus Coordinator.

Bambi Fisher, L.C.S.W., is a social work manager in pediatrics at Mount Sinai Medical Center and on the faculty at the Icahn School of Medicine at Mount Sinai, USA.

Jennifer D. Greenman, M.S.W., L.S.W., is a social worker at the Special Immunology Family Care Center at The Children's Hospital of Philadelphia, USA.

Anne P. Hahn, Ph.D., L.C.S.W.-C., is a social worker at Johns Hopkins Bayview Medical Center in Baltimore, MD, USA, where she works on the burn unit.

Phyllis Braudy Harris, Ph.D, A.C.S.W., L.I.S.W., is Professor and Chair of the Sociology & Criminology Department, Director of the Aging Studies at John Carroll University, USA, and is the founding co-editor of *Dementia*: *The International Journal of Social Research and Practice.*

Russell Healy, M.S.W., L.C.S.W., is a clinical social worker in private practice in central New Jersey, USA, and a doctoral student in the Rutgers School of Social Work's D.S.W. program.

Kathy Helzlsouer, M.D., M.H.S., is a medical oncologist and epidemiologist with a practice focus on cancer prevention and cancer survivorship. She is an adjunct professor at the Johns Hopkins University Bloomberg School of Public Health, USA, and founding Director of the Prevention and Research Center at Mercy Medical Center, Baltimore, MD, USA.

Jessica Hertzog, M.S.W., is a social worker at the Children's Hospital of Philadelphia, USA, and works in the Center for Fetal Diagnosis and Treatment, the Garbose Special Delivery Unit, and the NIICU.

Jennifer Diem Inglis, M.S.W., is a social worker at the Children's Hospital of Philadelphia, USA, and and works in the Fetal Heart Program and in the Garbose Special Delivery Unit.

Anne C. Jones, Ph.D., L.C.S.W., is a clinical professor at the University of North Carolina at Chapel Hill, USA, and and currently serves as the Co-Principal Investigator for the UNC-PrimeCare, an integrated behavioral health training grant funded by HRSA.

Toba Schwaber Kerson, D.S.W., Ph.D., is Mary Hale Chase Professor Emeritus in Social Science at the Graduate School of Social Work and Social Research, Bryn Mawr College, Bryn Mawr, Pennsylvania, USA, and a Fulbright Specialist.

John Krall, L.C.S.W., is the Program Manager of the Special Immunology Family Care Center at the Children's Hospital of Philadelphia, USA.

Jessica E. Lee, M.S.S., L.S.W., is a Ph.D. candidate at Bryn Mawr College Graduate School of Social Work, and she conducts research with and serves refugee communities in Philadelphia, USA.

Sue Livingston, B.S., began her career in education, teaching preschool, elementary, and middle school. She has spent the past 19 years at the Epilepsy Foundation Eastern Pennsylvania, USA, as education coordinator, and was instrumental in the development and management of Camp Achieve.

Sarah L. Maus, L.C.S.W., A.C.S.W., is a social worker at Abington Memorial Hospital, Jefferson Health, USA, where she is the manager of the Muller Institute for Senior Health.

Judith L. M. McCoyd, Ph.D., Q.C.S.W., L.C.S.W., is Associate Professor of Social Work at Rutgers University, The State University of New Jersey, School of Social Work, USA, with focus on clinical practice, loss and grief, and interprofessional education.

Shana L. Merrill, M.S., L.C.G.C., is a clinical genetic counselor at the Hospital of the University of Pennsylvania in Philadelphia, PA, USA, who specializes in rare tumor predisposition syndromes, cardiovascular genetic predispositions, and neurogenetic counseling.

Regina Miller, M.S.S., L.C.S.W., C.C.T.S.W., is a Social Work Team Leader at the Hospital of the University of Pennsylvania, USA, where she has worked for the past 11 years in Solid Organ Transplantation.

Arden Moulton, L.M.S.W., M.P.S., is a social worker at the Mount Sinai Hospital in New York City, USA, and Program Coordinator of the Woman to Woman Program.

Julianne Oktay, M.S.W, Ph.D., is Professor Emeritus at the University of Maryland, USA, School of Social Work. Dr. Oktay has done extensive research in social work in health, and has published two books on breast cancer: *Breast Cancer in the Life Course* and *Breast Cancer Daughters Tell Their Stories*.

Heather K. Ousley, M.S.S, M.S., is a social worker at the Children's Hospital of Philadelphia, USA, and works in the Center for Fetal Diagnosis and Treatment, the Garbose Special Delivery Unit, and the NIICU.

Kathleen Ray, Ph.D., L.C.S.W., is a social worker at the War Related Illness and Injury Study Center at the Veterans Administration in East Orange, NJ, USA.

Kathleen Rounds, Ph.D., M.P.H., M.S.W., is professor at the University of North Carolina, USA, at Chapel Hill School of Social Work.

Susan Scarvalone, M.S.W., L.C.S.W.-C., is a clinical research therapist at the Prevention and Research Center, Mercy Medical Center in Baltimore, MD, USA, where she works with cancer patients and their families to promote quality of life during and after treatment, and participates in clinical research initiatives.

Dasi Schlup, M.S.W., L.C.S.W., is a clinical social worker at Women's and Children's Hospital of the University of Missouri Health Care, USA. Her practice covers the Newborn Intensive Care Unit and High Risk Obstetrics.

Jessica Scott, M.G.H., C.G.C., is a certified genetic counselor specializing in hereditary cancer genetics at the University of Maryland Medical Center in Baltimore, MD, USA.

Cindy Sousa, Ph.D., M.S.W., M.P.H., is an assistant professor at the Graduate School of Social Work and Social Research at Bryn Mawr College, USA, where her work focuses on local and global dimensions of trauma, resilience, and health.

Laurie Stewart, M.S.S., L.S.W., is a social worker in the NICU at St. Christopher's Hospital for Children, USA.

Parangkush Subedi, M.S., M.P.H., is a resettled Bhutanese refugee and works at Philadelphia's Health Department. He initiated the Health Focal Point project with the Bhutanese American Organization Philadelphia.

Marikate Taylor, B.A., M.A., started her career in the nonprofit sector in 2012. She serves as the Information and Communications Coordinator for the Epilepsy Foundation Eastern PA, USA, contributing to efforts to improve qualitative measurement, reporting, and marketing efforts.

Rachel Warner, M.S.W, L.C.S.W., is a social at the Special Immunology Family Care Center at The Children's Hospital of Philadelphia, USA.

Allison Werner-Lin, Ph.D., L.C.S.W., Ed.M., is assistant professor at the School of Social Policy and Practice at the University of Pennsylvania, USA, where she conducts research addressing psychosocial aspects of genomic testing. She maintains a private practice with families affected by hereditary cancer syndromes and bereavement.

Traci Wike, Ph.D., M.S.W., is an assistant professor at Virginia Commonwealth University School of Social Work, USA.

Bonnie Fader Wilkenfeld, Ph.D., L.C.S.W., has extensive experience working in a variety of health care settings, most recently as a clinical social worker at a medical center consisting of a hospital, residential facility, and school for individuals with severe and profound multiple disabilities.

Nancy Xenakis, L.C.S.W., M.S., is Associate Director, Social Work Services at the Mount Sinai Hospital, New York City, USA.

Lisa de Saxe Zerden, M.S.W., Ph.D., is the Associate Dean for Academic Affairs at the University of North Carolina at Chapel Hill School of Social Work, USA, and is the Principal Investigator for UNC-PrimeCare, an integrated behavioral health training grant funded by HRSA.

Acknowledgments

Our immense gratitude goes first and foremost to our chapter contributors who shared their practice decisions with humility, humor, and honesty – this book obviously could not exist without these seasoned professionals. I am deeply grateful for Toba S. Kerson's mentorship and willingness to trust me to carry on her work with this casebook. My parents, Kathleen J. Moyer and Ivan W. Moyer, also deserve acknowledgment as they taught me by experience about many of the health issues covered here during the time we were working on this edition. Finally, I thank my "home team" – sons Ryan and Ian, Jim, the M.o.B., Anne and Corey – I could not have survived this year without you all.

Judith L. M. McCoyd

In some form, *Social Work in Health Settings: Practice in Context* has been a part of me since I became a social worker 50 years ago. It was a way to marry my sociological world view, my social worker's sensitivity to the pain of others, and my need to intervene in the most respectful ways possible. Also, it was a means to keep valued colleagues and former students with me. Many years ago, the excellent Judith L. M. McCoyd, then a doctoral student, assisted me the third time I wrote the book and contributed a case. Now, the book is hers.

This time around, edition four is for Jennie who sparkles plenty, Larry who loves a lot, and Leo who loves to learn.

Toba Schwaber Kerson

Chapter 1

Practice in Context

The framework

Toba Schwaber Kerson, Judith L. M. McCoyd, and Jessica Euna Lee

Social Work in Health Settings presents a framework called "Practice in Context," which the first author has used for the past 40 years as a tool for teaching and evaluation. The primary subject of the framework is the relationship between social worker and client because it is through trustworthy, strong, knowledgeable, and skill-based relationships with clients and others that social workers help clients to reach their goals (Beresford, Croft, & Adshead, 2007; Kerson & McCoyd, 2002). As a concept, "relationship" can be interpreted in diverse ways. It is an association or involvement, a connection by blood or marriage, or an emotional or other connection between people.

The definition of the social worker/client relationship used here is based in the work of others. Sociologist Erving Goffman, and anthropologist Gregory Bateson, theorize about some structural aspects of relationship such as the interactional focus, the connection of a relationship to its milieu, and the rules that inform or govern a relationship. Bateson uses the word *interaction*, and Goffman the word *encounter*, to be as precise as possible about their subjects. For this framework, *interaction* and *encounter* are seen as factors in a broader concept.

Goffman suggests that when studying interaction, the proper focus is not on the individual and his or her psychology, but rather the syntactical relations among the acts of different persons who are mutually present to one another (Goffman, 1981). To understand interaction, one must understand not the separate individuals but what occurs *between* them. Goffman (1966) further alludes to the special mutuality of immediate interaction:

> When two persons are together, at least some of their world will be made up out of the fact (and consideration for the fact) that an adaptive line of action must always be pursued in this intelligently helpful or hindering world. Individuals sympathetically take the attitude of others present, regardless of the end to which they put the information thus acquired. (p. 16)

Thus, in interaction, there is always a shared sense of situation and a capacity, in some way, to be in the place of the other, no matter what each participant's purpose in the interaction.

Goffman places relationship in context when he develops the notion of a "membrane" that "wraps" the interaction and, to some extent, separates it from its surroundings. "Any social encounter," he writes, "any focused gathering is to be understood, in the first instance, in terms of the functioning of the 'membrane' that encloses it cutting it off from a field of properties that could be given weight" (Goffman, 1961, p. 79). Still, while the relationship can be viewed and defined in its own right, it remains intimately related to the world outside of it.

Thus, Goffman says, "An encounter provides a world for its participants, but the character and stability of the world is intimately related to its selective relationship to the wider one" (Goffman, 1961, p. 80).

The rules that inform a relationship and the uses that the participants make of those rules are also part of Goffman's and Bateson's analyses of relationship. According to Bateson, interaction is the "process whereby people establish common rules for the creation and understanding of messages" (Bateson, 1971, p. 3). Goffman adds to this definition by noting that in encounters, rules are considered and managed rather than necessarily followed; that is, rules may shape interaction, but they also may be influenced by the participants. He writes:

> Since the domain of situational proprieties is wholly made up of what individuals can experience of each other while mutually present, and since channels of experience can be interfered with in so many ways, we deal not so much with a network of rules that must be followed as with rules that must be taken into consideration, whether as something to follow or carefully to circumvent. (Goffman, 1966, p. 42)

Social workers add a psychological dimension to these more structural views of relationship. We say that relationship has to do with people's emotional bonding. Also, the relationship between social workers and clients is a catalyst in that through understanding, support, nurturing, education, and the location of necessary resources, we help clients to address problems. Thus, the relationship affirms and motivates the client. In the same way, this forming of a helping relationship is not an end in itself but a means to help clients to reach their goals. In this book, the word *client* stands for any notion of a client unit, that is, an individual, family, program, organization, city, state, country, or advocacy effort that engages the services of a social worker who will help this entity to reach its goals.

Thus, for this framework, the relationship between social worker and client is defined using both sociological and psychological concepts. The sociological contributions have to do with structure; the focus is on interaction rather than on individual participants, on the use of rules, on the relationship's connection to (or separation from) its surroundings or context. The psychological contributions are the purposive, feeling, catalytic, and enabling dimensions. Here, the relationship of social worker and client means one or more purposive encounters intended to be catalytic and enabling whose structure and rules for interaction are set by dimensions of context as well as by decisions made by the participants.

Practice in Context framework

According to the Practice in Context (PiC) framework, the two basic elements that structure the relationship between social worker and client are (1) the "context" in which the relationship occurs and (2) the "practice decisions" that social worker and client make about the form and nature of the relationship. Context and practice decisions act as a matrix for the relationship, a supporting and enclosing structure. By determining many of the rules by which the work of social worker and client proceeds, context and practice decisions define the possibilities for relationship. Although elements such as personality, nature and degree of illness, psychosocial assessment, and cultural background contribute to the relationship, they are characteristics of the individuals involved and not the interaction.

This approach or framework is not a generic practice theory because it is not a system of ideas meant to explain certain phenomena or relations. Nor is it a model, because it does not show proportions or arrangements of all of its component parts. Here are simply described elements of context and practice that structure the relationship of social worker and client. Three overarching purposes help the social worker to: (1) clarify the work, (2) understand alterable and unalterable dimensions of practice and context, and (3) evaluate work in light of these dimensions. Each is meant to help the social worker reflect upon the decisions and actions of the social worker. With client participation, the social worker understands and tries to influence context and constructs the relationship in ways that will help meet client goals. Thus, PiC is about the craft of social work – the skills with which social workers manage dimensions of practice.

Context

To assume that possibilities for the work are completely determined within the social worker/client relationship is unrealistic, and may contribute to disappointment and a sense of failure on the part of the participants, evaluators of service, and funding sources. To a great extent, dimensions of context determine many of the rules for the helping relationship (Kerson, 2002). Context means the set of circumstances or facts that surround a particular event or situation, the surrounding conditions that form the environment within which something exists or takes place. Bateson defines context as a "collective term for all those events which tell the organism among what set of alternatives he must make his next choice" (Bateson, 1975, p. 289). He adds to this the notion that "however widely *context* be defined, there may always be wider contexts a knowledge of which would reverse or modify our understanding of particular items" (Bateson, 1971, p. 16). Although context is a limitless concept, and focusing on certain dimensions means ignoring others, to intervene effectively means that one has to be able to consider and assess the circumstances that constitute the situational conditions under which one is working.

The present framework addresses three dimensions of context that we continue to think have the most direct and describable consequences for the relationship between social workers and clients in health care settings: policy, technology, and organization. These elements are considered most important because of the ways each affects the structure of and possibilities for the social worker/client relationship. Policies increasingly provide rules specifying the services that clients may receive, who may provide them and under what conditions, and how services are to be evaluated. Organizations are also rule makers, setting the structure for service delivery and defining the nature of service often at the behest of policymakers. Finally, in this era when the means of communication continue to expand and change and technological interventions have us questioning definitions of life, death, gender, parenthood, etc., the impact of technology on the relationship between social worker and client is enormous. Social workers' understanding of and comfort with a great range of technologies enhance their roles as "translators" for their clients, their opportunities for empathy, as well as their general relational capacities. In addition, computer-assisted technologies and the internet have altered and expanded the ways in which social workers communicate, receive, and collect information. Thus, technology contributes to the content of the relationship, expands possibilities, and may also constrain it. The salience of each dimension and the ways those dimensions are related depend on the particular setting. In effect, these contextual factors may at most determine, or at least contribute to, the rules of the game, and as they change, the constraints and possibilities for action are altered as well.

Policy

Policies are explicit and definite sets of principles or courses of action that guide a range of actions in specific situations. They are always related to the political economy, that is, the ways by which a government manages its material resources. Policies address entitlements and restrictions; that is, they provide rightful claims, privileges or prerogatives, and/or they impose limitations and constraints. To think of policies in these ways demonstrates the need for social workers to understand the policies that may affect their clients. This understanding can help clients interpret policies and gain access to services. To be an effective client advocate one must excel at understanding the policies that shape clients' entitlements and restrictions.

The status of the populations with which social work is most concerned and the status of the social work profession itself are, to a great extent, reflections of the political economy and the social policies of any particular period in U.S. history (Mechanic, 2005). Understanding health disparities is critical in this regard (Barr, 2014; Schlesinger, 2011). Peter Drucker notes that every 10 years or so, society reorganizes its world view, basic values, political and social structure, arts, and major institutions (Drucker, 2004). Thus, social policy is dynamic, fluid, and responsive to many powerful forces within and outside of a particular community or society. This seems to be a time of enormous social reform in the United States, and hopes are high for reforming the health care system (Barr, 2011, 2014; Blank & Burau, 2014; Little, 2007).

For example, the Patient Protection and Affordable Care Act (ACA) was signed into law in 2010 (Congress, 2010). An aim of the ACA is to not only expand access to public health insurance but also improve the quality of health care provided through Medicare and Medicaid. Also referred to as ObamaCare, the ACA expands health care coverage to all U.S. citizens and aims to reduce U.S. health care spending. Many of its provisions took effect in 2014 and key enactments relevant to social work include:

- individual mandate to purchase insurance and requirement for most employers to offer coverage to workers;
- improved access to public health insurance (e.g., expanding Medicaid to people below 130% of the federal poverty line);
- reforms to improve health care quality and reduce health spending;
- regulation of the health insurance industry (e.g., setting minimum benefit standards for qualified health benefit plans and prohibiting health insurers from refusing coverage based on patients' medical histories (Congress, 2010; ObamaCare Facts, n.d.; Gorin, Pollack, Darnell, & Allen, 2014).

The base for policy is the law which in the form of legislation, administrative regulations, and/or court decisions affects every dimension and nuance of social work practice in any health setting (Kerson, 2002). Dickson (2014) identifies the following aspects of the health and human services that are permeated by the law:

1   the entrance into and exit from health and human services delivery systems;
2   the criteria used to determine eligibility for treatment, benefits, or services;
3   the rights to which patients and clients are entitled;
4   the rights to which professionals and staff are entitled;
5   the way in which health and human services programs are administered and regulated;
6   the relationship between the professional and the patient or client;
7   the practice of the health and human services professional (p. 3).

Therefore, in order to understand the policies that shape their practice, social workers must be able to understand the laws that affect the policies.

Another critical policy for social workers in health care settings is the Health Insurance Portability and Accountability Act of 1996 (HIPAA) that recognizes the importance of privacy of medical records. HIPAA regulations aim to assure the privacy and confidentiality of consumers' health information by defining (1) the rights of individuals, (2) administrative obligations of covered entities, and (3) the permitted uses and disclosures of protected information (NASW, 2001; U.S. Department of Health and Human Services, 2015). HIPAA defines "protected health information" as individually identifiable health information in any media that is held or transmitted by a covered entity (U.S. Department of Health and Human Services, 2015). Social workers are considered covered entities if they transmit protected health information for which HHS has a standard. HIPAA has implications for social workers working in public health, research, and direct practice. Such information can be as obvious as medical records and diagnoses or as seemingly "common" as whether a patient is indeed at the medical facility. The 2013 Omnibus rule provides updated guidance on HIPAA compliance. The revisions that HIPAA has undergone in the last decade demonstrate the need to respond to ever changing dimensions of technology (Morgan, 2013) and to be aware of the limits to information that can be shared when making referrals.

No matter what level they work on, social workers must be able to contribute to, interpret, and influence policy in order to advocate for their clients and the profession. Decisions regarding which populations to serve, allocation of resources, planning, and programming are too often made before social work practitioners become involved, and it is far easier to affect the structure of a program before it is instituted rather than after. These activities are also most beneficial to clients when clients and social workers advocate together. In addition, involvement in policy formulation helps the social work profession to broaden and strengthen its influence. When policy has a negative effect on clients or the profession, a united and concerted lobbying effort can stem the tide.

Historically, the presence of social work has been strongest in areas such as maternal and child health, as well as services to veterans, where social workers have been involved in developing policy on national, state, and local levels (Margolis & Kotch, 2013; Kerson, 1981, 1985). To a great extent, the policies social workers must familiarize themselves with depend on the populations with whom they work and the institutions for whom they work. Current foci of health-related social policy are on trying to control and/or cap costs and to incorporate new knowledge and the development of new technologies into the notion of cost control (Arrow et al., 2009; Mas & Seinfeld, 2008; Miller & West, 2009).

Controlling the costs of health care

In order to try to control health care costs, the federal government has created a series of responses. Many responses can be understood under the rubric of managed care. For several decades, managed care, which promises both service efficacy and cost containment, has been a focal point for influencing policy formulation and advocating for clients (Acker, 2010; Acker & Lawrence, 2009; Emanuel, 2012). At this point, the term managed care is used for almost any strategy or structure put forth to manage the quality or cost of health care. Broadly defined, managed care encompasses any measure that, from the perspective of the purchaser of health care, favorably affects the price of services, the site where the services are received, or their utilization. As such, it represents a continuum – from plans that, for example, do no more than require prior authorization of inpatient stays, to the staff model health maintenance organization that employs its doctors and assumes risk for delivering a comprehensive benefit package. Ideally, managed care should not simply seek to reduce costs; rather it should strive to maximize value, which includes a concern with quality and access.

A managed care system integrates the financing and delivery of appropriate medical care by contracting with selected providers who offer comprehensive health services to enrolled members for a predefined yearly or monthly premium, providing financial incentives for patients to stay within system for their care, instituting utilization and quality controls to which providers have agreed (and which increasingly seem to relate to patient satisfaction), and by requiring that the providers assume varying degrees of financial risk. More and more, providers are asked to balance the patients' needs with cost control (Summer & Hoadley, 2014).

Now, managed care is forcing social work to reexamine our practices and the values that support the missions of organizations. It is critical that social workers in health care see this current panacea-like solution as a series of complex strategies viewed by important and powerful interest groups as ways to control the costs of health care. Managed care is not the enemy of social work, nor is it a simple way to solve deep, complicated problems; in fact, it is not even an *it*. The fact that managed care is altering roles and tasks for social workers in many settings again underscores the importance of social workers being able to interpret policy and advocate for clients.

One early managed care schema was the development of diagnosis-related groups (DRGs). Formerly, the hospital charged the insurer what it decided it had spent to care for the patient, plus a small percentage in addition. Now, the insurer pays the hospital based on the patient's diagnosis (DRG). According to the DRG classification, if the diagnosis indicates 4 days of hospitalization, the hospital will be paid for 4 days of hospitalization only, even if the patient stays in the hospital longer. When the patient is hospitalized beyond the number of days indicated in the schema, the hospital must absorb the extra cost. Consequently, there is great pressure on the hospital to discharge the patient and great pressure on the social worker to make prompt and appropriate arrangements for the patient to return to the community. Thus, a social worker who previously may have had weeks to develop a relationship with, and an adequate discharge plan for, a patient, now may have a matter of days or hours in which to accomplish the same task. More and more, the focus of the health care facility is for the social worker to expedite the patient's discharge as soon as the physician can no longer justify the stay, or, even more important now, before the insurer denies payment for services rendered. However, an aim of the ACA is to expand access to public health insurance while also improving the quality of health care provided through Medicare and Medicaid.

Technology

For contemporary health care, the development and cost of technology relate directly to policy formulation. Technology and the organizations that house and/or distribute it account for a good deal of the astronomical costs of medical care today. The United States' passion for, rapid acceptance of, and diffusion of "high-tech" solutions means that hospitals, health professionals, patients, and families demand the best possible high-tech care, no matter what the cost. Technology circumscribes practice just as policy and the law provide parameters for practice. As Jasanoff (2008) says:

As prime custodians of the "is" and the "ought" of human experience, science and the law wield enormous power in society. Each plays a part in deciding how things are in the world, both cognitively and materially; each also helps shape how things and people should behave, by themselves and in combination. (p. 767)

Technology is applied science – the ways in which a social group satisfies its material needs. In the broadest sense, technology means the concrete, practical solutions people invent or discover; this can mean mechanical ventilation or Motivational Interviewing techniques, computer systems or new consumer-marketed genetic testing, anything that involves solving problems with specific techniques. In the present framework, technology primarily refers to medical/scientific inventions that are used for diagnosis or treatment: medication, surgical techniques, life-sustaining machinery, or ways of viewing or measuring bodily functions and, in addition, ways in which we collect, manage, and disseminate information and new possibilities for interaction in relation to both diagnosis and treatment. It is through the development of technology as well as management of lifestyle issues that we are expanding possibilities for treating illness and extending life (Steinbrook, 2009). Because of techno-logical development, for example, we are able to respond to conditions in-utero, keep people alive who would otherwise die, and redefine many conditions from fatal to chronic.

Technology also means information management, the rise of electronic record keeping, and the computerization of all imaginable kinds of data (Tjora & Scambler, 2009). It can also be said that new communication technology is transforming the social work profession just as it is affecting many others. For example, one only has to think of the enormous amount of research that Gary Holden has been able to present to social workers in health care from Gopher Resources for Social Workers to World Wide Web Resources for Social Workers, to the present day professional news services – Information for Practice (IP) (Holden, 2009). As National Association of Social Workers (NASW) web designer Ebony-Jackson says, "Social media technology, texting via phone and e-mail messaging are revolutionizing the way people communicate" (Sfiligoj, 2009). This means e-clinical work, e-therapy, social networking websites, chat rooms, distance learning, as well as other virtual efforts, etc. (Serafini, Damianakis, & Marziali, 2007) and new learning techniques such as e-health, tele-health, interactive video, video conferencing, and social work rooms on the Web (Groshong & Phillips, 2015; Matusitz & Breen, 2008).

Meanwhile, the development of life-sustaining and other technologies raise perplexing ethical and legal problems in health care (Morrison & Monagle, 2013). Sometimes, the extension of life can mean greatly diminished life quality. Invariably, life-sustaining technol-ogies and interventions develop prior to the development of ethical and normative guidance for dealing with outcomes of such technologies (full body scans and personalized genetic testing are examples; see McCoyd, 2009 for analysis of fetal diagnosis). In other situations, medical solutions may be dehumanizing and/or produce negative side effects. Each raises new questions related to confidentiality, privacy, and record keeping. Current concerns about confidentiality stem from these technological developments. Determining who has the right to access information – the individual or group paying for the care, the individual receiving the care, the individual with access to the computer system, etc. – has yet to be resolved satisfactorily. (See above for discussion of how the HIPAA Privacy Rule helps.)

For social workers, sometimes the lack of medical means to intervene in an illness cre-ates opportunities for psychosocial intervention. Historically, social workers had important roles in the care of people with venereal diseases and tuberculosis, in part because medical interventions were inadequate to treat the illnesses. Before the discovery of penicillin permitted treatment of syphilis at an early stage with a single injection, treatment required many outpatient visits over a period of 18 months. The social worker's role was to ensure that patients returned for prolonged outpatient treatment; they also educated patients and their consorts about the infection. Contemporary situations provide similar opportunities. With diseases such as AIDS and Alzheimer's, for which there are not yet adequate medical treatments, social workers help garner the social support needed to live with the illness. With other conditions, such as end-stage renal disease and severe burns, technology provides life support, and the social worker helps the patient and family to live with both the illness and the technology. Each of these circumstances provides opportunities for social work. In these ways, the presence or absence of technological solutions help to shape the parameters of the relationship between social worker and client.

Organization

Just as policy and technology structure practice, so does organization. An organization is defined here as a body of people structured for some end or work, and the administrative personnel or apparatus of that agency, business, or institution (Hasenfeld & Garrow, 2012). Increasingly, to understand organizational context means to be knowledgeable about multiple, complex systems involving varied funding streams, auspices, professional, and nonprofessional providers, and public, not-for-profit, and for profit agencies with varied degrees of authority. An insensitivity towards these demands or to contextual issues will inhibit service effectiveness. In the grand scheme of the delivery of health care, even the simplest organization has close ties to very large and complex networks of service. To compete in today's health care marketplace, most health care organizations are in the midst of transforming themselves in order to become more efficient and to control costs. For professional social workers, there can be no more hiding out in an office and ignoring all of the forces that affect the social worker/client relationship. It is also critical that social workers understand and have as much influence as possible on how their organizations, programs, and services are run and how they are evaluated (Kerson, 2002). We often find ourselves in the position of being evaluated from outside by others who may not understand or value our contributions as we do. Thus, part of understanding one's organization as an element of context shaping the relationship between social worker and client means incorporating evaluation into all of the work and engaging the evaluators if they, indeed, come from outside of the organization.

Organization also structures practice (Wike et al., 2014). For example, the role of a social worker in a burn unit is necessarily different from that in an adolescent parenting program. The attributes of each organization affect and often shape the social worker's relationship with the client. Furthermore, in each organization, the social worker may be working with clients whose care is paid for by a range of managed care alternatives, each of which has different rules about who is entitled to service and the conditions of the service itself. It is important for social workers to understand how the formal dimensions of their organizations affect health care delivery and the relationship between them and their clients. Here, we mean size, division of labor, degree of bureaucratization, degree of centralization of control, and role structure as well as the relationship of one's organization to others and to larger systems. Role structure is especially important in understanding social work's place and authority in the organization (Kerson, 2002). Changes in structure and design carried out in the name of efficiency and cost-effectiveness can enhance or restrict services and creativity. Informal dimensions include mores, the unwritten rules about behavior, which people know implicitly but rarely discuss, such as ways in which to relate to members of other professions or whether it is acceptable to have a meal at a client's home.

Also important are the networks, collaborative alliances, teamwork, and partnerships that people develop within and outside of the formal organizational structure in order to accomplish tasks (Solheim, McElmurry, & Kim, 2007). Often, the establishment of such a network means being able to enlist those with expertise or power for help in advocating for clients. Such power does not necessarily reside with high office. Sometimes it can be held by a chief of service, other times by a clerk. Although it is generally easier to make exceptions or bend the rules in a smaller organization, those who work for large, highly bureaucratized organizations also learn to develop informal networks. Intimate knowledge of an organization increases the possibility of making it more responsive to clients' needs. Social workers can leverage these outside relationships to assure that client's needs for their services are protected, as when several neonatal intensive care unit social workers used the Code of Ethics of the National Association of Perinatal Social Workers to advocate for staffing levels to ensure that all families with premature and ill infants would get social work services.

In conclusion, understanding context is about understanding the rules of the game. You cannot play the game without understanding the rules and you cannot take advantage of, exploit, bend, or go around the rules unless you fully understand them. For health-related social workers, the most critical elements of context are policy, technology, and organization – the regulations and laws, elements of technology, and organizational dimensions and issues that influence the work. Within context sits the relationship between social worker and client; so context determines parameters and also creates the nesting space within which the relationship that will help the clients to reach their goals is established.

Decisions about practice

Circumscribed by context, the relationship between social worker and client is where the work occurs. In the framework, the elements that provide structure and regulate the interaction are called practice decisions because they are guided by decisions made by social worker and client; these set the pattern for their relationship. Practice decisions means that the participants themselves have the power to create the vehicle that will enable them to accomplish their goals. The term stresses the dimensions of activity, judgment, and responsibility implicit in such choices.

In some situations, practice decisions may be constrained by elements of context. For example, in order to receive funding, an organization may have to adhere to policies set by a funding source regarding use of time or even goals. The organization would therefore constrain its social workers in those ways. Practice decisions are not always discrete and can recur as the relationship evolves. They are alterable and can act as a flexible structure that can guide the relationship and help the participants to judge the quality of their work. The 10 practice decisions in this framework are (1) definition of the client; (2) goals, objectives, and outcome measures; (3) use of contract; (4) meeting place; (5) use of time; (6) strategies and interventions; (7) stance of the social worker; (8) use of outside resources; (9) reassessment; and (10) transfer or termination.

Definition of the client

Defining the client involves the choice of a client unit, that is, deciding with whom one works in a situation (Turner & Shera, 2005). The client can be any unit, such as an individual, family, couple, parent and child, group, committee, housing project, or clinic. While a case is open, the definition of the client can change as its needs change. Sometimes the social worker intervenes with the most troubled people in the situation, and in other instances they may work on the client's behalf because that person is not available for work. For example, the person who is most dependent or most troubled may be too young, demented, or ill to be directly involved. At times, broadening the definition of the client from an individual to a larger unit enhances the social support of the ill person and strengthens the whole (Kerson, 2002).

Goals, objectives, and/or outcome measures

The words "goals," "objectives", and "outcome measures" all refer to aspirations that social workers, clients, programs, organizations, and funding sources want to attain (Walsh, 2013). As social workers, we hope that these reflect the needs and desires of the client. In the best of worlds, they should be owned by the client with the social worker collaborating to clarify, articulate, and help set the course for attainment. With the client's help, the social worker then makes practice decisions that help to structure the relationship in ways that will support the work. When this is not the case, when goals and objectives have been formulated by the funding sources or other stakeholders and not by the client, it is much more difficult to enlist the client. That, in itself, becomes an objective for the social worker because to work most effectively, this relationship has to be a partnership.

This work operates on two levels, at least. Overarching is the notion of "lending a vision," that is to say helping the client to envision a better life, better times, a more positive future. This frames the "goals" level, where wishes and dreams are articulated. It is the responsibility of the social worker to hold out hope, and sometimes it is only the social worker who lends this vision.

The second level is the more pragmatic one in which social worker and client divide the work into steps and objectives, that is, measurable outcomes that will tell them concretely about their progress in their work together. This work is the key to both assessment and evaluation (Kerson, 2002). Assessment in relation to measurable outcomes, to objectives, means that one has determined the criteria for evaluation.

The relationship between social work goals and objectives and certain diagnoses is also important here. Diagnosis is often made by another profession, usually medicine, with which social work collaborates. In some ways, when a diagnosis is imposed, it becomes part of context, an organizational issue that informs social work practice. However, a diagnostic term such as diabetes, arthritis, or epilepsy is a label that provides very little information about functional capacity, and it is often that capacity with which social work concerns itself. For example, the question for the social worker is not whether the patient has multiple sclerosis, but whether her symptoms make it impossible for her to care for her children. If social workers employ this kind of information to limit the use that they think a client can make of the relationship or even to discard certain clients into a category that receives no service, they are allowing diagnosis to restrict their work.

Objectives may be as concrete as obtaining an apartment or a prosthesis. Because objectives are, by definition, measurable, it is imperative that social workers think in these terms because they provide social workers, clients, funders, and the organization the means for assessing progress (Kerson, 2002). Being able to call attention to some success such as "arriving at work or school on time nearly every day" or "going to the senior center three times a week" is helpful in encouraging a client to continue to work in the relationship. Increasingly, funding sources are asking social workers and other helping professionals for outcome measures, which are the concrete means they will use to evaluate their work and the work of the clients. Although objectives for service provision had been acceptable in the past (e.g., "meet with the client twice in the week"), outcome measures related to the client's progress are now required for accountability. Through articulating objectives and outcome measures, and achieving success in reaching a certain percentage or number of these measures, social workers will be able to help clients to see their progress and will also be able to demonstrate their results and their economic value to the organization and the funding sources. Thus, goals are clients' wishes to which social workers and clients aspire and objectives and outcome measures are the realistic, attainable, concrete ways by which social workers and clients can measure their own progress and prove their worth to organizations and funding sources.

Use of contract

Contract means agreement between social worker and client about the means used to obtain goals, as well as the description of the goals themselves. It is the keystone, cynosure, and linchpin of the social worker/client relationship and of this framework. Composed of mutually agreed-upon obligations and expectations, a contract is a way of establishing norms for the relationship. Norms also exist for the relationship between client and agency. Increasingly, there are contracts between funding source, agency, and client.

Whether verbal or written contracts are more effective remains a matter for debate and most probably depends on the nature of the agency, work, and clients. Certainly, a written form clarifies the agreement, and having all participants sign adds formality and perhaps importance to the matters at hand. This written form is very common in drug and alcohol programs, and often the conditions for contract are set by the courts or the state. Some would argue that this very formality stultifies the interaction, interfering with creativity, transference, or other aspects of the relationship. Others would say that it lends a clarity that protects everyone involved. Because contracting requires that each party articulates his or her goals and norms, the contract includes each of the elements of relationship structure. Participants in a helping relationship always have some expectations of each other. Use of the dimensions of contract allows the expectations of all parties to be made explicit and helps prevent any misunderstanding.

Meeting place

Meeting place refers to the physical space where the relationship happens. Often, decisions about meeting place are determined by the rules of the setting and the needs of the clients. Most work occurs in the institution/agency or in the client's home. Increasingly, meeting place is determined by the organization rather than by the needs of the clients. The major portion of some services such as home care, foster care, and hospice is dispensed in the home, whereas other services such as discharge planning are generally offered in the institution. There is a renewed trend to place social work services back in the community with the increase in a range of case management services, intensive or otherwise, occurring wherever the client is.

Meeting place can influence assessment by limiting or increasing the amount of information made available about the client. A person's social scene provides some information about his or her identity. When meetings take place outside of the client's habitat, the social worker relies on the person's appearance and the details he or she provides about his or her life. The sight of an institutionally gowned person lying in bed in a hospital room provides few clues to individual identity. Personality, memories, experiences, and style are obscured. Often in such situations, it is easy for social workers to assume knowledge of their clients that, in fact, they do not have.

When clients are seen at home, social workers learn something about clients' means, organizational abilities, values, neighborhood, and, perhaps, their relationships with family members and neighbors (Paris, Genborys, Kaufman, & Whitehill, 2007). No other means compare to home visits for assessing the lives of clients or, sometimes, for empowering them. One sees the impact of problems, illnesses, and disabilities on daily living. Through home visits, social workers can help collaborating professionals and aides to understand a client's life and problems. Many organizations think that home visits are too expensive or intrusive and as a result do not allow them, but they remain a way to assess client capacities and resources. Household mementos and layout yield important information about how a client is faring and what help they may need.

The telephone and computers are other "places" to help people who cannot come to the organization and whom the social worker cannot visit. They have proven effective as a means of support and treatment for isolated clients. As was mentioned earlier, social work will continue to make greater use of "e" techniques as well (Santhiveeran, 2009) and social work support groups on-line have the ability to reach isolated caregivers in ways few support groups can (Green & Gray, 2013).

Two important aspects of meeting place are space and privacy, which in many institutional or agency settings are at a premium. Where none exists, social workers can create private space for themselves and their clients by using undivided attention, eye contact, voice quality, and body language. When other professionals ignore the need for privacy, social workers have to educate them in order to protect their clients and foster the work.

Use of time

Decisions about time relate to the duration of the relationship and the duration and spacing of each meeting. Since use of time is a means of structuring the relationship, sharing this information with clients empowers them. In the broadest sense, orientation in time and space "is felt as a protection rather than a straitjacket, and its loss can provoke extreme anxiety" (Mead & Bateson, 1942). The importance of time is no less diminished in single-encounter work in a hospital emergency room than it is in group work or long-term psychotherapy. In many instances, the use of time is determined by the organization or funding source. For example, policy may determine the duration of a session, how many sessions a client may be seen, or the number of days for which a patient is hospitalized, but, then, it is a question of how best to use the time that you have. Time is also an important dimension of contract. No matter who determines the duration of the session, the work is aided when the client is the sole focus for that time and when both client and worker understand how time will be used.

Strategies and interventions

Strategies and interventions refer to the selection of particular methods of care that are most appropriate for specific clients in particular situations (Kerson, 2002). In every situation, the social worker makes decisions about the ways the client can best be helped. These decisions involve choices about orientation, modality, technique, and intervention. To some degree, choice of strategies and interventions relates to definition of client and client unit. Thus, designating an individual as the client might indicate that one would do individual work, while designating the family as the client would indicate family work. However, the more general decision to work with a certain client unit opens the possibility for a plethora of decisions regarding particular theoretical orientations such as a psychodynamic, cognitive, or behavioral approach. Such orientations often reflect beliefs and world views of the social worker, which may relate little to particular client problems. For example, because it is common in our society to believe that elderly people are not amenable to psychodynamic work, these approaches are unusual in work with the elderly; yet, programs for the elderly report excellent work that is sometimes entirely psychodynamic and, other times, combines that with case management (Choi & Kimbell, 2009). This practice decision cautions social workers to choose treatment modalities that reflect needs and goals of clients rather than their own world views or beliefs. In turn, choice of a particular theoretical orientation and treatment modality brings one to decisions regarding specific techniques or interventions, such as the use of ritual, or some sort of narrative therapy. Techniques such as these are tools to bring a theoretical model into action. Monitoring their use offers the social worker another way to assess ongoing work because strategies such as these tend to have specified outcomes. At times, interventions that are used are different from ones that had been anticipated, because a client's needs may be redefined as the work progresses. Articulating practice interventions enhances social workers' control of their medium. Treatment method is also sometimes determined by dimensions of context such as organization or funding policy. For example, one facility may extol a particular form of family therapy to treat an illness such as bulimia and another may use a specific form of individual therapy to treat the same illness. These choices seem to arise from differing beliefs about etiology and/or cure.

In the United States and the United Kingdom, adoption of "evidence-based practice" has been part of the focus for accountability in health care and this can define what strategies and interventions are considered legitimate. Gambrill (2001) has asserted that using interventions that have not risen to the level of evidence-based practice (EBP) is unethical as they are based in authority ("my supervisor advised this") rather than research that empirically evaluated the intervention technique. Gilgun (2005) argues that evidence consists of more than evaluation of intervention techniques by researchers and suggests that theory and research are one "pillar" of evidence, but that practice wisdom, the social worker's intuited and learned knowledge of the situation, and the client's responses to the intervention are also legitimate "pillars" of knowledge/evidence. EBPs pervade both medicine and social work (Shdaimah, 2009) and the intersection of social work and science (Anastas, 2014) continues to be contentious: nevertheless, social workers in health settings must contend with calls for EBP or "best practices" calls for accountability and have the wherewithal to access literature about current best practices. When research is consistent and robust, it must inform the social worker's choice of strategies and interventions.

At times, the nature of the illness or disability affects the choice of modality. For example, an illness or disability that leaves an individual physically dependent, such as advanced rheumatoid arthritis or emphysema, may require that the social worker work with family members as well as the ill person. In the case of advanced Alzheimer's disease or with a seriously ill infant, the social worker may work only with family members. Use of time, another practice decision, sometimes may be a dimension of treatment modality. Since the 1960s, short-term, brief, and crisis-oriented work has been conventional, but within each of these orientations there are a myriad of practice decisions regarding modality and specific technique.

Case or care management

One modality that has resumed its important place in social work practice is case or care management, which is sometimes referred to as advanced or intensive case management (Walsh, 2013). The expression "care management" seems to be more palatable to clients because the word "case" suggests to some that they are passive in the role, without voice or full participation. Developed for client groups such as foster children, the frail elderly, chronically mentally ill, and the developmentally disabled, this modality is one response to the complexity of service delivery systems. It rests on what is promised as a full array of services, on service over a relatively long period of time, and on a special, dependable, therapeutic relationship with another individual. Case management can be used to organize the services of an entire agency, a national program of immense proportions, or a single caseload; but, properly defined, case management should never exclude clinical work. In fact, case management is both a concept and a process. One can view it as a system of relationships among direct service providers, administrators, funders, and clients. However, it is also an orderly, planned provision of a range of services that are directed at a specific problem area and are intended to help clients to function as normally as possible within their communities.

There are many approaches to case management as a strategy or intervention for the social work practitioner. These approaches vary in terms of the direct involvement of the social worker. They range from a brokering role, in which the social worker links clients to services, advocates for clients, and monitors client activities, to clinical or advanced case management, in which the managers act as primary therapists as well as monitors, advocates, and brokers. In these latter positions, the social workers carry a great deal of authority in the system of services that the client requires. Especially with those with serious and persistent chronic illness, such clinical case managers work in teams, although the special one-to-one relationship of clinical case manager and patient continues to be paramount. Case management has a special appeal to managed care approaches because such services are generally community-based rather than being based in institutions, and they can serve a utilization review function if given the authority to authorize or deny services to prevent their unreasonable or unnecessary use.

Integrative, pragmatic, and eclectic approaches

Practitioners generally suggest that their approaches are integrative, pragmatic, and eclectic; that is, they do what they must depending on the circumstances, needs, and capabilities of their clients, and they tend to draw from many modalities and techniques. Sometimes, it is difficult to distinguish between style of the social worker and choice of treatment modality. Those who are less active in their style and focus on listening/supporting may identify as more psychodynamic while those who are more active, structured, or directive may be following brief therapy models such as solution-focused or task-oriented modalities. Social workers may have styles with which they feel more comfortable, yet we must always be able to adapt to the needs of the client and the situation to use an approach most likely to help move the work in a way that benefits the client's well-being.

Stance of the social worker

Stance of the social worker refers to the "conscious use of self," that is, an understanding of one's self motivations and place in and impact on relationships. It implies that the social worker has sufficient self-awareness, experience, and discipline to be able to choose how to behave in a particular client situation. Unlike some other practice decisions shared with the client, the social worker is totally responsible for this choice. Experience and self-awareness provide the social worker greater mastery of stance so that, within realistic limits, the social worker can be what the client and situation need him or her to be. Just as an actor learns to assume a role, with professional education and experience, the social worker adapts and refines his or her stance according to the needs of the client situation. Some elements of stance are the worker's degree of activity or passivity, amount of advice-giving, use of authority, self-disclosure, and touch (Goffman, 1961). Other elements such as transference and counter-transference, prejudices, and false assumptions, which may support action that is different from the needs of the client situation, are part of the stance of the social worker as well.

Use of resources outside of the client/social worker relationship

Outside resources are the services used by client and social worker that are outside of the relationship, often external to the agency, and that further the work of the relationship. These services can range from the protective work of a child welfare or aging agency, to assistance with obtaining an apartment or walker, to referral to a mutual aid group. Determination of clients' ability to broker their own services is an issue here. Sometimes, clients and/or families can grow stronger by managing outside resources themselves; in some instances, the social worker can enhance the relationship by arranging services; and at other times, the social worker must procure outside resources because the client/family is unable to manage.

Mapping devices: ecomaps and organigraphs

Because it is helpful to visualize the clients' services and systems and the relationships that clients have with them, we have encouraged case chapter authors to include a mapping device that sets out the ecological system in which they are working and draws the boundaries that define a life space (Kerson, 2002). Such representations are useful for assessment, evaluation, and helping clients to set priorities and make decisions about altering relationships with individuals and organizations. One can present very complicated relationships on a single page, giving client and social worker some sense of control of a situation. Many chapters have chosen to use ecomaps, others have sought a more specific drawing tool, and a few, no device.

In the ecomap, a large center circle generally includes the client's nuclear family, with circles surrounding that one representing people and organizations with whom the client interacts. In this book, a strong relationship is drawn as an unbroken line. The flow of energy is either depicted as going back and forth between both parties, with an arrow at either end, or as going from only one to the other, with an arrow pointing at the party who is receiving the energy. A tenuous relationship is depicted as a light, broken line, while a stressful relationship is drawn as a heavy, broken line. A circle with a name in it and no line drawn to it means that there is no relationship between the client and the person or agency named in the circle. Like a snapshot, an ecomap captures a static moment in the client's life. Updated regularly,

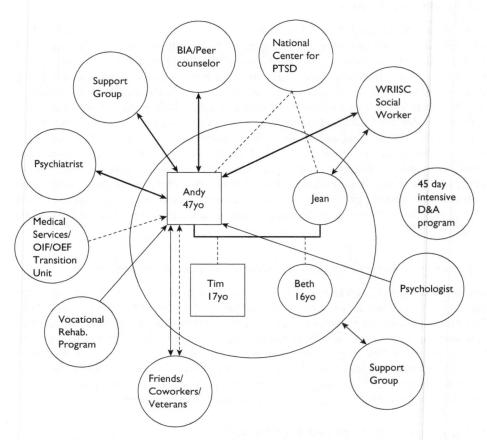

Figure 1.1 Ecomap for Andy Long. Example of an ecomap, in this case for a returning veteran with traumatic brain injury

the map suggests the direction of the work, can demonstrate progress, strengthen relationships, and can be used for evaluation. Figure 1.1 depicts an example drawn from Patricia Findley's chapter in the third edition.

Reassessment

Reassessment presents an opportunity for social worker and client to evaluate their work during the course of the relationship. Like artists, they are asked to step back and examine the work and evaluate it. Reassessment is the process of reexamining the dimensions of the framework as well as other issues that participants have deemed important. It can be made part of the pattern of each meeting or set aside to be brought into the work at certain intervals (see Wike, Rounds, & Dombalis, Chapter 24 for how reassessment is built in monthly). The technique can be as simple as discussing how the work is going or as sophisticated as using standardized measures of success (Fischer & Corcoran, 2013). Reassessment can also be a way to reactivate a stalled relationship or to slow one that seems to be speeding along almost out of control. William Schwartz's enduring questions, "Are we working?" and "What are we working on?" are helpful here. Finally, reassessment provides the social worker with an opportunity to assess and obtain feedback about his or her performance.

Transfer or termination and case conclusion

Transfer and termination mark the end of the relationship between client and social worker, that is, the fact that they will not be meeting in this way any longer. Greetings and farewells are ritual displays that mark a change in degree of access. Now, social worker and client will not have the same kind of access to each other as they would have had if the work continued. Ideally, termination is a decision that social worker and client have made together because goals have been accomplished and their work is finished. Often, when clients terminate before the social worker is ready, it can be because the client has perceived work more positively or more negatively than the social worker. Even when the client wants to terminate before the social worker thinks work is finished, it is important to end the relationship positively so that the client may return to the agency (or to another one) if he or she needs further help. Sometimes, termination signals the end of the relationship between client and agency. At other times, the social worker is leaving the organization, and the client will continue with another social worker. Vacations and other interruptions also evoke issues about termination. Often a difficult period, termination has great potential for growth through the use of the relationship. In any case, termination is ideally used to review the gains the client has made and to reinforce new coping strategies while also assuring that the client is aware of how to access assistance if it is required again in the future.

Conclusion refers primarily to outcomes and the current functioning of the client. Client and social worker summarize their work together so that each can leave the relationship with knowledge of accomplishments. In addition, they finish in a positive manner that will allow the client to seek help again, if necessary.

Differential discussion

In a differential discussion, all of the previous framework decisions are reviewed in order for the social worker to analyze his or her work (Figure 1.2). Differential discussion allows the social worker to be a Monday morning quarterback, that is, to look back on the case to decide which elements would remain the same the next time he or she worked with a client with similar capacity, personality, and problems. Differential discussion encourages the social worker to generalize from a specific client to a category of like cases with which he or she can use similar structure and techniques. It also makes a simple, case to case, project to project evaluation into a routine part of practice. For example, in retrospect, the social worker may decide he or she was too confrontational with a client, the coldness of the meeting place might have been a detriment, or the client may have been asked to coordinate more resources than he or she was able to manage. Emphasis on the social worker's ability to (1) generalize from a particular case and (2) alter elements in the relationship between social worker and client makes differential discussion the most useful dimension of the framework. This step moves the social worker out of the present relationship and on to the next, beginning with one strategy and ending with a test and adaptation process. See Figure 1.2 for differential discussion decision points.

Differential Discussion: Practice in Context Grid		
CONTEXT		
	Change	How
Policy		
Technology		
Organization		
PRACTICE DECISIONS		
	Change	How
Definition of the Client		
Objectives/Outcome Measures		
Contract		
Meeting Place		
Use of Time		
Strategies/Interventions		
Stanceof the social worker		
Use of outside resources		
Reassessment		
Transfer or termination		

Figure 1.2 The Practice in Context differential discussion grid

Practice in Context as a form of reflective learning

Older literature on being a reflective practitioner (Argyris & Schon, 1974; Schon, 1983) and recent literature from neurobiology support the idea that reflection on cases allows practitioners to learn how to handle future cases more effectively. Dreyfus (1986) and Flyvbjerg (2001) identify the trajectory of professional learning that involves repetition and reflection as key components in developing expertise, with Flyvbjerg (2011) particularly noting the importance of case study-based learning. Likewise, practitioner development research tells us that building professional confidence takes time, primarily time for reflecting on cases (Bischoff & Barton, 2002). Neurobiologists now inform us that this type of reflection is critical to deep learning and professional development (Epstein, Siegel, & Silberman, 2008). Over the many years the Practice in Context framework has been used in these casebooks and in classrooms, it is apparent that the enforced reflection on a case, particularly the differential discussion part of the framework, allows students and experienced practitioners to enhance their expertise and grow their awareness of ways that they may have improved case outcomes. This can then be applied in future cases. The use of these cases allows context-rich knowledge to be transmitted to newer practitioners while also challenging seasoned practitioners to think more deeply about how outcomes may have been improved. In short, the PiC provides a way to enhance practitioner's own expertise while also providing a vehicle (like this casebook) to transmit such expertise to other practitioners (McCoyd & Kerson, 2013).

A review of the overarching conception of PiC brings the framework full circle. Constraints on the setting, the influence that these constraints have had on the relationship, and the series of decisions that determine the structure of the relationship enable social workers to map their work and, as a result, enhance action. This review also helps to identify areas of advocacy and social action for the social worker.

Using the framework described above, *Social Work in Health Settings* acts as a casebook, a collection of real cases in settings described by and reflecting the style of each experienced social work practitioner. Our contributors often write in the first person as they report and reflect on true cases; sometimes those written by groups of social workers refer to the social worker in the third person, yet all are compelling in their immediacy. All client/patient names have been changed and many organizations are unnamed for purposes of confidentiality. Altogether, the settings are examples of the great range of health-related social work activity. Each article follows the PiC framework as its outline. The case chapters are organized in two sections: Part 1: Individual and family work in health settings and Part 2: Social work and public health, though, in fact, every setting and every case carries elements of both.

Ideally, the format for this book would be a three-ringed notebook in which case/setting articles and dimensions of context and practice could be arranged and rearranged for teaching purposes. One could then use these case/settings to discuss issues, such as short-term and long-term care; institutional and home care; physical and mental health; services for children, adults, and the elderly; public health exposures; or trauma and disease. In addition, one could examine a particular practice decision such as use of contract or stance of the social worker, across 30 practice settings. Overall, *Social Work in Health Settings* has one primary purpose: to help social workers to clarify and explicate Practice in Context in order to best ply their craft.

We sincerely hope you find the opportunities to reflect on each of these cases to enrich your knowledge, skills, values, and practice.

References

Acker, G. M. (2010). How social workers cope with managed care. *Administration in Social Work, 34*, 405–422. doi: 10.1080/03643107.2010.518125

Acker, G. M. & Lawrence, D. (2009). Social work and managed care measuring competence, burnout, and role stress of workers providing mental health services in a managed care era. *Journal of Social Work, 9*(3), 269–283. doi: 10.1177/1468017309334902

Anastas, J. (2014). The science of social work and its relationship to social work practice. *Research on Social Work Practice, 24*, 571–580. doi: 10.1177/1049731513511335

Argyris, C. & Schon, D. (1974). *Theory in practice: Increasing professional effectiveness.* San Francisco, CA: Jossey-Bass.

Arrow, K., Auerbach, A., Bertko, J., Brownlee, S., Casalino, L. P., Cooper, J., et al. (2009). Toward a 21st century health care system: Recommendations for health care reform. *Annals of Internal Medicine, 150*(7), 493–499. doi: 10.7326/0003-4819-150-7-200904070-00115

Barr, D. A. (2011). *Introduction to U. S. health policy: The organization, financing, and delivery of health care in America* (3rd edn.). Baltimore, MD: Johns Hopkins University Press.

Barr, D. A. (2014). *Health disparities in the United States: Social class, race, ethnicity and health* (2nd edn.). Baltimore, MD: Johns Hopkins University Press.

Bateson, G. (n.d.). Introduction. In *The natural history of an interview.* University of Chicago Library Microfilm Collection of Manuscripts in Cultural Anthropology, series 15, Nos, 95–98. 1971. Retrieved from http://varenne.tc.columbia.edu/bib/info/batsngrgr00comm0000.html

Bateson, G. (1975). *Steps to an ecology of mind.* New York: Ballantine.

Beresford, P., Croft, S., & Adshead, L. (2007). "We don't see her as a social worker": A service user case study of the importance of the social worker's relationship and humanity. *British Journal of Social Work, 38*, 1388–1407. doi: 10.1093/bjsw/bcm043

Bischoff, R. J. & Barton, M. (2002). The pathway toward clinical self confidence. *The American Journal of Family Therapy, 30*, 231–242. doi:10.1080/019261802753577557

Blank, R. H. & Burau, V. (2014). *Comparative health policy* (4nd edn.). New York: Palgrave Macmillan.

Choi, N. G. & Kimbell, K. (2009). Depression care need among low-income older adults: Views from agency service providers and family care givers. *Clinical Gerontologist, 32*, 60–76.

Congress (2010). *Compilation of Patient Protection and Affordable Care Act.* May 2010. 111th Congress 2d Session. Retrieved from http://housedocs.house.gov/energycommerce/ppacacon.pdf

Dickson, D. (2014). *Law in the health and human services: A guide for social workers, psychologists, psychiatrists and related professionals* (3rd edn.). New York: The Free Press.

Dreyfus, H. L. (1986). *Mind over machine: The power of human intuition and expertise in the era of the computer.* New York: Free Press.

Drucker, P. (2004). *Managing the non-profit organization: Practices and principles.* New York: Taylor & Francis.

Emanuel, E. J. (2012). Why accountable care organizations are not 1990s managed care redux. *JAMA, 307*(21), 2263–2264. doi: 10.1001/jama/2012.4313

Epstein, R. M., Siegel, D. J., & Silberman, J. (2008). Self-monitoring in clinical practice: A challenge for medical educators. *Journal of Continuing Education in the Health Professions, 28*, 5–13. doi: 10.1002/chp.149

Fischer, J. & Corcoran, K. (2013). *Measures for clinical practice* (5th edn.). New York: Oxford University Press.

Flyvbjerg, B. (2001). *Making social science matter.* London: Cambridge University Press.

Flyvbjerg, B. (2011). Case study. In N. K. Denzin & Y. S. Lincoln (Eds.), *The Sage handbook of qualitative research* (4th edn., pp. 301–316). Thousand Oaks, CA: Sage.

Gambrill, E. (2001). Social work: An authority-based profession. *Research on Social Work Practice, 11*, 166–175. doi: 10.1177/104973150101100203

Gilgun, J. (2005). The four cornerstones of evidence-based practice in social work. *Research on Social Work Practice, 15*, 52–61. doi: 10.1177/1049731504269581

Goffman, E. (1961). *Encounters: Two studies in the sociology of interaction.* New York: Macmillan.

Goffman, E. (1966). *Behavior in public places.* New York: The Free Press.

Goffman, E. (1981). *Interaction ritual: Essays in face-to-face behavior.* New York: Pantheon.

Gorin, S. H., Pollack, R., Darnell, J. S., & Allen, H. L. (2014). Affordable Care Act. *Encyclopedia of Social Work.* doi: 10.1093/acrefore/9780199975839.013.830 Retrieved from http://socialwork.oxfordre.com/oso/downloaddoclightbox/$002f10.1093$002facrefore$002f9780199975839.001.0001$002facrefore-9780199975839-e-830/Affordable$0020Care$0020Act?nojs=true

Groshong, L. & Phillips, D. (2015). The impact of electronic communication on confidentiality in clinical social work practice. *Clinical Social Work, 43*(2), 143–150. doi: 10.1007/s10615-015-0527-4

Green, Y. R. & Gray, M. (2013). Lessons learned from the Kinship Education and Support Program (KEPS): Developing effective support groups for formal kinship caregivers. *Social Work with Groups, 36*(1), 27–42. doi: 10.1080/01609513.2012.698384

Hasenfeld, Y. & Garrow, E. E. (2012). Nonprofit human-service organizations, social rights, and advocacy in a neoliberal welfare state. *Social Service Review, 86,* 295–322.

Holden, G. (2009). Information for Practice (IP). Retrieved from http://blogs.nyu.edu/socialwork/ip/ Information for Practice

Jasanoff, S. (2008). Making order: Law and science in action. In E. J. Hackett, O. Amsterdamska, M. Lynch, & J. Wajcman (Eds.), *The handbook of science and technology studies* (3rd edn., pp. 761–786). Cambridge, MA: The MIT Press.

Kerson, T. S. (1981). *Medical social work: The pre-professional paradox.* New York: Irvington.

Kerson, T. S. (1985). Responsiveness to need: Social work's impact on health care. *Health and Social Work, 10,* 300–307. doi: 10.1093/hsw/10.4.300

Kerson, T. S. (2002). *Boundary spanning: An ecological reinterpretation of social work practice in health and mental health.* New York: Columbia University Press.

Kerson, T. S. & McCoyd, J. L. M. (2002). The relationship between the social worker and the client system. In T. S. Kerson, *Boundary spanning: An ecological reinterpretation of social work practice in health and mental health* (pp. 143–198). New York: Columbia University Press.

Little, J. (Ed.). (2007). *Wanting it all: The challenge of reforming the U.S. health care system.* Boston, MA: Federal Reserve Bank of Boston. Retrieved from www.bos.frb.org

Margolis, L. & Kotch, J. B. (2013). Tracing the historical foundations of maternal and child health to contemporary times. In J. B. Kotch (Ed.), *Maternal and child health: Programs, problems, and policy in public health* (3rd edn., pp. 11–34). Burlington, VT: Jones & Bartlett.

Mas, N. & Seinfeld, J. (2008). Is managed care restraining the adoption of technology by hospitals? *Journal of Health Economics, 27*(4), 1026–1045. doi: 10.1016/j.jhealec0.2008.02.009

Matusitz, J. & Breen, G. M. (2008). E-health: A new kind of telemedicine. *Social Work in Public Health, 23*(1), 95–113. doi: 10.1300/J523v23n01_06

McCoyd, J. L. M. (2009). Discrepant feeling rules and unscripted emotion work: Women terminating desired pregnancies due to fetal anomaly (Lead Article). *American Journal of Orthopsychiatry, 79*(4), 441–451. doi:10.1037/a0010483

McCoyd, J. L. M. & Kerson, T. S. (2013). Teaching reflective social work practice in health care: Promoting best practices. *Journal of Social Work Education, 49*(4), 674–688. doi:10.1080/104377 97.2013.812892

Mead, M. & Bateson, G. (1942). *Balinese character.* New York: Academy of Sciences.

Mechanic, D. (2005). Policy challenges in addressing racial disparities and improving population health. *Health Affairs, 24*(2), 335–342. doi: 10.1377/hlthaff.24.2.335

Miller, E. A., & West, D. M. (2009). Where's the revolution: Digital technology & health care in the internet age. *Journal of Health Politics & Law, 34*(2), 261–284. doi: 10.1215/03616878-2008-046

Morgan, S. (2013). Social workers and the 2013 Omnibus HIPAA rule. *NASW Washington Chapter Newsletter.* Retrieved from https://nasw-wa.org/social-workers-and-the-2013-omnibus-hipaa-rule/

Morrison, E. E. & Monagle, J. F. (2013). *Health care ethics: Critical issues for the 21st century* (2nd edn.). Burlington, MA: Jones & Bartlett.

NASW (National Association of Social Workers) (2001). What social workers should know about the HIPAA Privacy Regulations. NASW practice and Professional Development: Practice Update from NASW. Volume 1(1). Retrieved from https://www.socialworkers.org/practice/behavioral_health/ mbh0101.asp

ObamaCare Facts (n.d.). Retrieved from http://obamacarefacts.com/

Paris, R., Genborys, M., Kaufman, P. H., & Whitehill, D. (2007). Reaching isolated new mothers: Insights from a home visiting program using paraprofessionals. *Families in Society, 88*(4), 616–626. doi: 10.1606/1044-3894.3684

Santhiveeran, J. (2009). Compliance of social work e-therapy websites to the NASW code of ethics. *Social Work in Health Care, 48*(1), 1–13. doi: 10.1080/00981380802231216

Schlesinger, M. (2011). Making the best of hard times: How the nation's economic circumstances shaped the public's embrace of health care reform. *Journal of Health Politics, Policy and Law, 36*, 989–1020. doi: 10.1215/03616878-1460560

Schon, D. A. (1983). *The reflective practitioner: How professionals think in action.* New York: Basic Books.

Serafini, J. D., Damianakis, T., & Marziali, E. (2007). Clinical practice standards and ethical issues applied to a virtual group intervention for spousal caregivers of people with Alzheimer's. *Social Work in Health Care, 44*(3), 225–243. doi: 10.1300/J010v44n03_07

Sfiligoj, H. (2009, April). New technology transforming profession: Evolving tools are changing how social workers and their clients communicate. *NASW News*: 4.

Shdaimah, C. S. (2009). What does social work have to offer evidence-based practice? *Ethics and Social Welfare, 3*(1), 18–31. doi: 10.1080/17496530902818732

Solheim, K., McElmurry, B. J., & Kim, M. J. (2007). Multidisciplinary teamwork in United States primary health care. *Social Science & Medicine, 65*, 622–634. doi: 10.1016/j.socscimed.2007.03.028

Steinbrook, R. (2009). Health care and the American Recovery & Reinvestment Act. *New England Journal of Medicine, 360*, 1057–1060. doi: 10.1056/NEJMp0900665

Summer, L. & Hoadley, J. (2014). The role of Medicaid managed care in health delivery system reform. *The Commonwealth Fund.* Retrieved from www.commonwealthfund.org/publications/fund-reports/2014/apr/role-of-medicaid-managed-care-in-health-delivery-system-innovation

Tjora, A. H. & Scambler, G. (2009). Square pegs in round holes: Information systems, hospitals and the significance of contextual awareness. *Social Science and Medicine, 68*, 519–525. doi: 10.1016/j.socscimed.2008.11.005

Turner, L. M. & Shera, W. (2005). Empowerment of human service workers: Beyond intra organizational strategies. *Administration in Social Work, 29*(3), 79–94. doi: 10.1300/J147v29n03_06

U.S. Department of Health and Human Services (2015). Health information privacy. Standards for privacy of individually identifiable health information. Retrieved from www.hhs.gov/ocr/privacy/

Walsh, J. (2013). *The recovery philosophy and direct social work practice.* Chicago, IL: Lyceum.

Wike, T., Bledsoe, S. F., Manuel, J. I., Despard, M., Johnson, L. V., Bellamy, J. L., & Killian-Farrell, C. (2014). Evidence-based practice for social work: Challenges and opportunities for clinicians and organizations. *Clinical Social Work, 42*, 161–170. doi: 10.1007/s10615-014-0492-3

Part 1

Individual and family work in health settings

Chapter 2

Primer on micro practice in social work in health care

Context, skills, interventions, and best practices

Judith L. M. McCoyd and Toba Schwaber Kerson

Context

Since the earliest days of the specialization, social work practice in health care has aimed to help patients and family members manage the symptoms of illness or trauma in ways that maximize their well-being and independence. Nevertheless, the world of social work practice in health settings (from health clinics and hospitals through community agencies) is changing as a result of rapid technological developments and subsequent changes in health policy and health care organization. New policies and organizational structures such as the "medical homes" established by the Patient Protection and Affordable Care Act (ACA, 2010) will create opportunities for health social workers as care navigators, behaviorists, and other roles that provide services long identified with health social work (McCabe & Sullivan, 2015). New catch phrases such as "integrated behavioral health" now label what medical social workers have been doing since the specialization began. Although new medical technologies have opened new areas for social work practice, such as genetic testing for cancer risk and work with individuals who are changing gender, traditional positions in social work departments in health systems have declined due to the challenges of defining social work's benefit in pure economic terms.

Almost 40 years ago, Kerson (1981) described medical social workers as caught in a "pre-professional paradox." That is, while medical social workers lived their values and did not assert professional privilege – they responded altruistically to need, honored the knowledge and skills of others less educated and with less status in health care organizations, and took care of those with the least status in our society – this actually interfered with the specialization's claims to professional status and autonomy based on specialized knowledge, skills, and a distinct code of ethics. In attempting to show professional status characteristics (autonomy, unique knowledge, and ethics) while at the same time deferring to others and associating with ill and low-status individuals within medical settings, paradoxically, medical social work was less able to establish its professional status. Despite the high level of need hospital and medical systems had for social work skills and knowledge and in spite of the value many physicians placed on their working relationships with social workers in health settings, social workers were viewed as helpers rather than professionals in their own right. This paradox continues to influence health social work today.

In this chapter, we use the term health social work because it connotes both physical and mental health expertise; avoids a focus on pathology; includes preventive efforts and concern with health and well-being; embraces a biopsychosocial model of care; and fulfills the National Association of Social Workers (NASW) Code of Ethics admonition to enhance clients' well-being. NASW (2011) identifies nearly 20 functions of health social work that can be synthesized as: (1) performing comprehensive psychosocial assessments that include the patient's understanding of the condition, barriers to care, and identification of strengths and resources; (2) addressing with concrete and mental health services (crisis intervention etc.) psychosocial conditions that negatively impact health; (3) intervening and advocating to assure that patients can access appropriate care and transition among levels of care in ways that maintain their health and quality of life; (4) helping individuals and their families to adjust to health conditions, make informed medical decisions, and achieve maximum social function; (5) educating and advocating with other health providers, community leaders and policymakers for appropriate service provision and resources to enable patients (especially vulnerable ones) to access care; and (6) encouraging healthy behaviors (physical and behavioral) for care and prevention.

In a secondary analysis of interviews with social work pioneers conducted by Kerson (1981), viewed together with 80 cases published in earlier editions of *Social Work in Health Settings*, Kerson and McCoyd (2013) found that health social workers continue to be animated by traditional ethical commitments to respond to need. In the face of new populations to be served (as new disease and other health threats emerge), and new organizational constraints (as insurers worked to control health care costs and move patients back to the community more quickly), health social workers continue to work to meet the needs of patients and their families, particularly at the "micro practice" level. Their commitment to amelioration and advocacy continues to honor the importance of social justice encoded in the NASW Code of Ethics (2008).

As insurers instigated quicker discharges over the last four decades, the use of the social work relationship became challenging, often limited to specialty health services (e.g., pediatrics, oncology, renal disease) and circumstances in which patients remained on the floors longer than a day or two. To promote the best outcomes for their patients/clients, health social workers had to build rapport quickly, assess and intervene rapidly, and advocate and refer efficiently. Ultimately, they needed to assist patients in the communities where they were discharged, opening new arenas for practice. In traditional hospital settings, the time crunch meant social workers had little time to attend to the psychosocial barriers to implementing the medical treatment plan, and often were reduced to ordering equipment or arranging home health services. Judd and Sheffield (2010) surveyed hospital social workers' time use and found:

> Providing specialized instruction so the patient and family can perform post hospital care constituted less than 25% of time for 81% ($n = 305$) of respondents with one-third (33.6%, $n = 113$) reportedly spending no time in this endeavor. Similarly, activities to assist the patient and family in understanding the diagnosis, anticipated level of functioning, prescribed treatment and planning for follow up was carried out by less than one-third of respondents (30.1%, $n = 128$) more than 25% of the time. Direct practice which includes counseling services or crisis intervention activities for patients within hospital settings was conducted only 20% of the time or less by 43.8% ($n = 165$) of respondents, with almost one-third (29.4%) indicating they spent 10% or less of their time in these activities. (Judd & Sheffield, 2010, pp. 863–864)

This sad state of practice is a function of economic and organizational forces rather than a result of changed client/patient needs or incompetence on the part of these social workers.

This chapter will review some of the skills necessary to practice effectively and ethically in such a difficult context.

Policy

As suggested above, the primary policies affecting health social work define how social work is funded and viewed within the agency/hospital where it is housed. Although some social workers practice privately in collaboration with health providers and can set their own fee-for-service (see, for instance, Healy in Chapter 12 and Werner-Lin and Merrill in Chapter 9), most are salaried workers within organizations and health systems that create the context of their work. As Maus and Kerson state in Chapter 20, "We often feel as if we are walking a tight rope between the goals of the hospital and those of the patient and family." Social workers must be able to provide rationales for their services and show their utility, efficiency, and effectiveness while also advocating service provision in ways that meet ethical standards of social work care.

Policies affecting medical insurance coverage circumscribe our work with patients in health settings. Medicaid (publicly funded health insurance for the poor) is administered differently in each state and just over half the states have expanded Medicaid for those with incomes up to 400% of the poverty line (ObamaCare Facts, n.d.) as encouraged by the ACA (2010). In the remaining states, a significant proportion of working poor and others are caught between the eligibility line for Medicaid and eligibility for subsidized insurance under the ACA. They are left without affordable health coverage. Care for disabled individuals or those over age 65 with the requisite work history is covered by Medicare, but policy now allows private insurers to offer Medicare policies that include prescription drugs or other benefits while offsetting these benefits with limited coverage for other medical services or out-of-network providers. ACA has set some minimum coverage levels for private policies, yet there is still tremendous variation in what services are covered and under what conditions, and the tradeoffs among policies are complex. This means that social workers must know and understand each client's coverage in order to best advocate for needed health services. It is incumbent on us to be able to call an insurer to push effectively for more days in a rehabilitation facility, for example, or for coverage for imaging when genetic testing indicates higher risk for oncologic conditions (see Scarvalone, Oktay, Scott, & Helzlsouer, Chapter 13, and Werner-Lin & Merrill, Chapter 9). We should be able to advise patients about which policies are more likely to meet their medical needs.

Technology

Technology drives how medical care is delivered in the United States in the twenty-first century. Developments in genomic technologies, robotic surgical interventions, and ever-more detailed imaging technologies create an incredibly expensive health system as large health organizations compete to draw patients with insurance to fund the technologies. Services that do not generate sufficient revenue often become marginalized. This creates the context for social work services: technological innovations combine with an aging population and a largely privatized insurance system to maintain high levels of class-based health disparities.

On a micro level, social work practice – practice is a form of technology – has always involved the ability to identify resources for patients. Early social workers canvassed neighborhoods and religious institutions to identify help for patients returning home from the hospital, while social workers today use the internet to identify resources for everything from durable medical equipment and home care through on-line support groups and legitimate medical information websites. Smartphone apps and texting are used broadly to monitor health conditions and share health information (see, for example, Text4Baby, www. text4baby.org/, or e-health apps, http://healthit.gov/patients-families/stay-well). In addition, as indicated in this casebook, nearly all health settings are moving to electronic medical records (EMR) and use of various e-health systems that promote less fragmented health care and more accurate information for patients. Competence with computers and smartphones is now a professional requirement. That said, such technologies are vulnerable. Recent case studies such as *Five Days at Memorial* (Fink, 2013) provide chilling accounts of what happens when electricity-dependent technologies fail after events like Hurricane Katrina. Our dependence on technology to enable medical care becomes a vulnerability when natural disasters hit.

Social work technologies also include the treatment tools or interventions we use. Social work is grounded in the Strengths Perspective (Saleebey, 2012) and uses various communicative therapeutic techniques in eclectic ways to quickly build rapport and promote assessment and intervention. Typical "technologies" in therapeutic communication used in health care social work include motivational interviewing (Rollnick, Miller, & Butler, 2008) and adaptations of cognitive behavioral therapy (CBT), especially stress management, relaxation techniques, and cognitive reframing (Gudenkauf et al., 2015; Karlin et al., 2012; Mannix et al., 2006). Likewise, the skills of solution-focused brief therapy (SFBT) combined with the strengths-based perspective (SB-SFBT) have demonstrated utility in health settings (Franklin, 2015). These evidence-based therapeutic techniques all require effective communication, especially the ability to adapt one's mode of interaction to fit the needs of patients, families, and health providers. As Cavanaugh and Konrad (2012, p. 294) put it:

> Effective communicators are capable of adapting their skills and rarely, if ever, assume full knowledge of the experience of a new patient/client. Instead, they view every individual as embodying illness or disability in a unique way. Effective communicators avoid assumptive thinking that may lead to the collection of insufficient information, misdiagnosis, risks to safety, and ultimately, poor patient/client care.

In short, the discrete technologies we use all depend on the fundamental skills of social work practice: active listening, open-ended questioning, paraphrasing and summarizing, partializing goals in stepwise problem-solving.

Organization

Dane and Simon (1991) argued that many of the tensions agency – and hospital-based social workers experienced during the 1980s were due to their status as "resident guests" within "host settings." This conceptualization explained the value conflicts and lack of power that social workers experience in medical settings. (Indeed, nearly all medical professionals are now "guests" within large health care organizations run as businesses.) As a result, social workers in health settings need to develop a "profession-in-environment" (Spitzer, Silverman, & Allen, 2015) approach similar to the 'person-in-environment' approach that animates micro practice.

Spitzer et al. (2015) have studied social work provision and leadership in health settings and observe that social work ideology (ethics and values) often conflicts with the business and practical health missions of hospitals and other health settings. They suggest that the ACA (2010) provides a push toward transdisciplinary care and the integration of behavioral and physical health that creates opportunities to rebuild social work roles in health settings. To do so, we must define our competencies clearly and assess and adjust our fit within the relevant organizations. They invoke the approach of Ida Maude Cannon (1877–1960), the mother of medical social work, who "rather than taking a radical position that challenged the medical model and the primacy of the physician in health care . . . instead attempted to accommodate social work within the prevailing hospital culture" (Spitzer et al., 2015, p. 197). This does NOT mean that social workers should modify professional ethics and values. "The ability to negotiate 'ideology' or ideal practice with practical realities without compromising professional ethics is a fundamental skill in host settings like health care" (Spitzer et al., 2015, p. 198). We wholeheartedly agree. We must be able to assess where we share the organization's positions on mission, service priorities, and preferred operational modalities (interventions). We must then focus on the commonalities and leverage them to support good social work practice. This requires skill in developing organizational competencies in addition to the typical clinical competencies. We must know how to assess organizational values, culture, and structural sources of power, and design interventions to modify them when necessary. This echoes Kerson's (2002) call to "boundary-spanning practice," which recognizes the political and organizational context for assessment and intervention.

Decisions about practice

Definition of the patient/client

We will refer to the "patient" here because most micro work in health settings is directed to individuals defined as patients rather than clients. As will quickly be apparent in the cases that follow in this book, the "client" is seldom just the patient who presents within the health care setting. Indeed, the identified patient may change or multiply, as Schlup reports in Chapter 3. She tried to negotiate the pregnant mother's needs (as the first patient) as well as the unborn triplets' needs (as future patients) and those of the mother's support person (who was key to resolving the case). Other times, the patient is so embedded within a system of care (see Chapter 16 for Ray's work with veterans) that the "client" is also the system itself. The definition of the client needs to be interrogated regularly by the social worker as it is important to be clear about the allegiances owed to patient-clients; it also define what responsibilities the social worker has for the support network of the patient, the population represented by the patient, the colleagues who constitute the health team, the society that may be funding the care, and other regulatory and legal bodies that may exert control over the patient. Until the social worker is clear about the full client constellation and the duties and responsibilities owed to each, the worker risks moving into roles of social control or unreflective intervention that may fail to recognize the ethical imperatives of work with vulnerable people. Therefore, an important skill of social work in health care, as with social work generally, is to adequately consider all the stakeholders who are involved in any particular case and to identify whose priorities must be managed and where allegiances lie. Much of this requires the ability to navigate on multiple levels as indicated by the discussion about organizational competence (Spitzer et al., 2015).

Goals, objectives, and contracting

Social work in health care requires critical assessment of who constitutes the client and what tensions exist among members of the primary client group or between the client and the health-provision team. Especially when there is tension, the worker needs well-honed skills for developing shared goals and objectives. Goals (for example, return to home safely) must be broken into smaller objectives (assure there is a caretaker, assess physical safety in the home, assure that the patient understands functional limitations, assist in emotional adjustment to new limitations). Each of these objectives needs a plan for accomplishment that involves at least informal contracting about who is responsible for what. (For instance, the daughter of a patient may enlist her relatives to develop a schedule for those who will care for the patient at home while the social worker may arrange for an occupational therapist to examine the home for mobility hazards and accessibility issues.) The social worker is the primary coordinator of these efforts and assures that each has been accomplished.

This process also applies to the support of informed decision-making (see Chapters 9 and 13). To promote informed decision-making about genetic diagnosis and/or treatment requires breaking that larger goal into objectives (collect information from the physician/ geneticist about the process of diagnosis; determine the patient's understanding of the available information; assess barriers to understanding the information; assess and address emotional responses and impulsivity) and a clear plan for which team member will address each objective with the patient/family.

To develop goals and objectives with a patient and support network requires skill at quick rapport-building, an ability to apply problem-solving techniques (including creativity about breaking large goals into discrete tasks), comfort with the medical material being addressed, and confidence that one has skills to help patients process complex and difficult information that has life-changing meaning for them. Arguably, part of this process is "lending a vision" (Schwartz & Zalba, 1971, p. 16) or carrying hope (Kerson, 2002): by identifying the goals and objectives, the social worker implicitly assures the patient that those goals can be met and that the patient's life will improve.

Meeting place and use of time

Many contributors to this book note how difficult it is to accomplish their work in the most complete and competent manner, primarily due to large caseloads and multiple responsibilities within their organizations. As the integration of behavioral health care into primary and other health settings continues, social workers will need to advocate for realistic caseloads and other responsibilities. Without such limits, we risk not only burnout and compassion fatigue for ourselves, but inadequate care for patients.

Similarly, social workers need private spaces in which to conduct assessments and interventions. Although many of our contributors note the use of patients' hospital rooms as the primary space for service provision, most also remark on the quickly arranged conversations in hallways and the challenges this practice entails for maintaining rapport and confidentiality. Learning to create private spaces by using one's body to shield the conversation and using a voice that does not carry are "soft skills" health social workers often develop to cope with their settings, but such workarounds are often unsatisfactory, particularly with aging patients and family members who have hearing and processing difficulties. Social workers must consider how space and time factors affect patients and their families, particularly as they convey disrespect and reinscribe oppressive historical patterns (Golden, 2014).

Strategies and interventions

To counteract the medical model's focus on pathology, health social workers need firm grounding in the strengths-based perspective. By assessing how problematic health patterns developed and are maintained in a particular individual, but focusing on the strengths that support change, the social worker establishes a collaborative, non-judging role from which to develop goals and objectives with the patient. It is very useful for a worker to be competent in motivational interviewing techniques that elicit the patient's own motivations/commitment for health changes within a collaborative empathic relationship (rather than prescribing or enforcing change, www.motivationalinterviewing.org/). A worker can elicit the patient's interest in change by asking paradoxically and provocatively why the patient would want to follow the health provider's advice/prescription for change anyway (Purath, Keck, & Fitzgerald, 2014). With the pressure of "shoulds" and "orders" removed, patients often can find their own motivation and commitment to change rather than reactively moving against others' judgments and prescriptions.

Health social workers also use the "Miracle Question" of solution-focused therapy originally developed by de Shazer (1988) ("Imagine that tonight as you sleep a miracle occurs in your life. Your problem is solved! . . . Think for a moment and tell me how you will know the problem has been solved. What behaviors/actions/events will you notice have changed?" www.unk.com/blog/miracle-question-examples/). This helps the patient, his or her family, and the social worker identify behaviors that can be changed to improve the health situation. It is also valuable to teach patients how to use CBT practices such as relaxation techniques and cognitive reframing. Likewise, mindfulness-based stress reduction (e.g., www.mindfullivingprograms.com/whatMBSR.php) can help many patients who are stressed by their health conditions and treatment.

Stance of the social worker

Social workers must be empathic and collaborative. They must approach new clients/patients with confidence in the benefits of collaboration and with curiosity and hopefulness. Repeatedly, research on the most effective therapeutic techniques has found that the effectiveness of any particular therapeutic modality is conflated with the characteristics of the therapist. The so-called "common factors" of elements that create the therapeutic alliance (such as authenticity, positive regard, and empathy (Drisko, 2004)), along with instilling hope, normalizing upsetting experiences (reframing), and helping the patient develop a meaningful explanation of her or his difficulties (meaning-making), are more important than the specific therapeutic technique (Budd & Hughes, 2009, p. 512).

This means that the social worker's empathy, hope, collaboration, advocacy, and authentic care undergird the strategies and interventions discussed above. Effective social workers also must project the confidence that one has something of value to bring to the relationship with the patient (not arrogance or domineering expertise); this in turn must be done in a manner that conveys warmth and respect while asking sometimes uncomfortable questions about sexual habits, relationship stresses, substance use, and other areas outside of "polite" conversation, topics often necessary to a helpful therapeutic alliance. Belief in the ability to help patients process health information, make medical decisions, navigate changed health care routines, and plan for new futures allows social workers to have the confidence to intervene, the respectful curiosity to explore how this particular individual is encountering his or her health condition, and faith that the collaboration will allow the patient to evolve to a better state of well-being.

Use of resources

The Practice in Context framework ensures that social workers think about the political, organizational, technological, and cultural contexts in which they work. Awareness of policies, community resources, social norms and customs/traditions, and health condition information is fundamental to the working knowledge of health social workers. In order to mobilize community resources in aid of patients, social workers must be willing to span disciplinary, geographical, and cultural boundaries (Kerson, 2002). Good practice in health social work requires thinking critically and creatively about how to leverage existing resources and create new ones. Even in settings dedicated to micro level work, the social worker is called upon constantly to reflect on the social sources of health disparities and to promote the resources necessary to minimize them.

Case evaluation and termination

The pace of work often leaves social workers little time to reflect, yet neurobiology and intuitive knowledge tell us that it is in reflection that learning occurs. In thoughtful case evaluation, we should compare original goals and objectives with how the case ended: Were objectives measurable? Were they accomplished? Did cultural differences, organizational or other structural barriers, or other elements of the case create difficult or even obdurate problems? How was this like other (perhaps only superficially) similar cases, and how was it different? Evaluating cases as part of systematic program evaluation or other research is a useful way to identify resources that might have made a difference, and sophisticated research programs can incorporate program changes in subsequent iterations of the evaluation design. Social workers are often the first to see that new medical technologies have created need for new or different resources (Scarvalone et al. in Chapter 13 reflect on the need for more peer support groups for women considering preventive surgeries due to *BRCA* mutations; Brooks suggests new ways of administering hospice benefits in Chapter 22). Although most hospitals and health settings gather data about patients' satisfaction with services, it is important for social workers to look at cases as indicators of needed services and resources both within the hospital or agency and across the community.

Termination requires the social worker to apprise the patient and family of future availability. It involves assuring that referrals are not only made, but followed up and connections made. Many health social workers are frustrated by the lack of time to follow up after patients are discharged, and although a point of pride in health social work is the ability to manage cases effectively within difficult time limits, workers need to stay aware of how the constant flow of intense relationships with often abrupt endings affects the patients and one's professional self. Schlup indicates (Chapter 3) that she made a special effort to reach out to her discharged client to be sure that the patient did not feel rejected or abandoned and to promote continuity of care. Patients' histories of rejection, abandonment, and stigmatization should inspire sensitive attention to the endings one has with patients to assure that they do not reopen old wounds. This aspect of trauma-informed care can be implemented with relative ease and avoids re-traumatizing patients by unplanned endings. Trauma-informed care principles such as awareness that many clients and staff have experienced trauma and that all deserve respect and a sense of physical, psychological, and emotional safety can go a long way toward making our health systems more humane. Indeed, working to challenge our hospitals, agencies, and other organizations to consider organizational changes mirroring the Sanctuary Movement (an early trauma-informed care model) might help to bring about therapeutic positive change for the patients we serve, as well as for the providers (including ourselves) who work in such settings (Esaki et al., 2013).

Differential discussion

As noted earlier, reflection on a case permits workers to learn how similar cases operate and to identify what interventions may allow the worker to promote better outcomes in subsequent cases. By considering the questions that constitute the PiC framework and then reflecting on how each of the decisions about practice might have been handled differently, one builds deliberative knowledge while adding to one's store of implicit knowledge. Mahan and Stein (2014) define the ways System 1 thinking and learning (fast, intuitive) and System 2 thinking and learning (deliberative, reflective) interact to reinforce learning. They define the interaction of Systems 1 and 2 as the modality for building neuronal pathways in the learner's brain when repetition, reflection, and engagement are part of the learning process. We believe that use of the PiC framework, joined with the reflection of the differential discussion (even if it is a discussion in one's own head or with a single colleague) allows deeper learning and promotes the evolution of Dreyfus' "expert" knowledge (1986). Within Dreyfus' model, the "competent performer" who feels personally involved and responsible for one's professional actions is transformed into an "expert" by virtue of repeated performance (case resolutions) to the point where they are able to spontaneously, holistically, and intuitively take action without the necessity of calculated problem-solving so much as enacting tacit knowledge about the best ways to intervene and interact given circumstance. As we said earlier, the differential discussion allows the social worker to reflect upon their work, that is, to consider each practice decision they made and then to consider whether they would make the same decision again or modify it. This helps guide their work if they encounter a similar practice decision in the future.

This promotes a way of thinking about cases that is nearly guaranteed to change brain pathways and build knowledge. The neurobiology of professional knowledge building was certainly not understood at the point where Kerson developed the PiC framework, but practice wisdom (Schon, 1983), medical education (Epstein, Siegel, & Silberman, 2008), and adult learning studies now provide additional rationales for why the PiC framework is so useful. As health social work evolves in response to new circumstances and needs, we expect that social workers who commit themselves to using the PiC framework and to deep reflection via the deliberation about how decisions about practice may have been handled differently will find that they develop knowledge for themselves and their patients/clients, as well as for the profession.

Conclusion

A recent qualitative study in Canada defined health social work roles as, variously, bouncer, janitor, glue, broker, firefighter, juggler, and challenger (Craig & Muskat, 2013). In a pilot project placing the social worker at the center of all communication for the health team and coordinating all care, Kitchen and Brook (2005) used the terms "hub" and "heart" to describe the social work role. In short, social work skills, values, and ethics prepare health social workers to take an active role in coordinating health team communications, working to help patients understand their diagnoses and plan of treatment, supporting patients as they process the emotional and structural barriers to treatment, mobilizing formal and informal supports, and attending to the ways patients' cultural characteristics help or impinge on care: social workers are the heart and glue of care for the patient.

References

ACA (2010). Patient Protection and Affordable Care Act. P. L. 111–148, 124 Stat. 119 (2010).

Budd, R. & Hughes, I. (2009). The Dodo Bird Verdict – Controversial, inevitable and important: A commentary on 30 years of meta-analyses. *Clinical Psychology & Psychotherapy, 16*(6), 510–522. doi: 10.1002/cpp.648

Cavanaugh, J. T. & Konrad, S. C. (2012). Fostering the development of effective person-centered healthcare communication skills: An interprofessional shared learning model. *Work, 41*(3), 293–301. doi: 10.3233/WOR-2012-1292

Craig, S. & Muskat, B. (2013). Bouncers, brokers, and glue: The self-described roles of social workers in urban hospitals. *Health Social Work, 38*(1), 7–16. doi: 10.1093/hsw/hls064

Dane, B. O. & Simon, B. L. (1991). Resident guests: Social workers in host settings. *Social Work, 36*(3), 208–213.

de Shazer, S. (1988). *Clues: Investigating solutions in brief therapy.* New York: W.W. Norton & Co.

Dreyfus, H. L. (1986). *Mind over machine: The power of human intuition and expertise in the era of the computer.* New York: Free Press.

Drisko, J. (2004). Common factors in psychotherapy outcome: Meta-analytic findings and their implications for practice and research. *Families in Society, 85*(1), 81–90.

Epstein, R. M., Siegel, D. J., & Silberman, J. (2008). Self-monitoring in clinical practice: A challenge for medical educators. *Journal of Continuing Education in the Health Professions, 28*, 5–13.

Esaki, N., Benamati, J., Yanosy, S., Middleton, J., Hopson, L., Hummer, V., & Bloom, S. (2013). The Sanctuary Model: Theoretical framework. *Families in Society: The Journal of Contemporary Social Services, 94*(2), 87–95. doi: 10.1606/1044-3894.4287

Fink, S. (2013). *Five days at Memorial.* New York: Crown Publishers.

Franklin, C. (2015). An update on strengths-based, solution-focused brief therapy. *Health Social Work, 40*(2), 73–76. doi: 10.1093/hsw/hlv022

Golden, A. G. (2014). Permeability of public and private spaces in reproductive healthcare seeking: Barriers to uptake of services among low income African American women in a smaller urban setting. *Social Science & Medicine, 108*, 137–146. doi: 10.1016/j.socscimed.2014.02.034

Gudenkauf, L. M., Antoni, M. H., Stagl, J. M., Lechner, S. C., Jutagir, D. R., Bouchard, L. C., et al. (2015). Brief cognitive-behavioral and relaxation training interventions for breast cancer: A randomized controlled trial. *Journal of Consulting and Clinical Psychology, 83*(4), 677–688. doi: 10.1037/ccp0000020

Judd, R. G. & Sheffield, S. (2010). Hospital social work: Contemporary roles and professional activities. *Social Work in Health Care, 49*(9), 856. doi: 10.1080/00981389.2010.499825

Karlin, B. E., Brown, G. K., Trockel, M., Cunning, D., Zeiss, A. M., & Taylor, C. B. (2012). National dissemination of cognitive behavioral therapy for depression in the Department of Veterans' Affairs health care system: Therapist and patient-level outcomes. *Journal of Consulting and Clinical Psychology, 80*(5), 707–718. doi: 10.1037/a0029328

Kerson, T. S. (1981). *Medical social work: The pre-professional paradox.* New York: Irvington.

Kerson, T. S. (2002). *Boundary spanning: An ecological reinterpretation of social work practice in health and mental health.* New York: Columbia University Press.

Kerson, T. S. & McCoyd, J. M. (2013). In response to need: An analysis of social work roles over time. *Social Work, 58*(4), 333–343. doi: 10.1093/sw/swt035

Kitchen, A. & Brook, J. (2005). Social work at the heart of the medical team. *Social Work in Health Care, 40*(4), 1–18. doi: 10.1300/J010v40n04_01

Mahan, J. D. & Stein, D. S. (2014). Teaching adults – Best practices that leverage the emerging under-standing of the neurobiology of learning. *Current Problems in Pediatric and Adolescent Health Care, 44* (Adult Education: New Concepts and Effective Methods for Today's Learners), 141–149. doi: 10.1016/j.cppeds.2014.01.003

Mannix, K. A., Blackburn, I. M., Garland, A., Gracie, J., Moorey, S., Reid, B., et al. (2006). Effectiveness of brief training in cognitive behaviour therapy techniques for palliative care practitioners. *Palliative Medicine, 20*(6), 579–584. doi:10.1177/0269216306071058

McCabe, H. A. & Sullivan, W. P. (2015). Social work expertise: An overlooked opportunity for cutting-edge system design under the Patient Protection and Affordable Care Act. *Health Social Work, 40*(2), 155–157. doi: 10.1093/hsw/hlv005

NASW (National Association of Social Workers) (2008/1996). Code of ethics. Retrieved from www. socialworkers.org/pubs/code/default.asp

NASW (2011). *Social workers in hospital and medical centers, occupational profile.* Washington, D.C.: Author. Retrieved from http://workforce.socialworkers.org/studies/profiles/Hospitals.pdf

ObamaCare Facts (n.d.). Retrieved from http://obamacarefacts.com/obamacare-sign-up/.

Purath, J., Keck, A., & Fitzgerald, C. E. (2014). Motivational interviewing for older adults in primary care: A systematic review. *Geriatric Nursing, 35*, 219–224. doi: 10.1016/j.gerinurse.2014.02.002

Rollnick, S., Miller, W. R., & Butler, C. (2008). *Motivational interviewing in health care: Helping patients change behavior.* Guilford, NC: Guilford Press.

Saleebey, D. (2012). *The Strengths Perspective in social work practice (Advancing core competencies)* (6th edn.). Boston: Pearson.

Schon, D. A. (1983). *The reflective practitioner: How professionals think in action.* New York: Basic Books.

Spitzer, W., Silverman, E., & Allen, K. (2015). From organizational awareness to organizational com-petency in health care social work: The importance of formulating a "Profession-in-Environment" fit. *Social Work in Health Care, 54*(3), 193–211. doi: 10.1080/00981389.2014.990131

Schwartz, W. & Zalba, S. R. (1971). *The practice of group work.* New York: Columbia University Press.

Maternal and child health settings

Chapter 3

Barriers for a mentally ill mother's adoption plan

Dasi Schlup

Context

Description of setting

The Women and Children's Hospital and Clinics (WCH) of the University of Missouri Health Care system is Mid-Missouri's largest health care facility, offering comprehensive care to women and children. It serves more than 60 counties and offers intensive care in neonatology and pediatrics, as well as over 30 sub-specialties and primary care pediatric care. The Newborn Intensive Care Unit (NICU) is a level 3, 48-bed nursery with 556 admissions annually. The Pediatric Service has a 53-bed unit. The Family Birth Center of WCH has 26 antepartum and postpartum rooms, 10 delivery rooms, and 2 surgical suites. In 2014 there were 1,785 births at the Family Birth Center.

The maternal–fetal medicine (MFM) clinic offers specialized care for high-risk pregnancies. The MFM perinatologists are obstetricians who specialize in the treatment of high-risk pregnancies. The typical high-risk patient has pregnancy complications including gestational diabetes, heart disease, kidney disease, congenital anomalies, a history of multiple miscarriages, and preeclampsia. Other high-risk pregnancies include multiple gestation pregnancies or those exposed to drugs and/or alcohol. Consulting specialists include cardiologists, radiologists, genetic counselors, pediatric surgeons, neonatology, and social work. In 2014 the clinic provided care to 14,556 patients and 25% of them had babies admitted to the NICU.

Policies

Several state and federal policies impact the multi-faceted case presented in this chapter. One role of a social worker is to facilitate the voluntary placement of an infant for adoption. Missouri Statute 453 sections 005–170, 315–325, 400, 500–503, and 600 define the state's adoption laws for court-approved legal transfer of a child and specify that a birth mother cannot initiate the process of placement until the infant is 48 hours of age. While this time frame varies from state to state, the intent is to provide the birth mother time to consider her decision after the birth of the child. The statute also states that once the adoption is finalized in the court, the birth mother cannot withdraw or revoke her consent. If an unwed mother names the biological father but he is not on the birth certificate, has not filed a paternity action, or filed with the Missouri Putative Father Registry, nor acted like a father, the law states that there is no obligation to serve him notice of adoption. If no action is taken, an adoption can proceed without the father's participation or consent. The WCH adoption policy requires a social work consult. The social worker conducts an assessment, provides support and counseling, and collaborates with the adoption agency or legal representative of the parties involved to facilitate the adoption plan. When a child is placed into foster care or with an adoptive family from another state, the process is protected by the Interstate Compact on Placement of Children Act (American Public Human Services Association, 2002; ICPC, 45ILCS15). This federal act protects children when moving from one state to another and protects the "jurisdiction, administrative and human rights obligations of all parties involved in an interstate placement." The ICPC requires a history and plan for the child and a home study which can take six weeks to process. Until that time the child must remain in the state of origin. The federal Child Abuse Prevention and Treatment Act (CAPTA) defines the act of child abuse and neglect as "Any recent act or failure to act on the part of a parent or caretaker, which results in death, serious physical or emotional harm, sexual abuse, or exploitation, or an act or failure to act which presents an imminent risk of serious harm" (CAPTA, 2010, Section 210.115.1). By law, the hospital social worker is a mandated reporter. In Missouri a medical professional can request a Newborn Crisis Assessment prior to a hospital discharge if there is concern for potential harm.

Assessments of the birth mother's physical and emotional health are the responsibility of the medical team. A concern for the patient's emotional stability prompts a psychiatric consultation. A psychiatrist can order a "96 hour hold" and immediate admission to a psychiatric facility for further evaluation and treatment. All employees of the Women's and Children's Hospital ensure a patient's privacy, especially in regards to their health information and medical records. In accordance with the Health Insurance Portability and Accountability Act of 1996 (HIPAA, 2013), information can only be released with the written consent of the patient. An exception to HIPAA is in the case of a report to the Child Abuse and Neglect Hotline. The Privacy Rule (see 45 C.F.R. 164.512(b) (1) (ii)) permits covered health care providers to provide medical information in situations of abuse or neglect to public health or appropriate government authorities.

Technology

Multiple methods of monitoring a high-risk pregnancy can result in improved outcomes for high-risk pregnancies. The most commonly used surveillance techniques include fetal movement counts. This low-tech approach is done at home and it helps the patient keep track of the activity of the fetus. The non-stress test measures the fetal heart rate in response to fetal movement over time. This test is done in the clinic or in the hospital. A "reactive" test is reassuring. If the fetus is not reactive, it may mean the fetus was asleep or it could indicate the fetus is not getting enough oxygen. A biophysical profile (BPP) scores fetal well-being by assessment of the heart rate, breathing movements, body movements, muscle tone, and amniotic fluid. Doppler ultrasound of the umbilical artery checks the blood flow in the umbilical artery and can indicate poor fetal growth.

High-risk pregnancies require frequent office visits to monitor and conduct tests that assess fetal health. It is often necessary to admit the patient to the hospital in order to perform testing daily or multiple times per day. The demands on the patient's time can be very disruptive to the patient's other responsibilities. The social worker helps to ensure that the patient understands the need for close surveillance of the fetus and addresses barriers to adherence. It is not unusual for an antepartum patient to become restless, anxious and depressed, and question the need for hospitalization. The social worker can facilitate a care meeting with the perinatologist and encourage the patient to explore coping strategies for adjustment to antepartum status.

Courtroom technology is an aspect of the case presented in this chapter. The introduction of advanced technologies in the courtroom includes the development of websites, interactive resources, remote assistance, e-filing, tools that can help the disabled persons have better access to information, and real-time video conferencing. Real-time video conferencing can be used when the witness cannot be present (Foster & Cihlar, 2014).

The internet offers patients the option of doing research on issues that affect their medical and personal situations. Patients may find statistical data or anecdotal information that can clarify or complicate their understanding of their medical information. The social worker will often review reputable internet resources and process with the patient the best approach to understanding the diagnosis and risks to her pregnancy. Some patients need to review and read all available information and some patients cope best with only the information given by the physician. The internet can also offer psychosocial information relevant to the case, including information on financial resources, housing, child care counseling, substance abuse rehabilitation, and adoption.

Organization

The clinical social worker plays an integral role in the multi-disciplinary team. When a diagnosis indicates the infant will be admitted to the NICU for treatment, the MFM outpatient clinic coordinates a consultation with a neonatologist and the social worker. Upon meeting the patient/family, the social worker and neonatologist ensure the patient's understanding of the diagnosis and range of expected outcomes of the pregnancy, including the prognosis and the expected plan of care. The neonatologist and social worker give the patient/family the opportunity to ask questions, explore options for intervention, clarify the information provided, and seek recommendations. The social worker also provides information about the operation of the NICU, including opportunities for parent time with the infant, visiting policies, and financial resources.

When a pregnant patient learns of medical complications, initially, the role of the social worker is to assess the patient's emotional response to the diagnosis. The patient may experience feelings of guilt, fear, grief, and anxiety. If the family expresses similar emotions, their needs will also be addressed. The social worker may provide crisis counseling, emotional support, and assistance with decision-making processes. Decisions may be needed on further testing, continuation of the pregnancy, and medical interventions upon delivery. A palliative care approach may be offered by the physician and the social worker. The social worker helps the patient/family process these difficult decisions. Early consultation with the social worker provides the opportunity to establish a rapport with the patient/family. The social worker begins the psychosocial assessment immediately and can address other factors unrelated to the medical complications, including domestic violence, illicit substance abuse, plans for relinquishment of the infant through adoption, depression or other mental illness, and prior history with Child Protective Services. As the social worker establishes a relationship of trust with the patient, he or she can begin to affect change and develop a plan with the patient as an active participant in the process. This provides the patient with some control of her situation and can alleviate further stress.

There are 2.5 full-time equivalent (FTE) maternal/child health master's prepared social workers in the Family Birth Center of WCH. The NICU has 1.5 FTE dedicated social workers and 1 FTE serves the MFM service. NICU admissions include an automatic social work consultation. The social worker is an integral part of the team, collaborating with the team for the best outcome for the family and the infant, and evaluating and planning for multi-cultural and psychosocial needs. This includes interventions such as: interventional and supportive counseling to adjust to illness, promotion of coping strategies, crisis intervention, brief therapy, grief counseling, and assistance with aspects of social and practical needs in the acute neonatal setting. The social worker collaborates with family, medical team, and community agencies. The social worker serves as a liaison for the family and providers, and coordinates conferences with the medical team in preparation for a successful transition home. Occasionally, the social worker may be required by the judicial system to offer testimony as an advocate for the parents and the infant. The social worker is in a position to provide the court with a professional assessment and recommendations that are based on an in-depth and multi-faceted relationship with the family system.

Decisions about practice

Case description

Chris presented to the MFM clinic of WCH as a 30-year-old single White female, 24 weeks gestation, with a triplet pregnancy. Her pregnancy was further complicated by late prenatal care and a minimal medical history. The MFM and neonatal physicians requested an in-depth psychosocial assessment of Chris. Chris was accompanied to the consultation by a counselor from Faith Maternity Home, a shelter for homeless pregnant women in a nearby community where she had been staying after relocating from North Carolina. Chris was recently divorced, unemployed with no stable source of income, had no family support, and was homeless. In addition, she had two birth children who were not in her custody. The current pregnancy was unplanned and undesired, with Chris stating, "I don't think about them as mine." She had researched shelters and came to Missouri specifically for the level of support provided by Faith Maternity Home. Chris planned to place the infants for adoption but refusing to appear in court, a mandate of Missouri adoption law.

I met with Chris briefly in the clinic upon her first visit but had more extended contact when she "fired" her obstetrician, Dr. F, because he would not deliver her at 27 weeks (about six months of pregnancy: full term is 40 weeks). She did not believe the infants were preterm. Goldenberg, McClure, Bhattacharya, Groat, and Stahl (2009) found that 75% of the women in their study believed an infant was full term after 34 weeks gestation. During this appointment, Chris agreed to a release of information between the Faith Maternity Home counselor and our facility.

My initial intake with Chris revealed a history of anxiety, depression, and sexual assault as a teen, in addition to fractured family relationships. The Faith Maternity Home counselor reported that Chris often exhibited "strange behaviors," such as using cooking oil on her skin and hair. They did not observe Chris having hallucinations, mania, or symptoms of depression. Throughout the hospitalization, Chris was needy, demanding, and uncomfortable around the staff caring for her.

Chris was admitted to labor and delivery and then to the antepartum service at 30 weeks with preterm labor and a shortened cervix. She was combative, uncooperative, and "fired" her first two nurses; the staff contacted me to intervene. I negotiated with Chris to work with one of the previous nurses and her doctor. Chris reported strange beliefs including her belief that rice she placed in her maternity belt was keeping the triplets from peeing on her skin. A psychiatric consultation was ordered due to questions about Chris' mental stability and competency. The psychiatrist interacted with her briefly and concluded that he did not observe any psychotic symptoms or behaviors, although he noted that she was vague and evasive which could indicate she was actively hiding an underlying psychotic mental illness. His final diagnosis was personality disorder with cluster A (odd, bizarre, strange) and cluster B (dramatic, erratic, volatile, narcissistic, and antisocial) traits. He believed that she was competent to make personal decisions.

Throughout her antepartum stay, Chris asked that I accompany her when she received medical information. This role of liaison and negotiator continued throughout the hospital stay. Chris continued to be a very difficult patient, often refusing recommended care of the infants as well as sharing her psychosocial history in fragmented pieces. Five days before Chris' scheduled cesarean section, she requested help in contacting her ex-stepmother, Sheila, in North Carolina, believing she might be supportive. Indeed, Sheila came to Missouri two days before surgery and displayed kindness, warmth, and empathy for Chris; they had maintained a relationship following her divorce from Chris' father. Chris signed a release of information between me and Sheila. Sheila produced copies of court papers from North Carolina stating that Chris' parental rights had been terminated to three other children due to physical and emotional harm including erratic behavior with hallucinations and delusions. Multiple psychiatric hospitalizations revealed incidences of bizarre behavior, and she was diagnosed with schizoaffective disorder, substance-induced psychosis, and major depressive disorder. Reportedly, Chris would be stable but then become medication non-compliant, resulting in acute deterioration of her mental state and ultimately alienation from her family. The only relationship she maintained was with Sheila, although at the time of hospitalization they had not spoken in several years.

Custody options were discussed with Chris who suggested keeping custody of the children upon discharge and accompanying Sheila to North Carolina in order to find an appropriate adoptive placement. I explained that the physicians would not discharge the infants to her care due to her inability to provide a stable home and in light of her expressed choice not to parent. An alternative plan to take legal steps to give Sheila temporary custody through the court was discussed. Sheila had not come to Missouri seeking any form of custody of the infants. She was in her mid-fifties living with her husband, also in his fifties, their 16-year-old daughter who had some developmental challenges, and her aged mother. Nonetheless, Sheila agreed to take on this responsibility. I contacted the county Juvenile Office to discuss the plan for temporary placement with Sheila and inquired about the role of Child Protective Services. The Juvenile Office endorsed the plan with the expectation that proper legal papers were filed with the court. They did not see the need for involvement with Children's Protective Services. This plan evolved into Chris' request that Sheila adopt the infants and Sheila agreed.

Upon delivery (at 34 weeks), Chris reiterated and confirmed her intention to place the triplets for adoption. The triplets were admitted to the NICU with respiratory distress. All three infants were stable, needing respiratory, thermal, and nutritional support. Chris declined any contact or pictures of the infants. She did ask about their health, weight, and general description. Sheila visited the infants and participated in their care. She developed a strong attachment to them and became a strong advocate for their interests. She continued to be an empathetic support person for Chris, whose behavior rapidly deteriorated within 24 hours of delivery. Chris became paranoid, germ phobic (cleaning all surfaces with alcohol swipes), walking on sheets, and refusing needed care. At one point she asked me to be sure and get the best home for the triplets if she dies, "because you know that doctor didn't put me together right."

According to Jones, Chandra, Dazzan, and Howard (2014), extensive studies of patients with a chronic psychotic condition show they often deteriorate in the postpartum period. "Childbirth is a powerful trigger of mania and psychosis with wild fluctuations in intensity of symptoms and severe swings of mood. It is estimated that postpartum admission rates to psychiatric hospitals are about 1–2 per 1000 births" (p. 1789). Psychiatric deterioration after delivery is not uncommon (McCullough, Coverdale, & Chervenak, 2002); we requested another psychiatric consultation.

Sheila retained a lawyer for herself and a separate lawyer for Chris. A petition for adoption was filed. Permission was obtained from the court to conduct a sworn videotaped testimony from Chris in the hospital testifying to her intent to terminate her parental rights without undue pressure. Just prior to the scheduled taping of the testimony, a second psychiatric consultation and assessment was completed. Despite some resistance in the interview, the psychiatrist was able to determine that Chris did not have the capacity to make decisions regarding the termination of her parental rights and placement for adoption. She diagnosed Chris as psychotic, with paranoid schizophrenia, and determined that Chris needed immediate psychiatric care and placed a "96 hour" hold and arranged for immediate admission to a psychiatric hospital. Chris was deemed incompetent to make the decision to terminate her parental rights. I consulted with the social worker at the psychiatric facility and explained the Juvenile Office's support of the adoption plan, nevertheless, she requested a Newborn Crisis Assessment from the Children's Division, making them a party to the case. Sheila's lawyer filed a motion to terminate Chris' parental rights and place the infants for adoption with Sheila and her husband based on my testimony confirming Chris' consistent request for this plan throughout the pregnancy. When Sheila's lawyer informed the judge that Chris was psychiatrically hospitalized, the judge stopped the proceedings. The judge instructed the lawyers and Children's Division to return to court within the next few days. If Chris remained hospitalized and unable to testify, the judge would rule that the infants should be placed in protective custody. This decision was based on the statue Missouri House Bill 343, 1997 which allows revocation of termination of parental rights due to undue duress. At that time, a guardian ad litem was appointed for the triplets.

Multiple court hearings ensued and the infants were placed in protective custody. The social worker for Children's Division, however, supported the plan to place the infants with Sheila until the adoption process could proceed. Sheila was advised that the Interstate Compact on Placement of Children Act: ICPC (45ILCS15) mandated filing a request to take infants out of the state and required completion of a home study by a licensed social worker in North Carolina. Children's Services was concerned that the home study and application for the ICPC could be lengthy and would not be complete before the infants' discharge. In that case, Sheila would have to remain in Missouri to complete the process, an untenable situation for Sheila as it would place her employment in jeopardy.

At the psychiatric hospital, Chris was diagnosed with delirium and paranoid schizophrenia but refused medication. She reportedly exhibited anxiety, paranoia, and depression. Chris was non-compliant and the psychiatrist filed for a 21-day hold, and consulted the probate court that ordered her medication to be administered by injection. Chris' psychiatrist noted that with treatment, her behavior, mood, concentration, coherence, and sleep pattern improved and her diagnosis was modified to schizoaffective disorder. Sheila continued to visit Chris and to provide support. The psychiatrist reported that she was stabilizing and Chris met with her lawyers and agreed to another court hearing. A teleconference testimony was arranged. Chris testified to her plan to terminate her rights and place the infants with Sheila. She was pleasant, articulate, and lucid as she explained her inability to parent. Chris' attorneys and the guardian ad litem were satisfied that Chris was able to make a sound decision to terminate her rights. Chris' psychiatrist testified that Chris had made progress and would be discharged soon. Despite the court's request for testimony that Chris was competent, the psychiatrist declined to assert that and Chris' testimony was not accepted. Chris was discharged several days after the hearing. She had hoped to be discharged to Sheila's care. This, however, was not possible as the Children's Division would not let her be in the presence of the triplets. Chris was discharged to Faith Maternity Home.

Chris made plans to return to North Carolina after the hearing. The attorneys met with Chris to sign papers of her intent to terminate her rights for adoption, but she unexpectedly refused to sign the papers. I speculated to Sheila that Chris understood that relinquishing the infants to Sheila might alter the supportive relationship Chris had with Sheila. Chris had hoped to live with Sheila in North Carolina. Sheila confronted Chris and explained that with great sorrow she would return to North Carolina without the infants and that their future would be determined by the courts. The following day, Chris contacted her lawyer and agreed to attend the hearing. The judge allowed all parties' testimonies to be entered into court documentation and instructed Chris to sign termination papers. Just as Chris put pen to paper, she turned to the judge and inquired whether she could "still change my mind, right?" The judge, clearly angered, ordered the attorneys and Chris to leave the courtroom and explain to Chris that her decision was irrevocable. Chris said she understood; however, she wanted reassurance that the triplets would be placed with Sheila and her husband. One hour later, Chris signed the papers, specifying relinquishment to Sheila and her husband and the court approved them. The triplets were discharged to Sheila and her husband the following week; the ICPC was filed and approved. Chris left the maternity home shortly after the hearing and returned to North Carolina.

Definition of client

In accordance with the standards set forth by the National Association of Perinatal Social Workers (n.d.) "The hospital social work services shall be provided to individuals involved with the relinquishment of an infant for adoption. Birth parents, adoptive parents and the adoptee are appropriately regarded as clients whose needs and rights shall be respected and considered." Services include "assessment, support, ongoing counseling and/or referral to an appropriate agency." The policy at WCH reflects this standard.

Goals, objectives, outcomes, and contracting

Chris' initial goal was to relinquish her infants without involving the Children's Division or the foster care system. She wanted to avoid appearing in court to testify to this intent. She was motivated to ensure the health of the infants and herself; this led to her attendance at the high-risk clinic and involvement with me. Chris and I agreed to pursue options for her relinquishment goals, in coordination with the MFM medical team. We did not establish a written contract; however, these objectives were documented in her electronic medical record. We agreed that social work continuity was important and, therefore, I would follow her throughout the pregnancy and the hospitalization of the triplets. It was important to educate Chris about the legal process of adoption and pursue options that allowed her to participate in the process of finding a family for her triplets. Chris had met with a social worker from a licensed adoption agency and did not feel comfortable working with the agency. We explored other agency and private adoption resources. Chris agreed to meet twice with a neonatologist who explained the importance of monitoring the pregnancy and Chris' compliance with care.

The initial psychiatric consultation led us to make decisions in practice that at times were disagreeable to Chris. Examples included her verbalized choices that would result in Children's Division taking protective custody (which she did not want) (i.e., "I can just leave them here after I give birth"). She also resisted procedures that would monitor the triplets, such as the non-stress tests. My role with Chris as my client was occasionally challenged by my commitment to ensure the best outcome for the triplets. Yet, I knew that maintaining the therapeutic alliance was important to Chris' well-being (Bender, 2005). This became an ethical dilemma, as ultimately the health and safety of the triplets took precedence over her personal goals. This required a balancing act in meeting all my standards of practice.

The measures of success of this case included medical compliance to ensure the best outcome of the pregnancy, a successful adoption plan for the triplets, and optimizing Chris' physical and mental health. The goal of medical compliance was evidenced by Chris' admission to the hospital at 30 weeks. Furthermore, though she did not consistently agree to interventions to monitor the pregnancy, she did cooperate adequately, resulting in the birth and the desired outcome of healthy triplets delivered at 34 weeks gestation. Her goal for placement of the infants was successful as they were placed for adoption with a family of her choice. Chris' physical and mental health was strengthened by her commitment to a psychiatric facility. Despite the disturbing change of course and her commitment to the psychiatric facility, this step gave her the best possible chance for improvement in her health and quality of life.

Meeting place and use of time

I met with Chris in the clinic exam room when she was on outpatient and in her private room once she was on the inpatient service. Nursing was only interrupted for immediate medical needs. After the triplets were born, I met with Sheila in the NICU, at the babies' bedside, or in a private conference room. Typically, the bulk of my time is spent in the NICU with families in crisis. My average time spent with antepartum patients is 2 hours a week. I spent an average of 5 hours a week with Chris as she had a difficult time adapting to the hospitalization. She was agitated and anxious, rude to the staff, and uncooperative. She relied on me to be her liaison and advocate to the care providers. A great deal of time was spent with the nursing staff providing guidance about how they could approach providing Chris' care. Chris needed intensive ongoing support, though Sheila's arrival offered some relief as she was able to reason with Chris and provide support. Prior to Chris' commitment to the psychiatric unit, there were multiple consultations with the obstetrical and psychiatric teams. With the birth of the triplets, my role as the NICU social worker required more focus on the triplet's discharge plans. Sheila's need for support continued with each new complication of the adoption. She was often depressed, defeated, and very anxious about her financial situation. Following Chris' involuntary commitment, I needed to coordinate services with Children's Services, Sheila, psychiatry, and the lawyers. I was subpoenaed multiple times, had multiple video conferences, and provided documentation for the ICPC application.

Strategies and interventions

My first meeting with Chris posed difficulty in conducting a basic assessment. She was suspicious and would only provide information that was directly related to her decision to place her infants for adoption. It was clear Chris had difficulty developing and maintaining inter-personal relationships. She had difficulty engaging with her health care providers, counse-lors, and residents in the maternity home. She mistrusted the legal system and foster care system. My strategy, therefore, was to develop a working relationship based on the theory of shared decision-making and therapeutic alliance. Chris' unplanned high-risk pregnancy, dependence on the staff of the maternity home, and lack of choice in her medical care pro-viders left little in her situation that she could control. It was important to establish an alli-ance with empathy and open communication, and provide supportive counseling. I reassured Chris that I would assist her in her decision-making process for the adoption and that I was committed to advocate for her rights and empower her with the ability to make choices.

The National Association of Social Workers (2008/2016) Code of Ethics states, "Social workers respect and promote the right of clients to self-determination and assist clients in their efforts to identify and clarify their goals." Laugharne and Priebe (2006) propose that establishing an alliance with patients who are resistant requires attention to trust, choice, and power, "with attunement to a patient's way of seeing the world" (p. 86). I ensured Chris' pri-vacy, was a liaison to the medical team and community resources, and was direct and honest with her. Laugharne and Priebe (2006) demonstrate that patient participation in choices about their care results in more engagement and cooperation. As part of the multi-disciplinary team, I recognized the ethical conflicts with which the nurses struggled. Simmonds (2008) elaborates: "it can interfere with the nurses' ability to exercise their professional judgment between the duty of care and the responsibility to act as a patient advocate" (p. 363). I strug-gled too. After delivery, Chris exhibited psychotic behavior and vehemently disagreed with our recommendation for the second psychiatric assessment and she resisted the commitment. My ethical challenge was acknowledging that shared decision-making was not in always in Chris' best interest.

Social work referrals are automatic for all admissions to the NICU. I provided support to Sheila as she adjusted to the triplets' preterm status and the stressful adoption process. I facilitated communication with the medical team. It was imperative that Sheila understood each infant's progress and plan of care. It was important for the team to understand the unique circumstances of the infants' placement, factors that could impact the discharge plans. I coordinated with Sheila's attorney and Children's Division to facilitate placement. I made referrals to appropriate community resources, testified in court hearings, and assisted with ICPC process. See Figure 3.1 for Chris' ecomap of involved people and services.

Stance of the social worker

I am an integral part of the multi-disciplinary team in the MFM and NICU service. Interactions take place throughout the day and consultation and processing plans for the patients are con-ducted in both a formal and informal fashion. My assessments and interventions are valued. I help the mother during high risk pregnancy, and later in the NICU, to navigate the complex medical system. I work to understand her perspective and needs. I provide her and her family with support, with counseling, facilitating communication with care providers, resources, and decision-making. This case was challenging as Chris' behavior resulted in alienating most of the medical team. I had to maintain a trusting relationship with her while also confronting her with the consequences of her behavior. I was in the position of interpreting her behavior and history to the team and normalizing the reaction of the medical team to Chris as a patient. The physicians' frustration after delivery meant they were reluctant to deal with Chris and I had

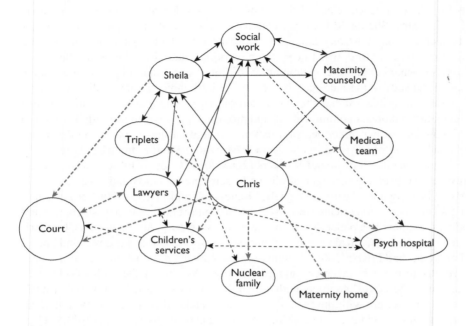

Figure 3.1 Ecomap of case study

to advocate for a second psychiatric consultation and Chris' commitment. These decisions were made in her best interest; even so, I felt I failed to deliver on my part of the contract with Chris for choice and self-determination. When Chris refused to sign the adoption papers, I struggled with the ethical dilemma of being true to Chris as I lost the perspective that Chris' manipulative behaviors towards Sheila were reflections of her mental disorder.

The complexities of the adoption process promoted a very close and intense relationship with Sheila and it required discipline to keep my role professional. This adoption process involved legal barriers, interstate adoption barriers, challenges of distance for Sheila and her family, and unusual and unexpected financial challenges for Sheila and her family.

Use of resources outside the helping relationship

Community resources are a valuable tool and every family situation is unique, requiring creative use of these services. These resources include home nursing visits after discharge, financial grants to help with gas, meals, and lodging, nutrition services, crib and car-seats, and to agencies that provide case management for outpatient services and follow-up for the continued development of the infant. The Ronald McDonald House is also available and helps house and serve families from long distances. This offers parents the ability to be close to the NICU.

I collaborated with multiple community resources in assisting Chris. The open communication with Faith Maternity Home was the most beneficial resource affecting this case. Their insight and observations of Chris provided a perspective that was not available to me. The home was also a safe and supportive environment for Chris after her release from the psychiatric facility and offered Chris help with long-term planning. I worked closely with the various legal teams, the Children's Division, and the Juvenile Office, agencies I work with on a regular basis. All these groups had the same goal: placement of the triplets with Sheila, though each entity often had differing paths to that goal.

Reassessment and evaluation

Throughout this case I was faced with issues I did not anticipate. Most days required creative problem solving and multi-disciplinary collaboration. The deterioration of Chris' mental status, the adoption process involving the court's decisions, the demands of the Interstate Compact Act, and the involvement of the Children's Division were very complicating factors. Nonetheless, the main objectives – a successful pregnancy, a safe placement of the triplets with a loving adoptive family of Chris' choice, and support and assistance for Chris – were met.

Transfer and termination

Chris' emergent transfer to the psychiatric facility resulted in an initial failure to terminate my relationship with Chris. This was very disturbing to me. I worried Chris would believe that I was another person in her life who dismissed her and abandoned her. After her discharge from the psychiatric facility, I was able to contact Chris by phone and express my disappointment that we could not process her feelings, process the change in our relationship, or work together on her future plans. I saw Chris at the final court hearing. She appeared notably different, well groomed, thinner, dressed in fancy clothes. We were able to talk about her relief that "this will finally be over" and she was responsive to my support as we awaited our summons into the courtroom.

Case conclusion

The triplets were discharged from the NICU, all very healthy with excellent prognoses. They were placed with Sheila and her husband. The adoption process is proceeding in North Carolina. Sheila recently sent pictures of the infants and they are beautiful, beloved, and growing. Chris returned to North Carolina shortly after the court hearing. She contacted Sheila twice; she told her that she was attending junior college and renting a room at a house near the school. She promised to follow up with counseling. Chris also told Sheila that she understood she could not come to see the infants or Sheila. It is unclear if Chris will continue to address her mental health issues in light of her prior history.

Differential discussion

My typical work day is focused on the families and patients in the NICU. Some days I may work intensively with a family in crisis and other days I am in constant motion addressing a multitude of issues for many families. Social workers in a medical setting utilize their counseling skills; however, mental illness is not the typical focus. Working with Chris pivoted me into that role and at times pulled me away from the needs of the families in the NICU. I knew it was important to maintain my working relationship with her to achieve the best outcome for her and the pregnancy. It was a constant concern of mine, her maternity counselor, and the medical team that she would leave against medical advice and put the infants at great risk. This case required much of my time and effort in order to keep Chris and her pregnancy safe and to help the staff deal with Chris' behaviors. Nonetheless, in retrospect, I took on too much responsibility trying to maintain those objectives and would have benefited from incorporating a primary care nursing team in the alliance I had formed with Chris. Involving them more directly may have given some of the nurses "buy in" to the challenge of working with Chris.

Upon reflection about my involvement with Sheila, I think I stretched my professional boundaries. She was very determined, savvy, and resourceful and did not need some of the legwork I provided. The complexity of Sheila's relationship with Chris, and Chris' manipulative behavior in the adoption process, fueled my determination to do anything I could to help make the adoption placement successful. I could not help Sheila with the usual resources available to my families as her needs were unique and geographically distant. Yet, I am glad that the children are with Sheila and that Chris has embarked on a productive path.

Discussion questions

1   When balancing the needs of the medical care plan, the desires of a pregnant woman, and the potential of a medically complicated pregnancy, how do you weigh the ethical obligations to each of the entities you must serve as a social worker?
2   How comfortable would you be in providing testimony for court proceedings? What ethical guidance do you believe you would need to manage this?
3   How might you manage time-intensive cases when the normal work requirements are already demanding?

References

American Public Human Services Association (2002). *Guide to the Interstate Compact on the Placement of Children*. Washington, DC: U.S. Department of Health and Human Services, Children's Bureau.

Bender, D. S. (2005). The therapeutic alliance in the treatment of personality disorders. *Journal of Psychiatric Practice, 11*(2), 73–87. doi: 10.1097/00131746-200503000-00002

CAPTA (2010). Child Abuse Prevention and Treatment Act of 1974, 42 U.S.C. § 5106 (2010).

Foster, R. S. & Cihlar, L. M. (2014). Technology and family law hearings. *Western Journal of Legal Studies, 5*(1), 1–17. Retrieved from: http://ir.lib.uwo.ca/uwojls/v015/iss1/2

Goldenberg, R., McClure, E., Bhattacharya, A., Groat, T., & Stahl, P. (2009). Women's perceptions regarding the safety of births at various gestational ages. *Obstetrics & Gynecology, 114*(6), 1254–1258. doi: 10.1097/AOG.0b013e3181c2d6a0

HIPAA (2013). Health Insurance and Portability and Accountability Act of 1996 (HIPAA), 42 U.S.C. §§ 104–191 (2013).

Jones, I., Chandra, P. S., Dazzan, P., & Howard, L. M. (2014). Bipolar disorder, affective psychosis, and schizophrenia in pregnancy and the post-partum period. *Lancet, 384*(9956), 1789–1799. doi: 10.1016/S0140–6736(14)61278-2

Laugharne, R. & Priebe, S. (2006). Trust, choice and power in mental health. *Social Psychiatry & Psychiatric Epidemiology, 41*(11), 843–852. doi: 10.1007/s00127-006-0123-6

McCullough, L. B., Coverdale, J. H., & Chervenak, F. A. (2002). Ethical challenges of decision making with pregnant patients who have schizophrenia. *American Journal of Obstetrics and Gynecology, 187*(3), 696–702.

National Association of Perinatal Social Workers. (n.d.). www.napsw.org/about/pdfs/

National Association of Social Workers (2008/1996). Code of ethics. Retrieved from www.socialwork ers.org/pubs/code/default.asp

Simmonds, A. H. (2008). Autonomy and advocacy in perinatal nursing practice. *Nursing Ethics, 15*(3), 360–370.

Missouri legal statutes

Adoption, Mo. Assemb. HB. 343 (1997).

Consent to an Adoption, Mo. Rev. Stat. § 453.030 (1997).

Interstate Compact on the Placement of Children, Mo. Rev. Stat §§ 210.620 to 210.700 (2005); Mo. Rev. Stat. §§ 632.305(2) to 632.305(3) (2011); Mo. Rev. Stat. §§ 453.005 to 453.600 (2012).

Mandatory Reporting of Child Abuse and Neglect, Mo. Rev. Stat. § 210.115.1 (1976).

Putative Father Registry, Mo. Rev. Stat. § 192.016 (1998).

Chapter 4

Fetal surgery

Jennifer Diem Inglis, Jessica Hertzog, and
Heather K. Ousley

Context

The use of sonography during pregnancy and its diagnostic benefits have been well documented (Leithner et al., 2004). For most women, the anatomical ultrasound offers them the first glimpse at their unborn child and the opportunity to learn the baby's gender. For some, however, this practice becomes anything but routine when a fetal anomaly is detected. The Center for Fetal Diagnosis and Treatment (CFDT) at the Children's Hospital of Philadelphia (CHOP) provides assessment of and care for pregnant women and their babies when a genetic or birth defect is identified.

Since its opening in 1995, the CFDT has evaluated over 17,000 women whose fetus potentially has a genetic or birth defect. Many of the conditions that are seen in the CFDT are ones that are best treated after the baby is born; however, they require close monitoring throughout the duration of the pregnancy. There are also conditions that may benefit from prenatal intervention, such as fetal surgery, followed by close monitoring for the duration of the pregnancy. Sadly, there are some conditions that are considered lethal and the fetus is likely to die while in utero or shortly after birth.

There are two different types of fetal surgery: fetoscopic procedures and open fetal surgery. During a fetoscopic procedure, a surgeon inserts a scope through a small incision in the uterus while using ultrasound guidance and either corrects or temporarily fixes the problematic condition. Examples of this would include laser placental division for twin-to-twin transfusion syndrome or the placement of a shunt in those fetuses who have complications with draining their bladder due to a urinary blockage. Open fetal surgery is much more complicated for both the fetus and the mother. It requires the mother to have a hysterotomy, an incision in the abdomen wall and into the uterus. From there the fetus, while still in utero, is exposed and the defect is fixed. Following surgery, the mother is on strict bed rest for the duration of her pregnancy. Examples of fetal surgery include a prenatal spina bifida closure or the removal of a lung mass when the baby is showing signs of hydrops.

Policy

Health insurance for prenatal, maternity, and newborn care became mandatory under the Affordable Care Act in 2014 (Patient Protection and Affordable Care Act, 2010). Prenatal care, including ultrasound, is covered by most private insurance carriers, and Medical Assistance. For patients who do not have coverage and who are not eligible for Medical Assistance, an application can be made for Charity Care coverage provided by the hospital.

Despite improved prenatal care coverage, barriers to care could include high out-of-pocket health costs, and travel and relocation costs. Coverage for fetal surgery is typically approved; however, prior authorization is almost always needed.

Ethical policies have been debated along with the advances in fetal procedures (American College of Obstetricians and Gynecologists, 2011; Smajdor, 2011). Even though fetal surgery is conducted to benefit the baby, the mother is considered the primary patient and surgery is not performed if the risk to the mother is too great. All the procedures are voluntary and the mother can decline them at any time. After a woman undergoes open fetal surgery, she is required to stay in the Philadelphia area for the duration of the pregnancy, with few exceptions.

Technology

The availability of advanced prenatal screening and diagnostic testing can provide a tremendous amount of information to a pregnant woman and may require her and her partner to make difficult decisions regarding the pregnancy. Most pregnant women typically have a first mid pregnancy ultrasound around 18–20 weeks estimated gestational age (EGA). Prenatal screening, including the use of ultrasound and maternal serum testing, can identify a fetus at higher risk for anomalies. Screening tests are non-invasive and require additional prenatal diagnostic testing for confirmation of the finding. Prenatal diagnosis, including amniocentesis and chronic villus sampling, use fetal cells to identify or confirm the existence of a genetic abnormality. Results of the testing may lead to a referral to the CFDT.

Once a referral is made, a nurse coordinator contacts the patient and the obstetrician's office to coordinate an evaluation and obtain a copy of the patient's records. Families who come to the center for an evaluation spend most of the day having medical tests to obtain the most accurate information about the baby. The evaluation consists of a 2-hour high-resolution ultrasound using three- and four-dimensional techniques with color and spectral Doppler that allow for precise visualization of the fetus. A fetal echocardiogram is performed to evaluate the heart structure and function. A fetal MRI evaluates the baby's brain and spinal cord and can identify defects such as masses in lungs, lower back, and neck.

Once the medical testing is complete, the family meets with a maternal–fetal medicine specialist and a nurse coordinator to review the results of the day's studies. During this time, the medical team discusses care options, answers any questions that the family might have, and provides a recommendation of where to deliver. Social work is consulted once these decisions are made. Anyone who will be having a procedure at CHOP or who will be delivering at CHOP has a social work consult on a follow-up visit.

There are several different types of anomalies evaluated at our center. They fall into the following categories: cardiac defects; congenital diaphragmatic hernias; lung lesions (CCAM, BPS, CHAOS); gastrointestinal disorders (gastroschisis, omphalocele, intestinal atresia); neurological malformations (hydrocephalus, spina bifida, brain anomalies); neck masses (cervical teratoma, cystic hygroma); sacrococcygeal teratoma (mass at lower spine); twins (twin to twin transfusion syndrome, TRAP sequence); urinary tract disorders (obstructions, renal anomalies); and miscellaneous conditions (chromosomal, skeletal, multiple anomalies).

Fetal surgery has been a major breakthrough in treatment; however, it carries significant risks for the mother. In both open procedures and fetoscopic procedures, there is a risk for chorioamniotic membrane separation where the amniotic fluid leaks into the space between the amnion and chorion. If this occurs, the mother is at further risk of having prematurely ruptured membranes and premature delivery. Prematurity of the baby, and its accompanying complications, is the most common risk factor in all fetal procedures. Due to this high risk factor, each mother who chooses to undergo fetal surgery must meet with a neonatologist prior to surgery to discuss complications of prematurity.

There are also long-term risks for future pregnancies. When a mother undergoes an open procedure, she is advised that she must have a planned cesarean section for all of her subsequent pregnancies. She is also at risk with her future pregnancies of having uterine rupture, therefore she is advised to wait at least 2 years after delivery before trying to conceive again. Families must understand these implications before they can make an informed decision about whether to pursue fetal surgery.

Organization

The CFDT provides unique and comprehensive prenatal care to women who are carrying babies with fetal anomalies, from the point of diagnosis through delivery and hospitalization (Howell, 2013). The CFDT operates within a children's hospital, with the ability to offer a family continuity of prenatal to neonatal care. A patient referred to the CFDT is contacted by a nurse coordinator who does a preliminary assessment by phone and schedules the appointment. The social worker may be enlisted at this point to assist a patient with resources needed to travel to CHOP. The CFDT has evaluated patients from all 50 states, Canada, Puerto Rico, and across the globe. Appointments can be scheduled as soon as the next day, especially in cases where there may be a limited time frame for fetal intervention. Time urgency is also present for families who might decide to terminate their pregnancy based on the findings from our evaluation. While the CFDT does not perform terminations, the practice is to give the patient accurate and detailed information so she can make an informed decision. Each of the three social workers available at the CFDT takes a very compassionate approach with a patient or couple who are considering termination. Frequently it is a heartbreaking decision that she/they are trying to make regarding a very wanted pregnancy. They are supported to express what they are thinking and feeling without the fear of judgment from our staff. Resources are offered for supportive services outside of CHOP such as therapy, internet websites, and telephone support. One of the support team members who worked closest with the family reaches out to follow up in about a week to see if they need any added support.

As seen above in the Technology section, each patient evaluated by the CFDT undergoes a full medical evaluation including an anatomical ultrasound, fetal echocardiogram, consultation with a genetic counselor and maternal fetal medicine specialist and nurse coordinator on the first day. If the patient is evaluated for fetal surgery, the social worker will meet the mother and her support person on the second day to conduct a full psychosocial assessment and make recommendations to the team. The assessment is a chance for the family to explore the impact of this surgical intervention on their family, support system, and physical health. An assessment, guided by a standardized tool, is conducted to gain knowledge about all areas of a patient's life: spouse, children, parents, work, church, other commitments, mental health, physical health, sleeping and eating habits, interest in future child bearing, etc. This conversation allows any needs of the patient and support system to be identified. Interventions and supports can then be planned to help make this pregnancy period memorable without being traumatic. Education about what to expect emotionally, physically, and financially is offered to help prepare the patient for the stressors that come with fetal surgery.

To be considered for fetal myelomeningocele (MMC) surgery, criteria have been adopted from the MOMS (Management of Myelomeningocele Study) trial to ensure the safety of both the mother and fetus (Adzick et al., 2011). One of the stipulations for fetal MMC surgery is that the patient (mother) and a support person must relocate to the local area for the remainder of the pregnancy. The mother must remain on strict to modified bed rest for the duration of the pregnancy. Additional psychosocial factors that may affect candidacy include the patient and support person's mental health and drug/alcohol use history. The social worker presents such concerns to the team for consideration. The results of the 2-day evaluation are then compiled and discussed to determine eligibility for surgery.

Decisions about practice

Definition of client

The Dobbins family came to the CFDT for evaluation and possible intervention. Stefanie, age 36, and her husband Andrew, age 35, are a middle class, White couple who live in a small town in Connecticut with their two children, ages 5 and 8. Stefanie and Andrew own their own home within walking distance of Stefanie's parents' house and a short drive from Andrew's parents. They identify as Roman Catholic and have a strong faith base. Stefanie works part time in a doctor's office and Andrew works full time as a manager at an auto repair shop.

Stefanie and Andrew were referred to the CFDT by their doctors in Connecticut for an evaluation of their male fetus after findings that were consistent with spina bifida. Spina bifida is "characterized by the extrusion of the spinal cord into a sac filled with cerebrospinal fluid, resulting in lifelong disability" (Adzick et al., 2011, p. 994). Surgery to repair the sac is available to some fetal patients before birth; however, the majority of children have the repair surgery after birth.

Stefanie's family had more knowledge about spina bifida than most of our patients; Stefanie's aunt has spina bifida. They were already familiar with the challenges associated with spina bifida and were not afraid to parent a child with this diagnosis. This couple struggled with the decision about whether to have prenatal surgery or wait until after birth. Many families are interested in prenatal surgery because it has shown a reduction in the rate of shunt placement, and improvements in the areas of mental development, motor function, and hindbrain herniation (Adzick, 2013).

Stefanie, Andrew, and Stefanie's parents came together for the two-day evaluation. In this circumstance, the suspected diagnosis was confirmed and both Stefanie and the fetus were found to meet the medical requirements for surgery. The second day was scheduled for a psychosocial assessment with a social worker to identify any challenges that could impact the outcome of fetal surgery. We should note that the three authors share the social work role and often share responsibilities for families and psychosocial support. Hence, we will talk about "social workers" or "we" rather than any one of us individually. The family was also scheduled to see the CFDT psychologist. This second day of appointments allows time in the patient's schedule to see the psychologist if concerns arise about coping throughout the recovery period. The psychologist meets with all patients who have a mental health diagnosis or drug/alcohol addiction. She assists the family with developing a treatment plan to cope with feelings about a fetal diagnosis that are compounded by their addiction or mental health. Referrals are made as needed to the other members of the psychosocial support team: the chaplain and the child life specialist. The patient and family also have a neonatology consult and a meeting with the surgeon who would perform the surgery.

During the social work assessment, we review the expectations about the surgical and post-surgical course and discuss the impact that the surgery will have on the family. We need to identify who will remain with the patient while she is in Philadelphia, for possibly up to five months. We discuss the financial strain the surgery places on families and the resources that are available to help assist them. The social worker assigned to the family gets to know their family context: family of origin for the pregnant woman and her partner; current family composition in the home; current work status; prior pregnancy losses or complications; and any other complicating factor for the family system. The social worker also assesses the family's resource networks at home, their other commitments in addition to work and family, their methods of coping with stress and anxiety, their history of mental health support in the past, and any trauma history or relationship abuse history for the mom or her partner. This practice is supported by Azri, Larmar, and Cartmel (2013) in their work, which describes ways in which social work provides support to a family receiving a prenatal diagnosis.

Stefanie described herself as having a history of both general anxiety and also mild postpartum depression that she described as "baby blues." She identified many concerns, including fears about not waking up from the surgery, relocating many hours away from her children for a long period of time, and the financial impact that this would have on their family. She was concerned about the emotional impact this experience could have on her relationship with her husband, as he would be home in Connecticut to work and manage the house and children while she was in Philadelphia. Andrew's supports at home were going to be limited because Stefanie's parents were relocating to Philadelphia to support her. She worried that the distance would result in Andrew feeling disconnected from the pregnancy and this baby. She anticipated feeling regret if she decided against the surgery and not doing everything possible to help her son have the best outcome. She was not-so-subtly polling both the staff and her family by asking "Do you think I should do it?"

It was evident that Stefanie was having a difficult time sorting through her emotions and heightened anxiety to come to a decision about fetal surgery. Feeling nervous is common. Her list of worries was extensive. The intensity warranted further exploration with the CFDT psychologist. She agreed to meet with the psychologist to help alleviate the anxiety about making the "wrong" decision. At the end of the evaluation, we recommended that she return home and discuss it further with her family. We agreed to connect with her in a few days to see if she had any further questions or had come to a decision. This allowed our team to review whether we believed surgery could be detrimental for this family in light of Stefanie's high level of anxiety.

Goals

The goals of the first meeting with a family considering fetal surgery include obtaining a full psychosocial history, assessing their coping skills, and informing them of resources available to help them through the long relocation period. The social worker assesses the family's understanding of the requirements and consequences of fetal surgery in contrast to a post-natal repair and supports them to make the decision that is best for them. Some families struggle with the decision to continue or terminate the pregnancy. Some families simply need to hear that they are not alone: there are other families who have had this experience, and they will be supported by a team who will be with them on this journey.

Contracting and developing objectives

Patients are often referred to the CFDT for evaluation shortly after finding out that the baby that they had hoped for has a fetal anomaly. They expect us to help guide them in the process of planning for the patient, her partner, and extended family including children. The CFDT recognizes the unique care needs of families who are expecting a baby with an anomaly (Howell, Johnson, & Adzick, 2006). The psychological effects of prenatal diagnosis are increasingly studied. One study "assume(s) a considerable number of women undergoing prenatal diagnostic procedures experience psychological distress" (Leithner et al., 2004, p. 240). Psychosocial support is provided by three social workers, a psychologist, a child life specialist, and a chaplain.

When the family has gathered the information they need to make a treatment decision, the role of the social worker is to assist the family in exploring their psychosocial needs. This can include providing anticipatory guidance about relocation and hospitalization, offering a blank calendar to map out a schedule of support people for the patient (or support people for the children at home), discussing housing options such as the Ronald McDonald House and Host for Hospitals host home program, and, of course, provision of psychosocial support. We also help explore other financial supports such as short-term disability eligibility or travel reimbursement available through some insurance companies.

Stefanie and Andrew returned home and called social work twice for information related to resources to help them through the surgery. They were interested in finding out how long they would have to wait for a bed at the Ronald McDonald House after the surgery and if we would be willing to write a letter to a local organization in their area that offers financial assistance to parents who have a child with a disability. After much careful thought and consideration, they decided they would like to move forward with surgery. The couple had a plan for Andrew and the children to visit at least once a month for a long weekend, and for Stefanie's mom to be her primary support person in Philadelphia. The team in the CFDT, including the maternal–fetal medicine specialist, nurse practitioner, psychologist, and the social worker, discussed the concerns around Stefanie's anxiety and concluded that we could provide adequate support for the family.

Meeting place

Patients initially meet with the medical team in one of two small consultation rooms outside of the Garbose Special Delivery Unit (SDU). In the room, there is a round table and chairs, a large flat screen on the wall for viewing images, and a desk with a phone and printer. These rooms are usually available for the social worker to use to meet with a patient and family during their initial assessment and at follow-up visits as needed. The social worker follows up with the patient several times during the prenatal period. E-mail, phone contact, and face-to-face contact occur throughout her care in the CFDT. The social worker will meet with a patient in her private or semi-private room on the SDU once she is admitted. When a baby is in the newborn/infant intensive care unit (N/IICU), the social worker will talk with a family at the baby's bedside or privately in the social work office located in the N/IICU.

Use of time

The social work assessment is typically scheduled during the patient's second appointment in the CFDT. If a patient is in crisis, or if the medical team determines that an immediate surgical intervention is necessary, social work meets with the patient on the first appointment day. For candidates for open fetal surgery, the social work assessment takes place on the second day of the two-day evaluation. The length of the relationship is determined by the diagnosis. For a fetoscopic procedure, the social worker may only be involved briefly to assist the patient and family in planning for the surgery. For those delivering in the SDU, including those who undergo an open fetal procedure, a more in-depth assessment occurs, to help the patient with practical and emotional preparation and to identify psychosocial needs that may require attention during the mother's or baby's hospital stay. The relationship continues throughout the course of care and can involve subsequent follow-up meetings prior to delivery. The same social worker follows a patient through delivery and often through the baby's hospitalization. The needs of the patient and family dictate the frequency of contact in the N/IICU.

Strategies and interventions

Once the plan for intervention is determined, the social worker helps the patient and family prepare for the demands of care. This can include planning for relocation during the pregnancy and arranging for the care of other children. Many families have limited social and financial resources, and relocation is costly. Even if finances are not problematic, they are faced with the challenge of isolation from their typical supports during relocation. These challenges are compounded for a single parent. Patients also arrive with pre-existing mental health needs that can impact their ability to cope. The social work role is to help the patient and her family navigate all of these issues while providing psychosocial support.

There were a few strategies used prior to Stefanie's relocation to Philadelphia to help reduce her worries. We put together schedules for her support people to rotate while she was in Philadelphia and another schedule for her children's care at home so that she could set aside any worries about not having enough support for both herself and her children. We also looked at the long weekends that would be coming up in her children's school schedule as times when they could come to Philadelphia to visit her. Social work consulted our child life specialist to ask for her help to alleviate some worry that Stefanie had about this negatively impacting her children. The Child Life Specialist suggested language that could be used to make it clear to the children that it would be a time-limited event with built-in visits and fun activities to stay connected. Two suggestions that Stefanie used while at home were to make a countdown calendar with the children to visually see the months and weeks that could be crossed off until she came home and allowing the children to create a list of "rules" that would help their substitute "mommies" know how to best care for them in special ways that are similar to how their actual mommy cares for them.

Once she came to Philadelphia, we worked on focusing on one small step at a time. The first focus was surgery. After surgery was recovery in the hospital. The next step would be discharge from the hospital to temporary housing in the hotel. Stefanie became too overwhelmed when thinking too far ahead. Once she was settled into the hotel, she started to become anxious about getting into the Ronald McDonald House. The financial impact on their family was stressful to her, although her extended family reassured her that they would assist the couple if needed. We communicated face to face at her weekly appointments and often would exchange one or two e-mails between appointments. I would reassure her that she would be offered a room as soon as possible and try to redirect her focus to a send-home project for her children or give her topics to research on the internet regarding spina bifida. She took to the tasks with full gusto!

Stance of the social worker

The initial assessment with a patient may involve crisis intervention, particularly for those who are newly diagnosed. The social work interview is informed by grief theory in the context of the loss of an expected, uneventful pregnancy. A strengths-based approach to the assessment helps the patient define her role in her care and can offer a sense of control, and assists the social worker in determining the additional support that may be needed. A somewhat directive approach is used to help patients and families prepare, as very few patients have had any prior experience with prenatal diagnosis and intervention. The focus shifts to problem-solving with the patient as plans are made for relocation and the details of the logistics must be determined. Following the initial assessment, ongoing support is offered in person, via telephone contact or via e-mail. A fetal surgery patient is seen in our obstetrics office every week between surgery and delivery. It allows for a social work visit to occur regularly, such as every other week, to reassess for coping and to further prepare for delivery and care of a newborn with a diagnosis. Many questions begin to arise a few weeks before delivery, and the regularity of social work contact leading up to that time lays a solid foundation for trust and openness.

Resources outside of the helping relationship

A multi-disciplinary model of care has been adopted by the CFDT. To that end, additional resources are available internally for the CFDT patient and her family. A chaplain can be consulted for families who identify a strong religious faith, who desire extra support during decision-making, or who request a blessing of the newborn. The social work assessment may identify the extent to which siblings have been informed of the fetal diagnosis and plan of care. The social worker will consult a child life specialist to meet with a family to discuss age-appropriate language for explanation and ways that siblings can be involved in mother's and baby's care. Families with children are often eager to speak with the child life specialist to help reassure them that separation from their children for up to six months will not harm development or attachment abilities (Cole, Ousley, & Shaughnessy, 2014). We reassure them that they will be able to navigate the needs of their other children and that our team will help provide ideas about how to stay connected at home.

Mental health treatment during a prenatally diagnosed pregnancy is a concern, particularly for those who relocate from out of the area whose insurance will not cover a local mental health provider. The CFDT psychologist is incorporated into prenatal care and can be consulted for assessment of mental health needs as well as for ongoing intervention through the pregnancy. Informal supports can take the form of online connections made with support groups or other parents. Patients who relocate prenatally to a local Ronald McDonald House often form informal supportive relationships with other patients undergoing a similar experience. Additional local supports can be accessed based on a family's needs, for example a crisis nursery for emergency child care or a methadone maintenance program.

Reassessment and evaluation

After surgery, Stefanie was discharged to a local hotel to wait until she moved up on the wait list at the Ronald McDonald House. She had expected the wait would be about one to two weeks, but as she entered the third week, she was very stressed and anxious about the financial impact this would have on their family. She was also very eager to get out of the hotel room and be able to move about more. We met weekly when she came in for medical follow-up. She was reassured that she would eventually be offered a room at the Ronald McDonald House. She sent e-mails to her social worker with questions, concerns, or ideas while on bed rest ranging in topic from housing, to spina bifida programs, to supports available for families with children with physical disabilities. Bed rest was not easy for this mom of two who was used to juggling work, parenting, and running a household. She was trying not to be critical of the job her husband and in-laws were doing with the children because she could not be there. She found it hard not to check in on every detail of what was happening at home because she had so much time on her hands. She reported relief in having an individual meeting with the social worker each week where she could express her frustrations in a safe, judgment-free setting. She felt buoyed by the supportive counseling and learning that she was not experiencing anything abnormal from other relocated mothers. She was encouraged to frame this experience as time-limited, as it would have a definite end when she and her son would go home after birth.

It is difficult for a patient to prepare for the struggle of those first few weeks during which they must remain primarily in bed with little time out of their room. There is often physical and emotional discomfort as she adjusts to this new environment outside of her home and family. Stress relief afforded by physical activity is not possible. An additional stressor is that the medicine patients must take every 6 hours can have anxiety-like side effects and interrupts any potential for 8 hours of continuous sleep.

Stefanie was relieved when she was able to move to the Ronald McDonald House. There, she had a built-in support group of moms who either recently delivered at our hospital or were preparing to deliver after fetal surgery. She had a quick bond with the other women and suddenly felt that she had a schedule and a purpose to her day. As a group, they took out an ad in the program for the fashion show fundraiser benefiting the CFDT to express appreciation for the work of the team. They supported one another through the difficult days of missing special events at home and were happy for each other when their families came to visit. Stefanie's move to the Ronald McDonald House coincided with her release from strict bed rest, which allowed her to get out a little more while in the wheelchair. At this point in her recovery and pregnancy, Stefanie was doing much better, but she had many more weeks to go.

The goal following fetal surgery is to reach 37 weeks EGA before delivery. Research has shown that for fetal surgery patients, the average gestational age at delivery is between 34 and 35 weeks (Moldenhauer, 2014; Moldenhauer et al., 2014). Stefanie came to the delivery unit in labor in her 35th week of pregnancy. It coincided with a visit from her husband and children, so the timing could not have been better! Her son, Nathan, was born and she and Andrew immediately bonded with him. Nathan stayed in the N/IICU approximately four weeks as he struggled with feeding and gaining weight, but he otherwise did well. The N/IICU follows a protocol that directs the care of infants who have had in utero spina bifida surgery. He had tests including an ultrasound of his kidneys and bladder and an MRI of his brain and spine. Nathan needed some orthopedic casting to help his legs and feet, but this was expected to be temporary. See Figure 4.1 for a graph of Stefanie's anxiety over time.

Termination and case conclusion

In preparation for leaving our care, we discussed Medical Assistance as a secondary insurance and follow-up appointments for the baby at a spina bifida center close to the family's home. We also discussed Stefanie's transition home and her return to the roles of mother and wife, and her

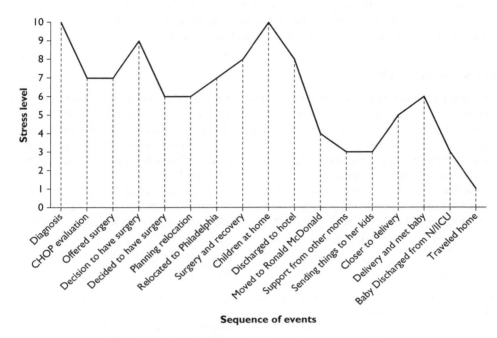

Figure 4.1 Level of anxiety during and after pregnancy

eventual return to work. She would need to give herself and her family time to readjust to life as a family of five. The relationship with social work ended on the discharge day from the N/IICU.

Differential discussion

Although we see patients from a variety of socioeconomic backgrounds, some self-selection likely occurs prior to a family's referral to the CFDT. Factors such as the financial resources and social support needed for the relocation necessary for care come into play and can limit those who can make use of fetal surgery. We continue to search for resources to assist families with the travel and lodging costs. Some patients, when faced with the additional financial responsibilities that are associated with a prenatal diagnosis, may choose not to continue the pregnancy prior to being evaluated for fetal intervention.

The patient highlighted in this chapter would likely have benefited from peer support throughout her pregnancy. Although an informal support network formed while she was staying at Ronald McDonald House, a defined support group for mothers who have undergone prenatal surgery does not exist. This mom needed regular support from our team and with that support she did very well. She was a good candidate for the surgery from the medical standpoint and with the layers of support available to her here (social work, child life, and psychology) she was able to do well and never needed any help outside of our team and her family. The CFDT has since initiated a prenatal psychoeducational group for mothers with a variety of fetal diagnoses. Stefanie would have benefited from it had it existed when she was a patient. We envision a mutual support group specifically for women who have undergone fetal surgery as we believe this population deserves ongoing support throughout their pregnancies. The social workers are considering how to feasibly create such a support group. A number of factors have prevented this group in the past, including space, staffing, and funding for what could be a very limited number of patients.

Discussion questions

1   What efforts can be made to ensure that advances in fetal care, such as fetal surgery, are available to all pregnant women regardless of socioeconomic status or location?
2   There are times when we see patients who have been told to terminate their pregnancy prior to coming to our experienced center and we are able to offer an intervention to improve the medical condition of the fetus. When is it ethical for a provider to recommend termination when there is a fetal anomaly detected?
3   How does a family weigh the quality of life issues for an unborn child against the quality of family life during an extended relocation, hospitalization, and potential life-long involvement with the medical system? What role does the social worker have in supporting the mother and her family?

References

Adzick, N. S. (2013). Prospects for fetal surgery. *Early Human Development, 89*(11), 881–886. doi: 10.1016/j.earlhumdev.2013.09.010

Adzick, N. S., Thom, E. A., Spong, C. Y., Brock, III, J. W., Burrows, P. K., Johnson, M. P., et al. for the MOMS Investigators (2011). A randomized trial of prenatal versus postnatal repair of myelomeningocele. *New England Journal of Medicine, 364*, 993–1004. doi: 10.1056/NEJMoa1014379

American College of Obstetricians and Gynecologists (2011). Committee on Ethics; American Academy of Pediatrics, Committee on Bioethics. Maternal-Fetal Intervention and Fetal Care Centers. *Pediatrics, 128*(2), 473–478. doi: 10.1542/peds.2011-1570

Azri, S., Larmar, S., & Cartmel, J. (2013). Social work's role in prenatal diagnosis and genetic services: Current practice and future potential. *Australian Social Work, 67*(3), 348–362. doi: 10.1080/0312407X.2013.848914

Cole, J., Ousley, H. K., & Shaughnessy, E. (2014). Promoting positive attachment *in utero*: Support families carrying a baby with a birth defect. Presented at the Pennsylvania Association for Infant Mental Health, October 2014, Harrisburg, PA.

Howell, L. J. (2013) The Garbose Family Special Delivery Unit: A new paradigm for maternal-fetal and neonatal care. *Seminars in Pediatric Surgery, 22*(1), 3–9. doi: 10.1053/j.sempedsurg.2012.10.002

Howell, L. J., Johnson, M. P., & Adzick, N. S. (2006). Creating a state-of-the-art center for fetal diagnosis and treatment: Importance of a multidisciplinary approach. *Progress in Pediatric Cardiology, 22*, 121–127. doi: 10.1016/j.ppedcard.2006.01.012

Leithner, K., Maar, A., Fischer-Kern, M., Hilger, E., Loffler-Stastkaand, H., & Ponocny-Seliger, E. (2004). Affective state of women following a prenatal diagnosis: predictors of a negative psychological outcome. *Ultrasound in Obstetrics and Gynecology, 23*(3), 240–246. doi: 10.1002/uog.978.

Moldenhauer, J. (2014). *In utero* repair of spina bifida. *American Journal of Perinatology, 31*(07), 595–604. doi: 10.1016/j.earlhumdev.2013.09.010

Moldenhauer, J. S., Soni, S., Rintoul, N. E., Spinner, S. S, Khalek, N., Martinez-Poyer J., et al. (2014). Fetal myelomeningocele repair: The post-MOMS experience at the Children's Hospital of Philadelphia. *Fetal Diagnosis Therapy, 37*(3), 235–240. doi: 10.1159/000365353

Patient Protection and Affordable Care Act ("ACA"), Pub. L. No. 111–148, 124 Stat. 119 (2010), amended by Health Care and Education Reconciliation Act, Pub. L. No. 111–152, 124 Stat. 1029 (2010), § 1001, 42 U. S. C. § 300gg-13 (amending § 2713 of the Public Health Services Act). Retrieved from healthlaw.org

Smajdor, A. (2011). Ethical challenges in fetal surgery. *Journal of Medical Ethics, 37*(2), 88–91. doi: 10.1136/jme.2010.039537

Websites

BedRest in Pregnancy, pregnancy from the shadows, http://pregnancy.about.com/cs/bedrest/a/bedrest
  htm
Better Bedrest, an outreach program for pregnancies at risk, betterbedrest.org
The Center for Fetal Diagnosis and Treatment, www.fetalsurgery.chop.edu
Fetal surgery video, www.chop.edu/video/birth-breakthrough-spina-bifida-video-series
Hosts for Hospitals, www.hostsforhospitals.org
Philadelphia Ronald McDonald House, www.philarmh.org
Postpartum Support International, www.postpartum.net
Sidelines National Support Network, sidelines.org

Chapter 5

Getting there
Decision-making in the NICU

Laurie Stewart

Context

St. Christopher's Hospital for Children is a non-sectarian, for-profit hospital that provides a full range of outpatient and inpatient services for infants, children, and young adults, and has 220 pediatric specialists (www.stchristophershospital.com). Currently, the hospital has 161 inpatient beds, 40 dedicated to the care of sick newborns. Thirty of the beds are for critically ill infants in the neonatal intensive care unit (NICU) and 10 are for stable infants in the continuing care nursery (CCN). Combined, these two units admit more than 300 patients a year. The average length of a NICU/CCN admission is 35 days.

St. Christopher's NICU is one of three Level IV (equipped to care for the sickest infants) nurseries in southeastern Pennsylvania. Most patients are from the Philadelphia area but the NICU also receives admissions from New Jersey and rural counties outside of the metropolitan area. On average, the NICU receives 285 admissions every year from referring hospitals. There are no deliveries (childbirth) at St. Christopher's – every patient is transferred from an outside hospital.

Policy

The First Congressional District encompasses St. Christopher's and is the second-most food insecure district in the United States. Many of our patients live in poverty, as do pregnant women (our patients' mothers) who often do not have access to adequate nutrition during pregnancy (Lubrano, 2010). Many do not know about the Woman's, Infants, Children's (WIC) program that provides supplemental nutrition for pregnant women and children under 5. If they do know and apply, they may wait for benefits until late in the pregnancy. In Pennsylvania for 2015, a family of three with a gross income less than US\$36,612 qualifies for WIC benefits.

Many NICU moms struggle to obtain comprehensive prenatal care. Poor prenatal care is correlated with adverse pregnancy outcomes, including premature delivery and maternal morbidity and mortality (Braveman et al., 2010; Ratzon, Sheiner, & Shoham-Vardi, 2010). In Philadelphia, 66 sites offer prenatal care to women with Medicaid. For the uninsured, there are 35 free city and community health centers. Waits for initial appointments have, at times, reportedly exceeded the duration of a pregnancy. On average, pregnant women on Medicaid wait 2.5 weeks for initial appointments in Philadelphia. Thus, low-income pregnant women are at increased risk of a pregnancy outcome that leads to a NICU hospitalization for their newborn (Maternity Care Coalition, 2011).

Infants and children in Pennsylvania have better access to medical care and coverage than do pregnant women. Children are able to obtain health insurance through the state regardless of income. As of January 1, 2015, under Pennsylvania's Medicaid expansion, infants and toddlers up to the age of 2 qualify for Medicaid if their family lives at or below 215% of the poverty line. Infants and toddlers above this line can qualify for the federally mandated Children's Health Insurance Program (CHIP), which requires parents to pay a sliding fee premium for coverage based on income.

Approximately 85% of NICU patients have insurance coverage under a Medicaid HMO and 10% have employer-based coverage or coverage through CHIP. The remaining 5% enter the NICU with no coverage at all. Parents apply for Medicaid or CHIP during their baby's NICU hospitalization. At the time of this writing, the Affordable Care Act marketplace (www.healthcare.gov/) has covered two NICU patients.

Caring for critically ill newborns raises ethical issues unique to the NICU population. The federal "Baby Doe Rules" initiated in 1982 and then formalized in the 1988 revision of the Child Abuse Prevention and Treatment Act, forbid the withholding of treatment for life-threatening conditions in infants. They prohibit withholding nutrition, hydration, and medication if such interventions would likely "be effective in ameliorating or correcting all such conditions" unless these interventions would be futile based on the infant's diagnoses or current medical status (White, 2011). Despite an initial flurry of attention in the late 1980s, few follow this standard. Instead, most neonatal settings follow the "best interest standard," where parents or guardians, presumed to be acting in their child's best interest, are presented with options for their child and make decisions about their care with the physicians. Case law upholds treating infants under the best interest standard, and as a result, Baby Doe is not, in actual practice, the standard of care (White, 2011).

St. Christopher's neonatology physicians follow the best interest standard, although different physicians have different thresholds in determining futility and, at times, differ in opinion on prognosis and which treatments should be offered. For example, some physicians working with a patient with a fatal diagnosis but with an uncertain life expectancy will offer long-term home ventilation, while others will not as they do not see this treatment as offering benefit to the patient.

Technology

St. Christopher's regularly invests in technologies that foster better patient outcomes. The NICU is a Level IV unit and is thus equipped to treat critically ill newborns. The unit offers extra-corporeal membrane oxygenation (ECMO), which allows oxygen to be delivered to blood outside of the body. Hypothermic neuroprotection (total body cooling) is available for babies who experience lack of oxygen and brain injury at birth.

The typical NICU technology includes ventilators, continuous positive airway pressure (CPAP), monitors that continuously evaluate pulse and respiratory rate, blood oxygenation and blood pressure, isolettes and pumps to administer medications and fluids. Monitors continuously monitor respiratory rate, oxygen saturation, blood pressure, and heart rate for every baby, from the moment of admission until the moment of discharge. Multiple leads and wires accompany this monitoring. This means that parents usually require the assistance of a member of the medical team in order to hold their babies, which at times presents a barrier to bonding.

The patients have electronic medical records that include all social work, case management and nursing documentation, and physician orders. Daily physician progress notes and physician consults are done by hand in a separate chart. This makes gaining a comprehensive understanding of a baby's medical and social issues a challenge as records are in multiple places.

The hospital prohibits the use of personal technology devices (cell phones, iPads, etc.) to convey any patient information. Many hospital employees, including the NICU social workers, have hospital-based cell phones to allow timely communication of patient information via text. Hospital staff cannot be "friends" via social media with patients and families or convey any patient-related information through these platforms.

Organization

St. Christopher's social work department includes 30 full-time and 6 per diem, part-time, and on-call workers. All social workers are master's prepared. Most outpatient clinics have a dedicated social worker and each inpatient unit has at least one full-time worker. The NICU and CCN have two social workers in alignment with the National Association of Perinatal Social Workers' guidelines that call for one full-time master's prepared social worker for every 20 beds (www.napsw.org/). In the NICU, social workers are part of a broad interdisciplinary team that includes physicians (attending, fellows, and residents), nurses, physical, occupational and speech therapists, child life specialists and case managers, and, when appropriate, the hospital's pediatric palliative care team.

The NICU team generally works well together in working toward the goal of a safe discharge for every NICU patient. Sometimes, this goal can be hindered by the legal limits of working in a for-profit hospital. A Medicaid law prohibits providing meals, and transportation for families in excess of US$50 a year. Anything beyond US$50 is considered an enticement and thus disallowed. This means the team must work together to develop creative solutions to many of the financial challenges faced by NICU families. For example, many parents cannot afford transportation to visit their newborn but we cannot offer transportation resources in excess of US$50 per family.

Description of the typical clients and situations

About half of the babies admitted to our NICU are born into two-parent households and half are headed by single moms (ages 14–50). Families are primarily African American, West African, Latino, or White and have varied levels of education, ranging from elementary school to having MDs and PhDs. Most NICU parents are high school graduates, are currently unemployed, and they typically struggle with food insecurity, housing, transportation, and child care. The trauma of having a newborn in the hospital makes life even more challenging.

St. Christopher's NICU treats babies with a wide range of medical issues and diagnoses. Some patients are born extremely premature, some are born full-term but experience serious birth injuries, and some babies are born with congenital or genetic conditions and diagnoses. Babies are in the NICU, on average, for a month. Most babies go home, some with long-term or life-long medical issues that require ongoing follow-up and care at home. Some babies (between 3 and 5% a year) die while in the NICU.

Every NICU family receives a social work consult within 24 hours of their baby's admission, per hospital policy, although sometimes scheduling conflicts or individual circumstances prevent this initial consult from occurring the first day. The social worker conducts a full biopsychosocial assessment in order to identify the immediate and long-term social work goals of the patient and family, and to develop, in conjunction with the parents and medical team, a plan to reach those goals.

Goals are wide-ranging. Some families focus on feeding their baby breast milk exclusively; some focus on obtaining emotional support to help them through their time in the NICU; others focus on issues related to housing and insurance. As their baby's hospitalization progresses, goals can shift, particularly when a child faces a diagnosis that is life-limiting or will lead to their baby's death. For example, some families who initially limited medical intervention shift toward more medical intervention to extend their child's life, while others decide to minimize medical intervention and focus on their child's comfort.

Decisions about practice

Description of the client

Baby Brooklyn Santiago was born prematurely at 33 weeks. She was transferred from her birth hospital's NICU to St. Christopher's due to stridor (a high-pitched sound with breathing, usually indicative of a blockage in the airway) and facial and skeletal features indicating an unspecified genetic diagnosis. Brooklyn's parents, Maribel and Joseph, both 20, are an intact, unmarried couple. Initially private about their relationship status, Maribel and Joseph ultimately disclosed to me that they lived with Maribel's parents but were concerned that hospital staff would judge them for living together and having a child while unmarried.

Upon initial examination, the medical team, led by a geneticist, thought Brooklyn had Trisomy 18, a diagnosis that is fatal within one week of birth in 90% of children. Doctors discussed this probable diagnosis and outcome with Maribel and Joseph on their first visit to the NICU. Within a day or two of the baby's admission, several doctors and nurses came to me with concerns that Maribel and Joseph were not bonding with their daughter. Their visits were brief and reportedly they did not engage with Brooklyn and declined to participate in her care. We wondered about their support system.

Initial goals, objectives, and contracting

During our initial meeting and assessment, my goal was to better determine Maribel's comprehension of her daughter's medical status and medical plan, and how she was bonding with her daughter. I wanted to assess her understanding of Brooklyn's condition and her reactions and feelings about her uncertain diagnosis. Maribel at first was confused about my role and I explained the role of the social worker in the NICU. She answered my questions briefly and quietly, until I asked how she felt about Brooklyn's hospitalization. She expressed frustration about not yet having a definitive diagnosis and about not knowing if her daughter would live or die. She wondered what her life might look like if she lived. She said she had been pumping breast milk but she stopped because the idea of having a milk supply for a baby who would never eat devastated her. She said she and Brooklyn's father were afraid to bond with a baby that they might never get to take home. Maribel's insight and honesty helped me better understand her major concerns. She began visiting more frequently, most often with Joseph, and sometimes with her mom and older sisters.

Meeting place and use of time

I met with Maribel most often at Brooklyn's bedside (as opposed to my office). Often, parents sacrifice the privacy of meeting in the office in order to remain with their baby. Generally, parents decide where they would prefer meeting. Depending on individual needs, I spend anywhere from 5 minutes to 2 hours with families each time we meet. With Brooklyn's family, our meetings averaged about 30 minutes on an as-needed basis.

Strategies and interventions

Genetic studies ruled out the possibility that Brooklyn had Trisomy 18. She remained unable to breathe without support; she was not gaining weight, and was unable eat from a bottle. While we awaited the results of a full genetic panel, an MRI of Brooklyn's brain showed severe anomalies in how her brain was formed. A meeting was held with the neurology team, the NICU medical team, social work and Maribel, Joseph, Maribel's three older sisters, and Brooklyn's grandmothers. A Spanish interpreter hired by the hospital also attended to interpret for the grandmothers.

The neurologic team explained that, due to the differences in Brooklyn's brain, she would likely have profound developmental challenges, including not being able to walk, talk, or feed herself. Brooklyn's aunts asked many questions focused on how sure the medical team was of their predictions. "Pretty certain, but we can never be 100% certain," was the reply. In this, the family found hope that Brooklyn would overcome her current issues and develop as most babies develop. Her parents said that they believed, with time, Brooklyn would be able to eat and breathe on her own.

Maribel and Joseph said that they wanted Brooklyn to remain in the NICU until she learned to eat and no longer required respiratory support. The physicians said, gently, that this was unlikely to happen and that she would require a g-tube (a feeding tube surgically inserted into the stomach). Brooklyn's parents asserted that their daughter should be given intensive speech therapy to help teach her to eat, just as any baby would had they not had such concerning MRI findings. The meeting ended when the medical team agreed to increase speech therapy sessions and the family agreed to meet again the following week to discuss Brooklyn's progress.

The same group met again the following week, and discussed Brooklyn's lack of progress with feeding and breathing. The medical team also explained that, due to lack of improvement in her respiratory status, she could require a tracheostomy in order to have a long-term stable airway. Maribel and Joseph, after discussing the benefits and risks at length, agreed to the g-tube.

Brooklyn underwent surgery for the g-tube. She tolerated the procedure well and was able to be fully fed via the tube soon after the surgery. Her respiratory status began to decline, however, and her parents felt that this was due to the surgery while the medical team believed that her disease process was evolving.

A few days later, the results of Brooklyn's genetic tests arrived. She had a duplication on one chromosome and a deletion on another. Individually, both were rare. The medical literature showed a poor outcome for each condition, with children ultimately dying of respiratory failure or aspiration pneumonia within the first six months of life. There were no documented instances of a child with Brooklyn's combined genetic findings. These conditions are inherited from the mother, meaning that, while Maribel was healthy, future pregnancies carried a

50% likelihood of producing a child with the same diagnoses as Brooklyn. Maribel's sisters were also at risk for being carriers.

I scheduled another meeting with Brooklyn's family, the geneticist, and the NICU team. The family did not arrive for the meeting. I called to check on them and they said that they could not come. I offered to reschedule at any time that worked for them. They declined. The NICU team encouraged me to convince them to come in as soon as possible to discuss the results of the genetic testing. Some members of the team began to become frustrated with Maribel and Joseph, claiming they were neglecting Brooklyn. The parents' visits to the NICU dropped off drastically during this time. Based on my previous interactions with the family, I strongly felt that they cared about Brooklyn and had bonded with her but were afraid of the information that would be given to them at the meeting. I believed they needed a bit of time without hospital staff pressuring them to accept the prognosis. I shared this opinion with the medical team and urged them to support the family's process. Not all agreed, leading to some tension among team members. A few team members thought that the Department of Human Services should be contacted for "medical neglect," but the full team did not support this approach.

After about a week, I called Maribel. I told her my concern that they were not visiting Brooklyn even though they wanted to do so because they feared being hit with hard information. Maribel essentially agreed that she and Joseph felt this way and I asked her to talk with Joseph about meeting and to call me with their decision. I was affirming their right to make their own decisions in this way. Maribel called me the following day and agreed to come in. A meeting with Maribel, Joseph, their families, genetics, neonatology, and an interpreter was scheduled.

The geneticist explained Brooklyn's genetic findings to the family, and that Maribel's sisters needed to be tested to determine if they too were carriers. The family was devastated – one aunt said that not only would Brooklyn likely die, this could mean that none of them should ever have children. We met at length and began discussing choices the family had, and what their hopes were for Brooklyn in light of her prognosis. The doctors estimated she could live for days to months but was unlikely to live until her first birthday. A tracheostomy would give her the best chance to live as long as possible, but the surgery presents significant risks. Additionally, Brooklyn would either have to be discharged to a long-term care facility or be taken care of around the clock at home by nurses and her parents after they spent weeks training to learn how to care for the trach. The NICU attending brought up a third approach – working with the hospital palliative care team (now called the CORE team, for Compassion, Options, Respect, and Education).

The CORE team works with families and patients who are facing a life-limiting or fatal diagnosis and explains medical choices and options, sometimes removing "cure" as the primary focus. Pain and symptom management are primary goals of the team, along with working with families to help carry out goals they have for their child, from having them travel to meet with important family members, to staying out of the hospital as much as possible. The CORE team helps some families to arrange in-home or inpatient hospice services. These CORE and family goals are usually wide-ranging and are implemented as quickly as possible.

Some families are immediately resistant when they hear about the CORE team. When doctors say the words "palliative care," sometimes families hear "hospice." We work with these families to explain that, while palliative care patients can also receive hospice services, the two are separate. A palliative care patient and family can approach the medical diagnosis aggressively, with surgery, multiple medications, inpatient hospitalizations, etc.

with the goal of having the patient remain alive as long as possible (Shah et al., 2008). Conversely, palliative care patients can also chose minimal or no intervention if intervention will just prolong their death and not "cure" the underlying disease. We try to change the view of hospice as a program that focuses on dying, framing it instead as a program that can help families and patients reach goals at the end of life and support patients and families through the physical and emotional pain of the dying process.

Stance of the social worker

As can be seen above, my stance is one of providing emotional support, interpretation of medical team findings to the parents and the parents' responses back to the medical team, and one of advocating for the family. Sometimes this can put me at odds with my colleagues, but I find that parents' fears often bring about behavior that is misinterpreted by many of the medical team. My stance involves maintaining support of the parents while also helping them move in the directions the medical team believes will bring about the most appropriate medical care.

Use of resources outside the helping relationship – the CORE team

Pediatric palliative care (PPC) teams are proliferating. As of 2013, 69% of pediatric hospitals had PPC teams. A 2008 survey found that 50% of pediatric hospitals had PPC teams (Feudtner et al., 2013). In 2006, the American Board of Medical Specialists first recognized PPC as a pediatric sub-specialty. However, most hospitals have minimal funding and staffing for PPC as PPC does not generate clinical revenue (Feudtner et al., 2011). Additionally, PPC is not without controversy. In 1982, so-called "Baby Doe" laws made withholding treatment illegal. Essentially, the Baby Doe laws would, if enforced, require that infants receive any and all possible treatment, regardless of how painful or risky and how unlikely treatment was to improve the baby's condition. However, "in nearly 30 years of deliberations about the Baby Doe case . . . only one case cites Baby Doe [and] the law has no history of enforcement, and, by inference, is not the standard of care" (White, 2011, p. 314). Instead, the "best interest" standard has evolved to be the standard of care in practice, allowing parents or legal guardians to make choices about interventions for their child. The American Academy of Pediatrics established the best interest standard in 2007 and further stressed the importance of the role of parents in decision-making. Case law also supports the use of the best interest standard (White, 2011).

The best interest standard is the approach the CORE team takes with its families and patients. The team is staffed by a chief physician, attending intensivist physician, social worker, child life specialist, chaplain, and nurse practitioner. All but the nurse practitioner have other professional responsibilities throughout the hospital in addition to the CORE team. Usually, when the NICU consults the CORE team, I work with the families in conjunction with the CORE social worker and then, upon NICU discharge, she is the family's primary social worker. On occasion, the CORE social worker works with the family independent of me if the family struggles to separate the medical goals of the NICU team with the life goals of the CORE team.

Brooklyn's family seemed to have an accurate understanding of palliative care and how the CORE team might be able to help them through the decision-making process. However, they were not yet ready to work with the team. Maribel and Joseph remained hopeful that the dire prognosis given to their daughter was wrong and wanted to give Brooklyn more time to improve. Maribel and Joseph asked if their parish priest could come to St. Christopher's and baptize Brooklyn. The baptism was arranged for a few days later. Maribel called me to ask how many guests could come – she said she was expecting 25–30 people. In the NICU, each baby is in a crib or isolette in about a 6 foot by 6 foot space. I told her I was concerned that there would not be room for everyone (and, privately, I was concerned that other families would ask why another family was allowed so many visitors) but that I would work with the NICU team toward a solution. Maribel was receptive to this, and so was the NICU team.

The NICU charge nurse suggested temporarily moving Brooklyn to the step-down nursery, a separate unit located above the NICU but staffed by the same doctors, nurses, and social workers as the NICU. This unit provided more privacy and more room. The family was receptive to this, and Brooklyn was transferred there an hour or two before the baptism. Soon, family began to arrive. Then more family, then more. There were at least 25 people circling Brooklyn. Godparents brought hand-made decorations, one grandmother brought a dress she purchased on a recent trip to Mexico. An aunt brought a cake. As I saw the dozens of people there for Brooklyn and to support Joseph and Maribel, I thought back to the initial concerns that Maribel and Joseph did not have a support system. See Figure 5.1 to see the supports available to Brooklyn's family.

Aside from the tubes, wires, and beeps from monitors, it seemed like any other baptism. One nurse agreed to silence the monitors and stand watch at the screens, monitoring the baby's vitals so the ceremony was not interrupted by beeps every few seconds. Another nurse helped position the baby and transfer her from the arms of one family member to another, while a third nurse and I took photographs that were printed and transferred to a CD for the family. When a patient is dying or has a poor prognosis, we try to arrange for professional volunteer photographers to take photos for the family, but none were available that day. This family was helped by a newly developed perspective that allowed them to meet the goals and hopes they had for their daughter.

Reassessment and evaluation

After the baptism, Maribel asked if she could speak with me in private. We went into a small lounge in the step-down nursery and she quietly said "I think we want to just take her home. How soon can we just take her home? Today?"

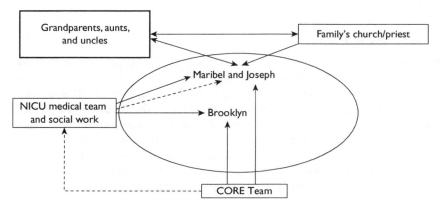

Figure 5.1 Ecomap of Brooklyn's family

I felt very surprised. I had expected the family to push on and to ultimately decide that Brooklyn should receive any intervention that would keep her alive. I know I stumbled over my words when I responded to Maribel. "So you are saying that you and Joseph don't want a lot of hospitals and doctors and surgeries? You want her to be with you at home as soon as possible?" I asked. Maribel said that the more she and Joseph spoke about Brooklyn, the more they realized that the dire prognosis they were given was right. She said that they could see her symptoms were evolving and they did not want her to suffer through more surgeries. They had a nursery fully ready for her at home, and the thought of her never being in it made them both cry, she said. "So, we just want her to be at home. Can you call that team if you think they can help us get her there fast?" Maribel asked. Joseph then joined us and confirmed that he wanted Brooklyn at home, too and that their families supported this plan.

The neonatologist made an official consult to the CORE team a few minutes later. Within the hour, the CORE physician and social worker met with the family. Maribel and Joseph said that they wanted hospice in the home to help with symptom and pain management. The CORE physician worked quickly with the NICU case management team to get insurance approval for hospice and g-tube and oxygen supplies. Nursing worked with Maribel and Joseph to teach them oxygen administration and how to use the g-tube.

Oxygen is delivered differently at home than it is in the hospital. The physicians had some concerns that Brooklyn would not tolerate the switch, and warned the family that Brooklyn could possibly die during transport or soon after arriving at home. The family debated whether they wanted Brooklyn to be resuscitated if she were to quickly deteriorate. They agreed that she was to be resuscitated while being transported via ambulance home but that, once she got home, she would not be resuscitated. Usually, babies discharged on oxygen are also discharged on a monitor. Because these monitors false alarm frequently and because Brooklyn would be allowed to die naturally if she began to decline, the CORE team, NICU team, and, most importantly, the family agreed that she would not go home with a monitor.

The CORE physician volunteered to come in on her day off and lead the ambulance transport home to help manage any complications during the ride. The family was receptive to this, so transport was arranged for early in the morning 2 days later. Usually, g-tube and oxygen training takes 3–5 days, as does insurance approval for supplies. Maribel, Joseph, an aunt, and a grandmother (again with an on-site interpreter) quickly learned how to administer oxygen and g-tube feeds.

Transfer and termination

Brooklyn was going home on a weekend so I met with the family the day before to make sure they knew that they would transition to working with the CORE team social worker. Maribel, Joseph, and their extended family were receptive to this transition. I told them that if at any point they needed or wanted to be in touch with me directly, they could. The next day, transfer home went perfectly. Brooklyn did well with the switch in oxygen and arrived to a house filled with friends and family eager to welcome her home. The family had food for the transport team and gave thank-you cards to the CORE physician to deliver to all who helped with Brooklyn's discharge. The transfer took place the day after Halloween and the family changed Brooklyn into a costume as soon as she got home and celebrated her first Halloween in conjunction with her first day home.

The CORE team checked in regularly with the family and hospice agency over the phone and visited the family a few times a month. After their first visit upon her transfer, the CORE social worker reported to me that the family seemed to be doing well, as did Brooklyn. Her medical status had not changed and Maribel, Joseph, and their extended family seemed to be enjoying caring for her, taking her to their favorite places, taking countless photographs – all the things most new parents enjoy. At Maribel and Joseph's request, Brooklyn had few follow-up appointments. For example, children with g-tubes generally follow up with surgery once or twice a month to ensure that the tube site is healing properly. We did not schedule these appointments, giving Brooklyn more time at home with her family. The CORE team visited her regularly and the physicians on the team served as her primary care provider, allowing for continuity of care.

After three months at home, Brooklyn's respiratory status deteriorated. Oxygen was no longer enough to keep her comfortable. Her parents faced another difficult decision – allow her to remain at home to die or to bring her to St. Christopher's for evaluation and possible escalation of respiratory support to keep her comfortable. Maribel and Joseph determined that Brooklyn was suffering and opted to bring her to St. Christopher's with the goal of keeping her as comfortable as possible. With Maribel and Joseph, the medical team decided that the utilization of CPAP (a method of respiratory support delivered via nasal cannula that provides continuous air pressure into the lungs) would mitigate, but not treat, her respiratory symptoms. Maribel and Joseph, with the support of their family, opted against further escalation of medical intervention. While seemingly more comfortable, Brooklyn's condition continued to deteriorate. She died surrounded by her parents and family about 36 hours after returning to the hospital.

During Brooklyn's readmission, the CORE team social worker supported the family. Brooklyn was readmitted on a weekend and she died surrounded by her parents and family before I returned to work on Monday. I called the family and spoke with Maribel. She was devastated, but confident in the decisions she and Joseph made. Since then, I have had no direct contact with the family, although the CORE team follows up regularly with families after the death of a child. Local grief and counseling resources are provided to every family whose child dies, and families are also encouraged to remain in contact with their social workers for support. Also, every year, St. Christopher's holds a memorial service for children who died during the previous year. I am hopeful that Brooklyn's family will attend.

Differential discussion

Working with Brooklyn and her family taught me that giving families time to process their child's diagnosis and prognosis can be helpful, perhaps even vital. Maribel and Joseph needed time to process the loss of having a healthy child before they could process the fact that she would likely die, regardless of medical interventions. In hindsight, giving the family time to make decisions and move forward with a plan for Brooklyn challenged me – I have realized I felt that they should be making decisions more quickly because I was worried they were not accepting the diagnosis. The team and I were afraid this would cause the baby to suffer as a result. Being an advocate for the family helped me to keep my personal bias in check – I found it easier to advocate for them when a few members of the team outwardly challenged giving the family more time to process information and make decisions.

In reflecting on Brooklyn's time at St. Christopher's, I think that consulting the CORE team earlier might have prevented her from having g-tube surgery – she could have been discharged with a NG (nasogastric) feeding tube that can be inserted painlessly at the bedside. Yet, they were probably more capable of managing the g-tube at home than the NG tube. It is possible that referring Maribel and Joseph to grief counseling before Brooklyn died might have helped them better cope with her prognosis earlier (Stroebe, Schut, & Finkenauer, 2013). Yet, in most ways, the outcome of Brooklyn dying surrounded by family was one I could not have envisioned early in this case.

Discussion questions

1   How might one advocate for better services, including nutrition and prenatal care during pregnancy, in a city with limited resources?
2   What ethical issues did Brooklyn's family face? What ethical issues did the medical team face? On a macro level, what ethical and social challenges do neonatal hospice and palliative care present?
3   How could the entire hospital team, social work, and the CORE team included, work together to better communicate with the family and help them accept CORE's services earlier to enable them to meet their goals for Brooklyn?

References

Braveman, P., Marchi, K., Egerter, S., Soowon, K., Metzler, M., Stancil, T., & Libet, M. (2010). Poverty, near-poverty, and hardship around the time of pregnancy. *Maternal & Child Health Journal, 14*(1), 20–35. doi: 10.1007/s10995-008-0427-0

Feudtner, C., Kang, T. I., Hexem, K. R., Friedrichsdorf, S. J., Osenga, K., Siden, H., et al. (2011). Pediatric palliative care patients: A prospective multicenter cohort study. *Pediatrics, 127*(6), 1094–1101. doi: 10.1542/peds.2010-3225

Feudtner, C., Womer, J., Augustin, R., Remke, S., Wolfe, J., Friebert, S., & Weissman, D. (2013). Pediatric palliative care programs in children's hospitals: A cross-sectional national survey. *Pediatrics, 132*(6), 1063–1070. doi: 10.1542/peds.2013-1286

Lubrano, A. (2010, October 10). A portrait of hunger. *The Philadelphia Inquirer*. Retrieved from www. philly.com/philly/news/special_packages/20101008_hunger_one.html?c=r

Maternity Care Coalition (2011). Survey of prenatal care availability for Medicaid managed care recipients. Retrieved from http://maternitycarecoalition.org/wp-content/uploads/2012/02/Phil-Prental-Care-Report-2011.pdf

Ratzon, R., Sheiner, E., & Shoham-Vardi, I. (2010). The role of prenatal care in recurrent preterm birth. *European Journal of Obstetrics and Gynecology and Reproductive Biology, 154*(1), 40–44. doi: 10.1016/j.ejogrb.2010.08.011

Shah, M., Quill, T., Norton, S., Sada, Y., Buckley, M., & Fridd, C. (2008). "What bothers you the most?" Initial responses from patients receiving palliative care consultation. *American Journal of Hospice and Palliative Medicine, 25*(2), 88–92. doi: 10.1177/1049909107310138

Stroebe, M., Schut, H., & Finkenauer, C. (2013). Parents coping with the death of their child: From individual to interpersonal to interactive perspectives. *Family Science, 4*(1), 28–36. doi: 10.1080/19424620.2013.819229

White, M. (2011). The end at the beginning. *The Ochsner Journal, 11*(4), 309–316. doi: 10.1043/1524-5012-11.4.309

Web and community resources

A short video about a family who decided to care for their newborn with a fatal diagnosis at home with the support of hospice, https://www.youtube.com/watch?v=ToNWquoXqJI

Online support and in-person support groups for parents whose infant has died, www.nationalshare.org

A non-profit that organizes volunteer professional photographers to take portraits of fatally ill infants or infants who have died without leaving the hospital, www.nowilaymedowntosleep.org

A blog written by professional writers whose infants have died, www.glowinthewoods.com

A non-profit organization that works with children and teenagers experiencing the death of a loved one, www.grievingchildren.org

Children and youth

Chapter 6

Working with families with HIV-positive children

Juli E. Birmingham, Deborah A. Calvert,
Jennifer D. Greenman, John Krall, and Rachel Warner

Context

The Special Immunology/Family Care Center (FCC) at the Children's Hospital of Philadelphia (CHOP) was established in 1988 to address the growing human immunodeficiency virus (HIV) epidemic among children who were exposed to or infected with HIV at birth. The program was designed to provide wrap-around and co-located services for these children and their families. The design was based on the understanding that HIV is more than just a medical condition and that a holistic, family-centered approach would better serve clients. The FCC's mission is accomplished through four major functions: medical care, psychosocial services, testing to monitor growth and development, and research. Medical care encompasses on-going primary medical and HIV specialized care. Psychosocial services are specially designed to address barriers inhibiting access and utilization of medical services and improve overall quality of life. We monitor physical and cognitive growth including educational and developmental testing and offer nutritional counseling. The FCC also engages in clinical and behavioral research to advance the quality of available care. In addition, FCC has established a cooperative agreement with an adult HIV provider, which allows parents living with HIV to receive their medical care at the program at the same time their child is receiving theirs.

Perhaps the most important change in the field of HIV care since the FCC's inception is the improved medication for HIV treatment, which has enabled clients to live longer and more symptom-free lives. New medications have drastically reduced the incidence of HIV transmission from mother to child at birth. Since 1994, protocols have been established that have substantially reduced the incidence of perinatal HIV transmission. According to the National Institutes for Health website (2014), "With the implementation of recommendations for universal prenatal HIV counseling and testing, antiretroviral (ARV) prophylaxis, scheduled cesarean delivery, and avoidance of breastfeeding, the rate of perinatal transmission of HIV has dramatically diminished to less than 2% in the United States and Europe." Since 1996, there has been an increase in the number and types of ARV medications available to treat HIV and it has been shown that a combination of medications can reduce viral levels, maintain immune system functioning, and decrease symptoms and opportunistic infections (Centers for Disease Control and Prevention, 2013). The results of the implementation of combination ARV therapy can be seen in the fact that no client has died due to HIV at CHOP since 2011, and only 2 out of 238 of the HIV-exposed infants seen at CHOP between 2010 and 2015 were infected with HIV. Our expectation is that if clients continue to participate in

HIV medical care and remain adherent to their ARV regimens, the virus will remain under control and they will eventually transition to adult care.

Thanks to these advances in medical care, the average age of the clients perinatally infected with HIV seen at the FCC is now 16 years old. Our clinic has shifted from serving primarily children to working with teens and young adults. Actively engaging with adolescents is particularly important in facilitating a successful transition to adult care. The approach used by FCC works well with clients as they grow into adulthood. In particular, youth can benefit from consistent outreach and support to attend medical appointments, adhere to medication regimens, and help navigate complex systems of services and public benefits (HRSA, 2012; Higa, Marks, Crepaz, Liau, & Lyles, 2012). In addition, co-locating medical care and supportive services is fundamental to program success and has long been the model for HIV medical care (HRSA, 2007, 2012), yielding more success in engaging and retaining youth in services (Higa et al., 2012).

Policy

The FCC has received federal grants to support its services for over two decades. This support comes from funds authorized by the Ryan White Comprehensive AIDS Resources Emergency (CARE) Act, which first passed in 1990. This Act funds medical and other services to low-income people living with HIV. In addition, Ryan White funds can be accessed to provide emergency food assistance, transportation costs to services, and ARV medications. The funding enables the provision of care without regard to a client's ability to pay (HRSA, n.d.). Programs like FCC are expected to bill for services whenever possible, but the CARE Act set up a system to ensure HIV care provision to anyone living with HIV who does not have other means to engage in and utilize care.

With the passage of the Patient Protection and Affordable Care Act (ACA), the long-term need for the Ryan White CARE Act has been called into question. More specifically, if everyone can access affordable health insurance or publicly supported care through Medicare or Medicaid, then some have argued that a discretionary fund to support HIV care is no longer needed. In particular, expanded Medicaid based solely on income would enable low-income people living with HIV to access insurance coverage for medical care and medication. Although expanded insurance coverage is an important step forward for people living with HIV, a more holistic approach to HIV care includes many services that are not covered by insurance, especially case management and counseling (Kates, 2013).

Technology

Aside from advances in medical and medication technology discussed above, technology is also used to maintain and keep regular contact with clients and staff. We follow up with clients and families using telephone calls, text messages, and occasionally through social media, as we found that these approaches are more widely used by adolescents and young adults. Staff use e-mail to communicate regarding client issues when we do not have face-to-face meetings.

Our clinic makes use of electronic medical records to track and collect data, monitor client care, and report data collected. We run reports on client attendance enabling us to keep track of clients who have not been seen in over four months in order to reengage them in care. Our clinic also has a drop-in space for clients to come and use computers and meet with social workers or other staff to work on job/school applications, scholarships, or other computer-based needs.

Organization

At FCC, we work as an interdisciplinary team that includes doctors, nurses, a dietician, a medical assistant, a developmental psychologist, and an adolescent counselor, in addition to social workers. The team meets three times a week to discuss details of current cases and formulate plans to best assist clients and coordinate care. We primarily see clients during clinic visits which are scheduled every one to three months, though clients may come in to see a social worker or the counselor at other times. During the medical visit, the client sees the medical provider, social worker, adolescent counselor, nursing staff, and other team members as needed.

A unique aspect of our interdisciplinary team is the amount of time we spend together. We generally eat lunch together, regularly celebrate important staff milestones through in-office potlucks, and hold two annual out of the office parties for staff and our families. This time spent together outside of the daily work context enables staff members to develop positive relationships, decreases compassion fatigue, and increases investment in work relationships.

There are many benefits when working on an interdisciplinary team in a shared office space such as continuity of care, shared knowledge of client information, decreased patient triangulation of staff, and the ability for all staff to see each client holistically. However, this also brings with it some challenges. Social workers start from a client-centered approach to support client needs and goals, which may not be health related, such as finding housing or obtaining a job. Goals of the medical establishment are primarily focused on overall health of the client, such as medication adherence or follow-up appointments. The role of the social worker in a medical setting is to advocate for client needs and support medical providers in understanding the complex issues that the client is facing. In a setting such as ours, it is important to work together to provide consistency for our clients and families.

Description of typical clients/situations

The FCC serves children and youth from birth to age 25. Clients are evenly distributed by sex. Most live in Philadelphia, but FCC has clients who live throughout the surrounding counties. In the United States, racial and ethnic minorities, particularly African-Americans, are the group most severely impacted by perinatal HIV. At FCC, approximately 65% of the clients living with HIV are African-American, followed by Africans (15%), (who are recent immigrants or international adoptees), Whites (11%), Latinos (5%), Asians, Haitians, and mixed heritage (4%). The large majority of FCC clients live at or below the federal poverty line, and almost 80% have Medicaid as their primary insurance.

The clients living with HIV who are seen at FCC require frequent medical visits, daily medications, and support for living with a chronic and, potentially, life-threatening illness. It can be very difficult to sustain this level of care, especially for teens and young adults, as taking daily medications is difficult (Gardiner & Dvorkin, 2006). In addition, youth living with HIV face many challenges that can significantly impact their willingness and ability to remain in care, including economic instability, mental health symptoms, and lack of family support. Without efforts to address the complex needs of youth, many will not receive the care and services they need.

Poverty and inadequate community resources often place youth in a position where they have little opportunity for a good education or support for occupational/vocational training and success (HRSA, 2012). Lack of opportunity is discouraging to youth and places them at higher risk of dropping out of school, abusing substances, and practicing risky sexual behaviors (AIDS Alliance, 2005). Young adult clients have difficulty finding work, especially work that pays a living wage and includes benefits such as health insurance and sick paid time off. Resources for learning a trade are limited and most clients have difficulty being able to identify a profession or career that they would like to pursue.

Nationally, youth living with HIV report high levels of mental illness, which are intensified by stigma associated with HIV (HRSA, 2007, 2012). At our clinic, very high rates of mental health problems have been identified among the youth being treated for HIV infection, particularly depression, anxiety, and adjustment associated with learning their HIV diagnosis. A study at CHOP found that 93% of clients 18–24 years of age reported that they felt traumatized by learning about their HIV diagnosis and that over 30% of study participants have post-traumatic stress symptoms (Radcliffe et al., 2007). Mental health problems have long been associated with poor retention in care and adherence to appointments and medication regimens (Wagner et al., 2011).

Decisions about practice

Definition of the client

We first met Christina when she was 3 years old. Her mother entered a drug and alcohol recovery program where she tested positive for HIV. This led to Christina's mother's children being tested, and her youngest, Christina, tested positive for HIV and was referred to FCC for primary and HIV care. Christina and her mother were both prescribed ARV medications and it soon became apparent that the family had a difficult time providing the necessary care for a child with a chronic illness.

During Christina's early years the family regularly missed appointments and it was difficult to engage them in care. When Christina's mother brought her to the FCC, Christina was underweight and had elevated HIV loads, and her mother provided an inconsistent medical history. When staff discussed their concerns with Christina's mother, she became irate and often left without completing Christina's medical visit. Staff informed her that if she was unable to meet Christina's needs and attend all medical appointments, a referral to Child Protective Services (CPS) would be made. Unfortunately, Christina's mother's mental health and substance abuse continued to pose a major barrier to Christina's care and CPS was contacted. Upon investigation, CPS decided that Christina needed to be removed from her mother's care and she was placed in medical foster care. Eventually, parental rights were terminated and Christina was adopted by her foster family when she was about 6 years old.

Over the years, Christina struggled academically and her educational challenges were discovered through testing at our clinic. The social worker advocated for Christina by attending the school Individual Educational Planning meeting (IEP). She worked to coordinate additional services for Christina in the areas where she struggled most. Although Christina's issues initially presented themselves as educational, staff soon became aware that there were other concerns. Christina's adoptive mother frequently called the social worker reporting behaviors Christina exhibited that were concerning. Christina isolated herself from the family, refused to shower, hid food and medications under her bed, and occasionally stole from family members. After further discussion between the social worker and the adoptive mother, it came to light that the family was struggling with integrating Christina into their family. For example, the adoptive family went on vacation stating that they needed their own family time and left Christina with another relative. Her adoptive mom was able to verbalize the struggles she and her family had with integrating Christina in their family and it was clear that they often felt resentful about the disruptions Christina's presence caused. In addition to these challenges, there were concerns about the use of corporal punishment and/or physical abuse in the home.

In order to support the family, FCC provided weekly individual counseling and home nursing visits to improve medication adherence. Christina attended regular support groups at FCC and had frequent contact with her social worker. The social worker also referred the family to a community-based organization for family therapy to address issues related to attachment and to improve the family dynamic. Unfortunately, Christina's adoptive family struggled to follow through with these appointments. They asserted that Christina was old enough to be responsible for her own medication adherence, health care, and behaviors. The family eventually was unable to care for her and by the time she was a teenager, she had been through two more foster families. Coordinating these moves, assuring some continuity to her education, and supporting Christina were all major challenges for our work together.

Christina's mental health continued to decompensate through her teen years and her behaviors became even more concerning. She was experiencing symptoms consistent with post-traumatic stress disorder, including periods of dissociation, self-harm, explosive and suppressed anger, disruption in relationships with family, friends, and FCC staff, and frequent periods of despair. On many occasions, Christina would call to schedule medical visits, show up to clinic, and then refuse to engage with staff. There were times where she would begin the medical visit and in a matter of minutes her affect would shift and she would abruptly leave with no explanation, which was frustrating for all involved. At one medical visit when she was about 16, Christina reported that she was feeling suicidal. After a thorough assessment by the social worker, the team decided that it was best to take Christina to a Crisis Response Center, where she was admitted for psychiatric care.

Christina spent the next 2 years in and out of inpatient psychiatric hospitals. During this time, the social worker initiated meetings with all of the community agencies involved (school, CPS, mental health services) in order to develop the best care plan for Christina. Although the family was invited to these meetings, they chose not to come. The meetings consisted of FCC staff, the inpatient social worker and psychiatrist, and CPS. Due to the family's lack of involvement during these 2 years and their refusal to welcome Christina back into their home, it was decided that a group home would be the best option for her. The group home assisted Christina in taking her HIV and psychiatric medications regularly, which helped to stabilize her medical and mental health. She began accessing more services available to her at FCC, such as individual counseling, assistance with job searches, tutoring, and group events.

Goals

The HIV-positive young adults in our program have goals typical of most individuals at this developmental stage. We work to help them balance personal and health goals. Our attempts to help our clients identify their goals and break them down into measurable objectives. Young adults typically wish to graduate from high school or obtain a GED (General Educational Development), attend educational programs such as college or technical training, advance in jobs or careers, and create and maintain fulfilling relationships. Our clients' hopes and dreams are complicated by their need for medical care and mental health treatment.

Many of our clients, Christina included, are challenged by loss and instability in their lives, and therefore their goals may change frequently. Focusing on school and mental health care may be primary goals for one visit, while the next visit they may need support around obtaining a job in order to maintain housing. This turmoil makes it difficult to stay focused on some of the long-term goals. The maintenance of both physical and mental health can be overwhelming and time consuming at a time when they believe their peers are free to explore and enjoy life. The social workers help our clients find consistencies in their immediate, short-term, and long-term goals in order to create a realistic care plan, and we help to promote motivation to continue working towards health, career, and relationship goals in developmentally appropriate ways.

Christina's goals revolved around obtaining a part-time job and earning her college degree. Christina and the team also talk about long-term self-sufficiency in regards to housing and finances. She also hopes to develop healthy, stable relationships in the community. Physical health and emotional well-being are part of her long-term goals and she understands that without them she will not be able to take care of her daily needs and work towards other life goals. See Figure 6.1 to see the many family constellations and services interacting with Christina.

Strategies and interventions

Our clinic has moved to implement aspects of trauma-informed care. A trauma-informed care model has increasingly been utilized in social service and medical settings, as research continues to show how common a history of trauma is in the general population. This approach was partially informed by the Adverse Childhood Experiences (ACE) study, which provides a lens through which to view our clients' challenges. Researchers interviewed adults regarding their experiences as children with adverse events such as physical, sexual, and emotional abuse, and neglect as well as events that disrupt the family. The study found a correlation between the number of adverse childhood experiences and the participants' long-term mental and physical health (Felitti et al., 1998). More recent research indicates that people living with HIV have high rates of trauma, the combination of HIV and trauma being labeled as syndemic (co-occurring and mutually problematic), and a trauma-informed model of care is suggested (Brezing, Ferrara, & Freudenreich, 2015).

Recognizing the huge impact of trauma throughout the lifespan, trauma-informed care focuses on an understanding of current behavior and problems as a result of past experiences. Traumatized individuals can behave in ways that push people away, causing self-isolation, and reinforcing core beliefs that they are not worthy of care. Traumatized individuals often reject support from those who offer consistency and stability. In the Sanctuary Model, Dr. Sandra Bloom (2013) has shown that trauma affects brain development, social development, and contributes to risky behaviors, which may in turn lead to chronic health issues. In a trauma-informed care model, trauma is recognized and treated, openness and communication are emphasized, and everyone is respected. This can be thought of in terms of "What happened to you?" versus "What is wrong with you?" The model views everyone's unique

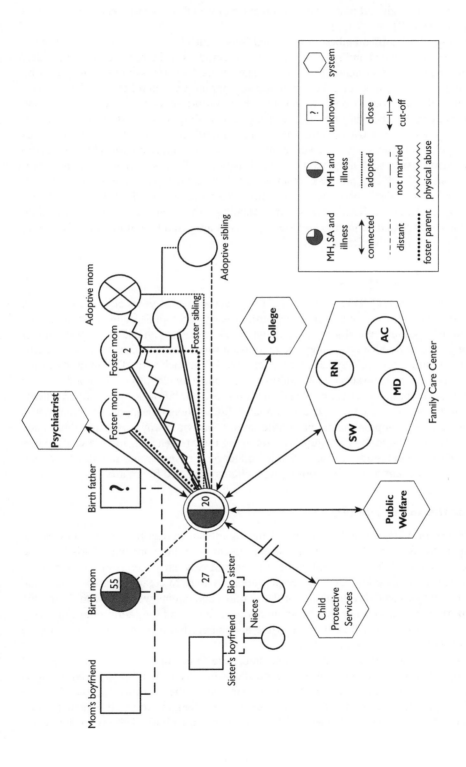

Figure 6.1 Christina's ecomap. MH, mental health; SA, substance abuse

perspective as important and places value on working through issues to create cohesiveness and mutual respect (Bloom, 2013).

Clinicians and all staff members respect and honor our clients, recognizing the trauma that they have experienced and survived. Often, this respect can be reflected in simple acts of thoughtfulness towards clients. FCC staff make themselves accessible to our clients by returning their calls or connecting them with the appropriate staff member. If a client misses a visit, staff will reach out in order to get them back on the schedule as soon as possible. We respect clients by checking first to see if they are willing to see a student or resident. Additionally, clients meet with doctors fully clothed until the physical exam necessitates undressing (which it often does not). This allows clients to feel more comfortable and secure while discussing issues with the doctor. All staff members discuss a client's health holistically. For instance, a doctor may ask about a client's relationships just as a social worker may check in with a client about their medication adherence. We work in transdisciplinary ways to support the client. Staff work towards creating a safe space for clients by avoiding assumptions about sexual behaviors and identity. These are just a few of the things we do to create a safe space for our clients.

Meeting place and use of time

The FCC works with our HIV-positive population over a span of years and, in most cases, clients have been coming to our clinic since birth or early childhood. Visits most often take place in our offices within the clinic space, though quick contacts with clients in the computer room, lobby area, and hallways as they move to exam rooms are common too. Most clients are on a three-month schedule and see their social worker at each visit. The amount of time spent depends on what issues need to be addressed and client availability. Scheduled meeting times can be set up based on client need and our clinic also has "drop-in" times where clients can come in for a quick issue or to use a computer. Some clients disappear for months at a time, miss scheduled appointments, or conflict arises, but we always welcome them back and support them through their struggles (encouraging return even after missed visits is part of the trauma-informed model of care). While boundaries are important, this flexibility and openness is an excellent model for working with clients impacted by trauma.

Stance of the social worker

Trauma theory provides an understanding of the significant impact that trauma has on the families and clients with whom we work. It was essential in the work with Christina, who experienced prolonged and repeated trauma starting at a very early age, resulting in a sense of helplessness and powerlessness. As social workers, we try to create an environment that supports optimal personal development for the families and clients we work with. Using the trauma-informed model, we are able to set up realistic short- and long-term goals, knowing they will change over time. Remaining flexible and supportive is an integral aspect of the stance of the social worker in our setting.

In working with a traumatized population, staff need to be supportive of each other and have appropriate boundaries in order to reduce staff turnover and secondary trauma. With Christina, our team struggled with how to balance supporting the client while protecting ourselves. Her rages, rejections, and disappearances were challenging to us all. Understanding that some clients come to us with a long history of trauma and a limited ability to cope when things get stressful helps us better meet their needs and to set up a plan that also works for the team. It also allows us to support one another as a team to help us maintain the respect and care that we know is vital to our clients' well-being.

Use of resources outside the helping relationship

As indicated, there were many outside resources mobilized over the course of Christina's care. Child Protective Services was very involved with Christina over the years as they terminated her parents' rights, moved her to her first foster home where she was eventually adopted, and then moved her to two other foster homes during her adolescence, eventually assisting with the group home placement. Even so, it was often the role of the FCC social worker to coordinate the school and mental health services that Christina was using. As Christina resided within a large urban school district and her "home school" kept changing, managing to get appropriate school work and educational intervention was a major challenge. Much of the social work intervention at that time was with community agencies, advocating for Christina's educational continuity, on-going mental health services, and support for stable housing.

Transition and case conclusion

Transition from pediatric to adult care is a process that happens over a long period of time for clients with a chronic illness. In childhood, the focus of a transition plan for this population is patient education, laying the groundwork for patients to have the knowledge needed as they move into adult care. This process is something our clinic continues to focus on in order to make it easier for our clients to have a successful transition. At an early age, we begin to teach how the immune system works and how to keep one's body healthy. Once our clients know their diagnosis, we talk with them about what their lab work means and about the medications that they take and why. During their teen years, we address various aspects of being HIV-positive, including HIV transmission, sexual health, HIV within a relationship, and coping with their diagnosis. As their transition to adult care nears, we teach clients how to navigate insurance and the health care system. We assist them in searching for appropriate adult HIV health care options. Although it is ultimately up to the client to choose where to go, we try to pair them with a clinic that will best meet their needs. Before transition, we refer clients to a community case manager to help bridge the gap between pediatric and adult care.

Today, at age 21, Christina is taking her psychiatric and HIV medications, working hard to find a part-time job, is enrolled in college, developing relationships, and is more stable. This journey into adulthood is complicated by her mental illness and extensive history of trauma. As Christina's case with us comes to a close, it is only the beginning of her life as an adult. As advances in HIV medical care have made it possible for our patients to live a full adult life, Christina's on-going trauma and stigma of being a person living with HIV may remain challenging for her.

For many of our clients, transition is seen as another loss and can be a barrier to their retention in care. As Christina nears the time where she will need to transition to adult care, FCC staff is working with her on ways to make this loss manageable while assisting her in creating a support system to take her through adulthood. The FCC has done its best to provide appropriate levels of support and guidance to Christina throughout her development, partly to keep her healthy during childhood and partly to prepare her for her transition into adult care. Historically, programs that cater to adults are not able to provide patients the same type of supportive services that pediatric programs can offer to younger patients. Over the next few years, our team will assist Christina in taking more ownership of her health care needs. She should be able to access community resources and coordinate her own care, including making appointments and refilling her medications. By the time of her transition, we want Christina to have a good understanding of her health care and wellness needs. With the support of the services provided by FCC, along with her own growth and resilience, Christina has a strong foundation to move forward.

Differential discussion

Writing this chapter allowed us to examine Christina's life and all of the significant events she has experienced. This provided us with a greater perspective on the compounded effect that trauma has on her and many of our patients. Although it can be difficult for us as providers, we have learned some hard lessons. Namely, sometimes we must take a step back and acknowledge that we cannot fix a situation. This takes the pressure off and enables us to better support our clients when we are frustrated about their housing, economic situation, schooling, etc. There is no simple answer to fixing Christina's situation then or now. All of the systems involved with many of our client's lives are interwoven with poverty and institutional racism. As disheartening as this all sounds, we continue to do this work because we see the impact that we make on individual lives every day by being their advocate and helping to connect them to resources that are available. We believe our model of care helps to send a message of worth to our clients to enable them to meet their challenges with more support and stamina. Ideally, we could assure that all individuals were safely housed, supported with excellent schooling and mental health services, and had stable family situations, but we must function within the current reality. Despite the lack of effective resources available to meet all of Christina's needs, she has continued to make progress in her life goals. As we write this case conclusion, it astounds us how resilient Christina, and other clients who have experienced trauma, can be. The resiliency of our patients inspires us to continue to do this work every day.

Discussion questions

1   When community agencies are each functioning in independent ways, how might the health social worker leverage authority to ensure that care is coordinated?
2   What do you believe you would find most challenging in implementing a trauma-informed model of care? How might you respond to repeated missed appointments? Verbal outbursts and rejection?
3   Pediatric care typically allows intensive social work intervention while most adult care is provided with few social work or other allied health professionals. With the new sanction for integrated behavioral health, how might you make a case for adult care to have similar levels of allied health team members?

References

AIDS Alliance for Children, Youth & Families (2005). *Finding HIV-positive youth and bringing them into care.* Retrieved from https://careacttarget.org/library/finding-hiv-positive-youth-and-bringing-them-care

Bloom, S. L. (2013). *Creating sanctuary: Toward the evolution of sane societies* (revised edition). New York: Routledge.

Brezing, C., Ferrara, M., & Freudenreich, O. (2015). Review articles: The syndemic illness of HIV and trauma: Implications for a trauma-informed model of care. *Psychosomatics, 56*, 107–118. doi: 10.1016/j.psym.2014.10.006

Centers for Disease Control and Prevention (2013). *Prevention benefits of HIV treatment.* Retrieved from www.cdc.gov/hiv/prevention/research/tap/

Felitti, V., Anda, R., Nordenberg, D., Williamson, D., Spitz, A., Edwards, V., et al. (1998). Relationship of childhood abuse and household dysfunction to many of the leading causes of death in adults. *American Journal of Preventive Medicine, 14*(4), 245–258.

Gardiner, P. & Dvorkin, L. (2006). Promoting medication adherence in children. *American Family Physician, 74*(5), 793–798. PMID: 16970023

Higa, D. H., Marks, G., Crepaz, N., Liau, A., & Lyles, C. M. (2012). Interventions to improve retention in HIV primary care: A systematic review of US studies. *Current HIV/AIDS Reports, 9*(4), 313–325. doi: 10.1007/s11904-012-0136-6

HRSA (Human Resources and Administration) (n.d.). *The Ryan White HIV/AIDs Program: A living history.* Retrieved from http://hab.hrsa.gov/livinghistory/timeline/1990.htm

HRSA (2007, June). Transitioning from adolescent to adult care. *HRSA Care Action.* Retrieved from http://hab.hrsa.gov/newspublications/careactionnewsletter/june2007.pdf.pdf

HRSA (2012, June). Delivering culturally competent care to the young adult client. *HRSA Care Action.* Retrieved from http://hab.hrsa.gov/newspublications/careactionnewsletter/junecareaction2012.pdf

Kates, J. (2013). Implications of the Affordable Care Act for people with HIV infection and the Ryan White HIV/AIDS program: What does the future hold? *Topics in Antiviral Medicine, 21*(4). Retrieved from https://www.iasusa.org/sites/default/files/tam/21-4-138.pdf

National Institutes for Health (2014, March 28). Recommendations for use of antiretroviral drugs in pregnant HIV-1-infected women for maternal health and interventions to reduce perinatal HIV transmission in the United States. Retrieved from http://aidsinfo.nih.gov/contentfiles/lvguidelines/perinatalgl.pdf

Radcliffe, J., Fleisher, C. L., Hawkins, L. A., Tanney, M., Kassam-Adams, N., Ambrose, C., & Rudy, B. J. (2007). Posttraumatic stress and trauma history in adolescents and young adults with HIV. *AIDS Patient Care and STDs, 21*(7), 501–508. PMID: 17651031

Wagner, G. J., Goggin, K., Remien, R. H., Rosen, M. I., Simoni, J., Bangsberg, D. R., & Liu, H. (2011). A closer look at depression and its relationship to HIV antiretroviral adherence. *Annals of Behavioral Medicine, 42*(3), 352–360. doi: 10.1007/s12160-011-9295-8

Chapter 7

Social work in a pediatric hospital
Managing a medically complex patient

Jennifer Fenstermacher

Context

Description of setting

Alfred I. duPont Hospital for Children (AIDHC), USA, part of Nemours Health System, is dedicated to the health of children. The newly expanded hospital has single rooms for all patients and has been designed "by families for families." It is committed to compassionate, comprehensive care and excellence in patient care, education and research (www.nemours. org/locations/nemours-dupont.html). Specialist inpatient and outpatient services are available to children from birth through age 21 (to age 18 for primary care). Every social worker in the Patient and Family Services Department is master's level, assigned to a specific service, and responsible for both the inpatient and outpatient needs of that service.

Policy

Three important policies affecting our work are the re-accreditation process through the Joint Commission (formerly known as JCAHO – Joint Commission on the Accreditation of Healthcare Organizations), HIPAA (Health Insurance Portability and Accountability Act), and the Affordable Care Act (often referred to as Obamacare). The Joint Commission (JC) is an independent, non-profit group that determines and upholds standards for hospitals; it accredits facilities based on compliance with regulations and efforts to improve (www.joint-commission.org). The JC team surveys hospitals regularly to ensure that the hospital complies with standards and regulations for safety in health care. As part of the inspection, social workers are expected to be aware of and able to answer questions regarding key standards. Social workers are often included in "tracer" cases, where the surveyors follow a patient over the course of several hours and interview every team member who interacts with the patient. When the inspection is complete, the hospital is re-accredited and receives a report suggesting areas for improvement.

The Health Insurance Portability and Accountability Act of 1996 (HIPAA) primarily affects the social worker in the area of protected health information (PHI). Title II of HIPAA includes the Privacy Rule, which states that:

> a major goal of the Privacy Rule is to assure that individual's health information is properly protected while allowing the flow of health information needed to provide and

promote high quality health care and to protect the public's health and well being. The Rule strikes a balance that permits important uses of information, while protecting the privacy of people who seek care and healing. (U.S. Department of Health and Human Services, 2015)

A hospital may use and disclose PHI without an individual's authorization in three areas: treatment, payment, and health care operations. For social work, the relevant issue is treatment because social workers may work with family members who must sign a release of information (ROI) form to enable the treatment team to share information or make referrals. This form is not necessary for referrals for durable medical equipment or home care; however, it is necessary for work with community agencies and schools unless parents request that school nurses have access to the medical chart. Treatment includes the provision, coordination, and management of health care and related services, including consultations and referrals

The Affordable Care Act (ACA, www.hhs.gov/healthcare/rights/) comprises two pieces of legislation: the Patient Protection and Affordable Care Act (P.L. 111-148) and the Health Care and Education Reconciliation Act of 2010 (P.L. 111-152). Prior to ACA, efforts to contain health care costs included paying hospitals based on patients' diagnosis codes. Social workers were responsible for discharging patients expeditiously even if necessary services or resources were not available. ACA continues to try to contain costs, but protections are in place to align lower costs with quality care. An ongoing challenge for duPont is that although parents from neighboring states wish the children to receive care from us, ACA insurers often will not cover out-of-state care.

Significant dimensions of the ACA are the expansion of Medicaid to cover more individuals with limited financial resources and not allowing insurance companies to deny coverage to those with pre-existing conditions (Health Care Rights, www.hhs.gov/healthcare/rights/). The development of "medical homes" for provision of comprehensive health care is a focus of the ACA, and development of Accountable Care Organizations has been an outgrowth of these efforts (Shortell, Wu, Lewis, Colla, & Fisher, 2014). Nemours embraces this effort.

Technology

Technology is ever-present and always changing in a pediatric hospital. The social worker's responsibilities are to be aware of the technology (medications, equipment, etc.), to help patients and families to make informed decisions about technology use, and to support communications among the medical team, patient and family about such use. We also assist in obtaining equipment/technologies for patients' home use, if appropriate. We may help a family navigate a financial assistance program in order to obtain medications, advocate with an insurer to get coverage for a new technology previously not (yet) covered, use the internet to locate resources for the family, and consult with supporting agencies such as those supplying durable medical equipment and home care. While social workers know that this type of work is valuable to the patient and family, it sometimes feels thankless because patients, families, and colleagues are often unaware of the enormous effort it requires.

Another area of technology that affects a social worker's daily routine is the electronic medical record (EMR). With the advent of HIPAA and ACA, electronic documentation has become the norm. Documentation in social work serves several functions: (1) assessment and planning; (2) service delivery; (3) continuity and coordination of services; (4) supervision;

(5) service evaluation; and (6) accountability to clients, insurers, agencies, other providers, courts, and utilization review bodies (Kagle, 2008; Reamer, 2003). Children's hospitals have had a spotty record of adoption of EMR as many of the early products were designed for general hospitals and not well adapted to pediatric care (Teufel, Kazley, Andrews, Ebeling, & Basco, 2013), but Nemours has worked to assure adoption of the EMR to facilitate comprehensive care. It is critical that the social worker be aware of the content of the documentation, the language and terminology, and the credibility of the document (Reamer, 2005). Social workers often joke that if it is not written down, then it did not happen.

Organization

The AIDHC motto is doing "whatever it takes" to ensure the best treatment for the children in our care. It is sometimes difficult to live up to that motto when expectations of families, colleagues, and ourselves seem impossible. Yet, we keep trying. The hospital is divided into divisions, departments, services, and teams; the outpatient primary care units are now "medical homes" as recommended by ACA.

Patient and Family Services staff members have an ethos of teamwork. Social workers attend an interdisciplinary team meeting each morning (known as screening) with a member of the utilization review team, nursing, and an attending physician to discuss the patients and their needs (medical, social, financial, etc.). This provides each social worker with a comprehensive picture of the daily census and allows the social worker to ask any questions or share important information with the members of the team. Early identification of patients who need a social work assessment is integral to effective discharge planning. It is important to recognize that while the overall goal is the maximization of health for each patient, each team members' objectives and responsibilities vary in terms of achieving that goal.

I am the social worker assigned to the General Pediatrics Service. I am responsible for all of the general pediatric patients on a 24-bed unit, meaning I could be actively working with up to 24 patients at any given time. My typical caseload is around 15 patients and their diagnoses range from asthma to gastroenteritis, cyclic vomiting to failure to thrive, or meningitis to an ear infection. The patients' and families' needs vary just as widely: nebulizers to enteral feeding set-ups, assessment of individual stressors to assessment of psychosocial family situation, applying for insurance to arranging transportation home. I also am the one to sit with a parent after a child has received a difficult diagnosis or help a child think about what his or her favorite things are so we can use that as a way to personalize the care. It is a fast-paced service with many short stays and quick responses required. I also have a handful of patients on the Diagnostic Referral Service (DRS) who have more complex diagnoses that require longer hospital stays, a slower pace, and more social work involvement. These are rewarding for the relationships developed and frustrating for the difficulties of finding a plan of treatment that works. The patient described in the rest of this chapter comes from the DRS.

Description of typical clients and situations

We serve a wide variety of pediatric patients, many of whom are relatively short-stay, acute-care patients whose families are distressed. We serve these patients well and send them on their way healed. We also care for children whose chronic complex conditions require intensive intervention to help provide the comprehensive and compassionate service we promise.

Decisions about practice

Definition of the client and description of the client situation

Ned is an 18-year-old man who has been treated at AIDHC for the past 13 years. He now lives in a residential care facility and visits his mother, father, and younger brother on weekends. Our DRS team saw Ned because of his complex diagnosis and multi-system disorder. I have been his social worker on and off for over a decade. He has Tetrasomy 18p, a rare chromosomal disorder. Symptoms include craniofacial malformations, varying degrees of developmental delays, speech difficulties, malformation of the spine, hands, and feet, difficulty coordinating movements, and altered muscle tone. In addition to his genetic condition, Ned also has cyclic vomiting syndrome (CVS). His particular type is called Sato's variant and involves elevated blood pressure and behavior changes. There is a large anxiety component to CVS, and because of Ned's developmental delays, it has been difficult to use stress reduction/relaxation techniques with him. Ned was in the hospital almost continuously for 2½ years when he was younger. Despite numerous adjustments in medications, implantation of a vagal nerve stimulator, and a medically induced prolonged sedation, he showed little improvement at that time.

Due to his anxiety and the behavioral issues associated with his diagnoses, Ned responds to stress with agitation and requires constant one-to-one care. His hospitalizations provide a bit of respite for the family. Ned was not able to attend school from about age 9–12. He was unable to handle even the most restrictive environment that his school district could provide due to his anxiety and behavioral issues. He was not home often enough for home-bound instruction and seldom felt well enough for in-hospital school during his numerous admissions.

His family and I searched unsuccessfully for residential placements that would be appropriate for Ned for many years and only found such a placement when he was about 13. Many facilities rejected him saying he was either not technology-dependent enough or that they were unable to handle his behavioral needs. Funding a placement was also challenging as state agencies pointed fingers at one another and none would take responsibility. Having him admitted to an appropriate residential care facility was a major accomplishment.

Ned was referred for social work services due to his complex medical diagnosis. One might assume that would make him the client. I have discovered over the course of my involvement with him that the client has changed from him, to his family, to the medical team working with him, to the staff caring for him, and back to the patient himself. When Ned is feeling well, he is a delightful, funny, engaging young man who loves vacuum cleaners, laughing, dogs, and 1980s dance music. When he is ill and active in a vomiting cycle, his family becomes the focus of my attention and support. Due to the lack of effective treatment and outside resources when he was younger, his family has needed someone to listen to their concerns, frustration, and anger about what their loved one was going through, their questions about when it might stop, and their fears about how they will handle his disorder as he ages.

Understandably, his family are and have been discouraged, and so have the medical team members and staff who care for him. I have seen team members with their heads in their hands and tears in their eyes wondering why the latest treatment was not working and if there is more they can do. This continues to be my opportunity to support them and reflect back that they are doing the very best they can with what they know and what they have available to them.

Goals

The goals in pediatric hospital discharge planning vary from the small and concrete (obtaining a home nebulizer) to the large and intangible (avoiding social isolation). The treatment team and Ned's family established three goals for him during the long hospitalization from ages 9–13: (1) increase independence; (2) avoid social isolation; and (3) remain at home or in a residential setting, instead of being an inpatient at the hospital. Ned's parents have additional responsibilities outside of the hospital, including working and caring for their other child, Alan, now age 14. Their goal is to achieve a balance between Ned's illness and the needs of their family. This is not easy and is often accompanied by guilt. See Figure 7.1 for Ned's family ecomap.

Contracting and developing objectives

Utilizing the goals mentioned above, the family and I created a plan that is flexible and changes with each admission or new development/challenge. This has not been a stress-free process. Objectives to help Ned increase his independence have included learning to dress

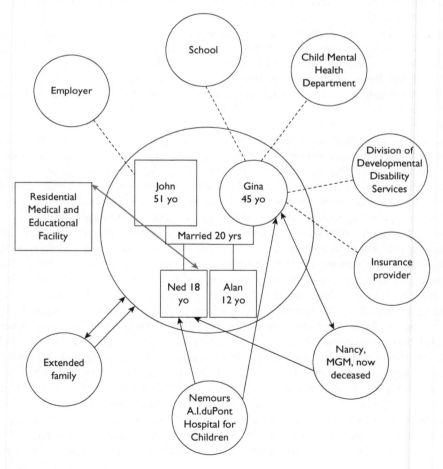

Figure 7.1 Ecomap for Ned

himself and walking on his own. Physical and occupational therapy help Ned achieve these goals and objectives during his inpatient stays and work with him on an outpatient basis on those rare occasions when he is home long enough for services to get into place.

In order to avoid social isolation, our objective has been to enroll Ned in an appropriate educational program. This was quite difficult due to his anxiety issues and inability to utilize stress reduction/coping techniques due to his developmental delays. When Ned has been placed in a new situation with too many people, he becomes anxious, feels the physical sensations in his stomach and starts vomiting, at which point another vomiting cycle starts. We were finally able to find him a residential and educational placement at about the same time he and his family went to another facility for a second opinion when he was nearly 13.

The third goal was keeping Ned out of the hospital for as long as possible. From ages 9 through 12, Ned was never home for more than two months at a time. I spent a large portion of my time working to acquire private duty home nursing for Ned. Having a nurse 12 hours per day, 7 days per week would allow the family more freedom and enable them to see Ned as a family member, not a patient. Insurance benefits cover this service but the nursing agencies were unwilling to take his case because they could not guarantee their nurses consistent hours due to his history of short home stays.

Meeting place

Meeting places take on many shapes and sizes in a hospital. They range from large lecture halls to huddling in a hallway trying to form an area of privacy in a public space. Sometimes there are things that need to be expressed out of Ned's earshot, and that is when we utilize my office, the attending physician's office, and the cafeteria, wherever the family feels most comfortable at the time. The telephone is a very important tool in my practice. Ned's mother knows that she can call anytime, and I will respond promptly. The hospital's new private rooms have enhanced everyone's comfort level, control over their environment, and have improved the quality of interaction and communication, yet there are still some conversations that take place elsewhere to communicate with parents separately from the patient/child.

Use of time

The majority of my discharge planning cases are short-term, brief interventions with patients I may never see again. These revolve around obtaining a piece of medical equipment, a nursing visit, or other services. There is a marked difference in the investment of time, self, and energy between these cases and my work with Ned and his family.

Working with a patient and his family for several years has many positives but there are areas to be sensitive to as well. Spacing and duration of visits is one such area. When Ned was younger and in the hospital, I saw him and his family every day and sometimes several times per day from an hour in his room discussing plans with his family to a few minutes in the hallway when he went to physical therapy. This can create too much familiarity and boundaries can become diffuse. I had to be very careful as Ned's mother and I are the same age and could easily be friends outside of the hospital. I admit that the lines have blurred on occasion and sometimes our conversations have become too intimate. We are both aware of this. It is my responsibility to pull back and gently put the boundaries in place again when it happens.

Another consideration is the length of the relationship. I have known this family for over a decade and at times, have seen them more than I see my own family. When Ned was going on 13, his family decided to take him to another hospital for a second opinion as they were feeling frustrated and thought maybe the medical team could no longer be objective because they were so comfortable with Ned, his condition, his behaviors, and his family. The hospital from which the family sought a second opinion agreed with our treatment plan. Ultimately, we found a good residential placement for Ned, and he returned to us for follow-up care.

Strategies and interventions

According to the National Association of Social Workers (NASW) Standards for Social Work Practice in Health Care Settings (2005), intervention and treatment plans are steps identified by the health social worker, in collaboration with the client and with other members of the team, to achieve the objectives identified during assessment (pp. 21–22). These intervention or treatment plans may include: information, referral, and education; individual, family, or group counseling; psychoeducational support groups; financial counseling; case management and discharge planning; interdisciplinary care planning and collaboration; and client and systems advocacy.

I consider myself to be an advanced generalist and use developmental systems theory (DST) as a conceptual lens that allows me to focus on the complex interactions of the patient, family and medical system within a community (Greenfield, 2011). DST incorporates a strong focus on strengths-based perspectives and guides me to look at the strengths of the entire system to work for the benefit of the patient. In the hospital setting, I must be prepared to work with a variety of different clients: one-on-one with an individual, a whole family, a support group, hospital committees and teams, and outside resources, just to name a few. The strategies and interventions that I use are determined by the needs of my clients and the needs of the hospital.

Interventions I use the most include active listening, self-disclosure, and humor. Active listening involves paying close attention to both the verbal and non-verbal messages that the client is sending and reflecting those messages back to the client so that he knows he is being understood. There are several skills utilized during the active listening process: (1) using verbal and non-verbal prompts to encourage the client to continue talking; (2) asking questions that encourage the client to clarify his statements; (3) paraphrasing or rephrasing the literal meaning of the client's statement; (4) reflecting the feelings of the client's statements; (5) summarizing the literal and feeling components of several statements; and (6) exploring extended silences without changing the topic (Shulman, 2006).

Another helping skill is self-disclosure where a social worker makes statements that reveal some of her own thoughts, feelings, or life experiences (Knight, 2012). This nuanced skill can be used with great care after rapport is established and always relating disclosed material to the client's current concern. Positive effects of self-disclosure include making it easier for clients to discuss sensitive things and putting clients at ease when they feel that they know something about the social worker as a person and not just a professional. If too much is shared, self-disclosure can cause clients to question a worker's emotional stability and professional competence and it can cause a client to feel manipulated. Self-disclosure can be tricky when patients or their families are similar as it may lead to lower boundaries and difficulty maintaining professional roles. The general guideline is that we self-disclose only after we assess that the self-disclosure is helpful for meeting the client's need, not our own.

Humor is my favorite helping tool and one that can be used with clients or colleagues (Digney, 2013). People need to have fun. As social workers, we see clients who are in truly dire circumstances and our resources are sometimes inadequate, leading to frustration.

Humor can be used to defuse the frustration and sadness we experience in our daily work. Social workers are often concerned that our expressions of humor could be misunderstood as insensitivity and we must take care to use humor that is not demeaning. There are risks associated with using humor at work, but without it, social work practice can be unbearable.

Using humor with clients can also be risky and should be viewed like any other technique, realizing that what may be helpful, appropriate, and effective with one client may be offensive to another. Digney (2013) argues that shared humor with youth can help defuse anger and mistrust and can help to connect workers to youth. It is of the utmost importance that social workers never laugh *at* a client, although laughing *with* a client may be helpful. A client or family's sense of humor should always be affirmed and supported, no matter how odd it might seem to you as the social worker.

Stance of the social worker

After introducing myself to a patient and his or her family and explaining the function of social work in the hospital, my goal is to partner with them in seeking and enabling the best care for their child. Partnering can be accomplished through several different roles: advocate, discharge planner, counselor, and mediator, to name a few.

As an advocate, I speak up and reach out to other resources to access the most appropriate services for what the patient and family need. As a discharge planner, I research insurance benefits, locate in-network providers, obtain the necessary services from said providers, arrange for the delivery of equipment and supplies, and ensure that training happens. As a counselor, I listen to the patient and family and provide emotional support during the hospital stay. As a mediator, I am the bridge between the patient, family, and the medical team. I seek clarification and try to interpret the family's concerns and questions to the treatment team while also interpreting the team's medical messages to the family in ways they can understand.

In all of these roles it is important to have an understanding of one's self, motivations, place, and impact on relationships (Reupert, 2007). It is a conscious use of self that allows me to bring my personality to each of these roles and interactions. For me that includes organization, teamwork, and a large dose of humor.

Use of resources outside the helping relationship

I have been a hospital social worker for almost 15 years and in that time I have compiled a notebook of resources and useful information. By referring to my notebook, I may save myself or a colleague valuable time in resolving an issue. Part of my job is to learn to navigate systems and services as effectively as possible. In Ned's case, I reached out to many different sources including his school and state agencies. I continue to try to be creative in finding resources and answers for all my clients, sometimes even reaching out to media figures to enlist help.

The internet has proven to be a great source of information. It can link families with support groups, such as the Cyclic Vomiting Syndrome Association (www.cvsaonline.org). Ned's mother has been open to the opportunity to speak with other parents at our hospital whose children are diagnosed with CVS. She has shared her experience and knowledge with other families who are just beginning their journey. Linking families to others in similar situations is often a helpful intervention when done sensitively.

Using outside resources is part of the bigger case management picture. Strengths-based case management combines a focus on client strengths and self-direction with three other principles: (1) promoting the use of informal helping networks, (2) offering assertive community involvement by case managers, and (3) emphasizing the relationship between client and case manager. Each principle supports the resource acquisition activities that characterize case management (Brun & Rapp, 2001). Others envision the case management role as promoting treatment adherence through the use of the case management relationship via service integration, cultural competence, individualized service, multi-systems interventions, and quality improvement (Vourlekis & Ell, 2007). The power of the relationship is key in helping the patient and family utilize care and resources most effectively. My use of self, along with the resource notebook and family-to-family support, are examples of informal helping networks that allow me to provide individualized service and multi-systems intervention aspects of case management. Maintaining the relationship with my patients' families is the central factor in being a positive and successful hospital social worker.

Sometimes with longer term complex patients, I help the family transition from pediatric services to adult care providers along with the Transition of Care team who are charged with this responsibility. This is a stressful time for families as they leave familiar health care providers and often have concerns about the way their now adult child will be able to manage health care provision more independently (Shanske, Arnold, Carvalho, & Rein, 2012). Good relationships now combine with a solid discharge plan to make managing these future transitions a bit easier. Ned's family has been working with the Transition of Care team to plan for this transition.

Reassessment and evaluation

When reviewing our objectives, it is rewarding to look back and see how far we came. When Ned was younger, it seemed he would never find stability and yet he is now a tall young man with a deep voice who has adjusted to his residential placement. Even so, before, our unofficial motto was "Two steps forward, one step back." Ned's frequent admissions allowed ample time for reassessment and evaluation. Through the process of looking back, I can see the way the second opinion was a catalyst that brought growth and change over time.

Transfer and termination

Prior to the request for a second opinion, I had considered asking my supervisor to reassign this case. I felt that I had become too close and comfortable with the situation and issues and was unable to see other options. I wondered if a new worker would see fresh options, and yet I was reluctant to leave this family I had worked with for so long and about whom I truly cared. The thought of switching them to a new worker weighed heavily on me.

Luckily for me, Ned's family decided to have him admitted to another hospital for a second opinion when he was 12. Ned's transfer was difficult for all involved. His mother had a lot of guilt about going somewhere else and said she felt like she was betraying all of the people who had taken such good care of her son. I was able to listen to her and give her what she needed – permission to do what she thought was best for her son and assurance that we would continue to be a support to her and her family even if he was not technically our patient. After the second opinion affirmed our treatment plan and we helped locate an appropriate residential placement, Ned began to receive his follow-up care with us again.

Ned's mother continues to stay in touch with me and his attending physician, and it has been rewarding to watch Ned become more stable and healthy over the years.

I did not realize how much I needed a respite from this case until Ned went for the second opinion. Looking back, I know that short break from Ned's care allowed his physician and me to renew ourselves and return to his care with more hope and validation.

Case conclusion

Ned is living in a very wonderful, supportive residential and educational setting, and his parents have guardianship of him. His medical condition stabilized during his adolescence and he seldom has lengthy hospitalizations. His mother keeps me up to date and we remain friendly, with professional boundaries in place.

Differential discussion

Being a hospital social worker can be an overwhelming job. There are moments of great joy and great sadness. Being present during intimate family times is a privilege but can become a burden. Occupational stress is real in the social work profession, especially in hospitals. In stressful hospital organizational cultures, social workers often experience high-volume and high-acuity caseloads, quick patient turnaround (leaving little time for intervention and planning), devaluation of social work within a medical model, and professional territory and responsibility disputes. We are also exposed to patients who have experienced traumatic events or illnesses, and we need to address our patients' pain and trauma as well as our own reactions and feelings. This can be difficult in a hospital environment that allows little time for processing these reactions and frequently precludes meeting personal needs because of the fast pace of the job (Gregorian, 2005; Pockett, 2003).

I believe these typical social work problems are exacerbated because my patients are children who have not had the opportunity to live a life of their choosing, only a life that their diagnosis allows. It is often harder for us, the treatment team, because we are aware of all that life has to offer and have something to compare it to; Ned's life revolved around vomiting and frequent admissions to the hospital. Feeling responsible for trying to bridge the space between a fulfilling childhood and a patient's condition is challenging, especially in situations like Ned's.

The majority of my caseload is high-volume and fast-paced, which presents a different stress than what I experienced in Ned's case. With Ned, there was a chronic, constant, pervasive stress, which even crept into my dreams. I did not always keep my boundaries firm and that only increased the level of my discomfort. Ned became very ill one summer and was admitted to the PICU (pediatric intensive care unit) where he was intubated and remained on a ventilator for almost two weeks. During this time, there were moments of crisis where Ned's future was uncertain and I provided his mother with my personal cell phone number in case something happened while I was not in the hospital. Luckily, Ned came through that episode but his mother did call my cell phone number on several occasions. It became an unnecessary stress I placed on myself and I felt obligated to answer her calls. I could not be upset with her for calling because I was the one who had crossed the boundary. I had good reasons for doing this: I wanted to be informed and support the family. Yet, it was also selfish of me to think that I was the only one who would be able to provide Ned and his family with what they needed when any of my colleagues would have done a fine job. I intend to avoid ever doing this again, but one cannot predict what the future holds.

My empathy for Ned's family came at the price of my own self-protection. Even though I am able to cognitively "put myself in another's shoes," it does not mean I should take that so literally. Feeling physically exhausted and emotionally drained can be side effects of social work. It is paramount to remember that the work is what you do and not who you are. It is okay, and necessary, to leave your patients at the hospital. Self-care has to be consistent and includes anything that recharges your physical, mental, and emotional batteries. Most social workers learn this lesson early in their careers. I guess that I was due for a refresher course. I am glad Ned returned and that I have been able to see his improvement. It has been my honor and privilege to know Ned and his family.

Even as I write this, I am asking myself whether I should maintain this level of involvement with Ned and his family. They are no longer on my unit, so what am I really offering? Do I want updates on his condition and discharge plan, or is it that I want to maintain contact with this family? These are interesting questions to ask and difficult ones to answer. I saw Ned and his family almost every day for 2½ years and it was easy to become too familiar and part of their family system. I experienced a loss when they left, albeit briefly. Yet, I learned to give more thought to the information I disclose to families and am more aware of the amount of time that I spend with any one patient. The line between professional and personal boundaries can be very thin at times. Ned and his family helped me learn to be conscious of this at all times.

Discussion questions

1   How might you work to reset a boundary that you have breached with the parents of a child who is seriously ill? How would you balance maintaining the rapport and relationship while defining the boundary?
2   When a child is seriously ill, how might you work with the sibling to bring their needs into focus for the family?
3   When a child has lived with chronic illness through childhood, what do you believe are some of the issues related to helping them to transition to adult health care providers?

References

Brun, C. & Rapp, R (2001). Strengths-based case management: Individuals' perspectives on strengths and the case manager relationship. *Social Work, 46*(3), 278–300.

Digney, J. (2013). Lightening the load? Humour and the therapeutic use of daily life events. *Relational Child & Youth Care Practice, 26*(2), 12–17.

Greenfield, E. A. (2011). Developmental systems theory as a conceptual anchor for generalist curriculum on human behavior and the social environment. *Social Work Education, 30*(5), 529–540. doi: 10.1080/02615479.2010.503237

Gregorian, C. (2005). A career in hospital social work: Do you have what it takes? *Social Work in Health Care, 40*(3), 1–14.

Kagle, J. (2008). *Social work records* (3rd edn.). Long Grove, IL: Waveland Press.

Knight, C. (2012). Social workers' attitudes towards and engagement in self-disclosure. *Clinical Social Work Journal, 40*(3), 297–306. doi: http://dx.doi.org/10.1007/s10615-012-0408-z

National Association of Social Workers (2005). *NASW standards for social work practice in health care settings*. Washington, DC: Author.

Pockett, R. (2003). Staying in hospital social work. *Social Work in Health Care, 36*(3), 1–24.

Reamer, F. (2003). *Social work malpractice and liability: Strategies for prevention* (2nd edn.). New York: Columbia University Press.

Reamer, F. (2005). Documentation in social work: Evolving ethical and risk-management standards. *Social Work, 50*(4), 325–334.

Reupert, A. (2007). Social worker's use of self. *Clinical Social Work Journal, 35(2),* 107–116.

Shanske, S., Arnold, J., Carvalho, M., & Rein, J. (2012). Social workers as transition brokers: Facilitating the transition from pediatric to adult medical care. *Social Work in Health Care, 51,* 279–295. doi: 10.1080/00981389.2011.638419

Shortell, S. M., Wu, F. M., Lewis, V. A., Colla, C. H., & Fisher, E. S. (2014). A taxonomy of accountable care organizations for policy and practice. *Health Services Research, 49*(6), 1883–1899. doi: 10.1111/1475-6773.12234

Shulman, L. (2006). *The skills of helping: Individuals, families and groups* (7th edn.). Belmont, CA: Brooks/Cole.

Teufel, I. J., Kazley, A. S., Andrews, A. L., Ebeling, M. D., & Basco, J. T. (2013). Health care in the digital age: Electronic Medical Record adoption in hospitals that care for children. *Academic Pediatrics, 13,* 259–263. doi: 10.1016/j.acap.2013.01.010

U.S. Department of Health and Human Services (2015). Health information privacy. Standards for privacy of individually identifiable health information. Retrieved from www.hhs.gov/ocr/privacy/

Vourlekis, B. & Ell, K. (2007). Best practice case management for improved medical adherence. *Social Work in Health Care, 44,* 161–177. doi: 10.1300/J010v44n03_03

Chapter 8

Assistive technology and developmental disability

Helping Gina find her voice

Bonnie Fader Wilkenfeld

Context

Description of setting

Our residential care facility (RCF) was founded in 1946 as a special school for children with cerebral palsy (CP) in response to a lack of appropriate educational facilities able to accommodate children with special needs. The effort was spearheaded by a private family who discovered there were no acceptable educational options for their child who was born with CP. The special school was the first step in what transformed into a commitment to provide comprehensive services to people with varied physical and developmental disabilities. Our residents' diagnoses include: CP, spina bifida, Lesch–Nyhan disease (LND), and a wide range of rare genetic disorders including Rett syndrome, Angelman syndrome, Cornelia De Lange syndrome, Wolf–Hirshorn syndrome, and 4Q deletion syndrome.

Initially, the programs offered within this special school focused on special education, physical and speech therapies, and recreation. As enrollment increased, staffing and the variety of service offered increased and the RCF became state certified. Currently, the RCF is a model comprehensive medical and educational center devoted to the delivery of state of the art services for individuals with developmental disabilities (IWDDs). We are home to 101 children and adults from across the nation and we provide the following services: outpatient health clinics; a modern, technologically sophisticated educational program; a facilitated arts program; and an adult day program serving individuals with complex medical conditions and developmental disabilities. Our RCF attracts participants nationwide.

Policy

The Americans with Disabilities Act (ADA) of 1990 guaranteed that people with disabilities were granted certain civil rights under the law; this law prohibits discrimination against individuals who have a physical or mental impairment. Discrimination against IWDDs involves denying them access to the public services, transportation, goods, and services that are offered to the general public. According to the ADA provisions, environmental accommodations (e.g., ramps, braille signs, elevators) must be made by public places to ensure that individuals with disability can access and utilize those areas in order for them to become fully integrated in those physical environments.

Developmental disability, a specific category of disability, has been defined as a chronic disability, which is attributable to a severe mental or physical impairment and manifests before the age of 22 years (Brown & Radford, 2007). This impairment is likely to continue indefinitely, and results in functional limitations in three or more major life activities such as: self-care, receptive/expressive language, learning, mobility, self-direction, capacity for independent living, and economic self-sufficiency (World Health Organization, 2001).

The Individuals with Disabilities Education Act 1990 (IDEA) established core curriculum content standards for all children with developmental disabilities regardless of their cognitive or physical capacities. This law states that all children with disabilities should be integrated into the public school system and have the opportunity to be exposed to the same curriculum content that children without disabilities are expected to master. The curriculum content is administered to children with disabilities in a manner tailored to meet their specific needs. Legislation for IDEA came about when it was discovered that many school systems lacked adequate physical and technical resources and staff to enable appropriate education for children with disabilities. Subsequently, the Developmental Disabilities Act (2000) stipulates that:

> Disability is a natural part of the human experience that does not diminish the right of individuals with developmental disabilities to enjoy the opportunity to live independently, enjoy self-determination, make choices, contribute to society, and experience full integration and inclusion in the economic, political, social, cultural, and educational mainstream of society. (P.L. 106–402, October 30, 2000)

The Social Model of Disability drives the enactment of the previously described legislation and places emphasis on modifications in the environment to afford IWDDs access to everyday society (Burkhardt, 2004; Race, Boxall, & Carson, 2005). Assistive technology (AT) and other accommodations may bridge gaps arising from the IWDD's functional limitations to allow easier involvement and integration (McNaughton & Bryen, 2007). Information technology, computerized voice output devices, and motorized wheelchairs provide opportunities for participation in many previously unforeseen arenas. They allow IWDDs to be mobile in their communities and to interact with others in ways that were previously impossible. While of unprecedented benefit in facilitating access and enhancement of quality of life for IWDDs, there are many issues that need to be identified and addressed for AT to be of maximum benefit for IWDDs.

Technology

Assistive technology

Assistive technology (AT), also referred to as assistive augmentative technology, consists of adaptations and devices that run the gamut from off-the-shelf, readily available devices such as car seats, strollers, baby spoons and, bowls, to those that are specifically adapted to meet the needs of a particular individual with disabilities (Campbell, Milbourne, Dugan, & Wilcox, 2006). These complex, technology-based items include: specialized switch devices, power wheelchairs, adapted speech augmentation devices, and computers. Specialized variations in these devices with ongoing technological developments create new options almost on a daily basis. When tailored to an IWDD's needs, AT may be the difference between more independent function and remaining dependent on caregivers.

AT has the potential to be of great benefit, but may also be misused. Unforeseen ethical issues can arise at many different levels which need to be anticipated and addressed.

For instance, when a technology is made available and then not repaired as needed, IWDD may experience more frustration than they had using earlier technologies. Hence, it is important to look at the pros and cons of any new tool that becomes available in our quest to help vulnerable populations achieve and progress. With the acceleration of technological developments, new devices and methodology become available at a rapid fire pace with implications for their usage that could not have been previously envisioned.

Organization

Today's RCF has a special hospital for children and adults with medically complex developmental disabilities, a special education school providing academics, and training in functional life skills for students ages 3–21. In addition, the RCF houses a comprehensive outpatient center meeting the health care needs of people from the surrounding community who have disabilities. The RCF also trains health care professionals, therapists, and educators in how to work effectively with people who have developmental disabilities. There are a variety of young interns within each area of therapeutic specialization and young volunteers who interact with the population regularly (particularly in after-hours recreation programs and on weekends).

The school is one of a constellation of services offered within the RCF. It provides a comprehensive educational program with instruction in all academic areas. The school serves students from preschool through grade 12 (ages 3–21) who have medically complex developmental disabilities. Teachers are fully certified in special education and highly qualified to teach the core curriculum content areas. Students' needs are met through truly individualized educational plans (IEPs), which focus on strengths and developing skills through best practices. Related student services include therapies, social work, psychology, and medical care. The RCF school is approved through the state department of education and is accredited by the Middle States Association of Colleges and Schools.

Decisions about practice

Description of the client

Gina is a cute, 16-year-old girl with big brown eyes and short brown hair, who has spastic quadriplegia associated with her primary diagnosis of CP. She is dependent on care assistants for all aspects of daily living. She is able to independently navigate her environment using a motorized wheelchair. She has the cognitive functioning/developmental level of a 3- to 5-year-old child. Gina has resided in the RCF since she was 8 years old. Her family lives several hours' drive away. Due to her specialized level of care, her parents placed her in the RCF despite the fact that they were limited in their ability to visit or take her home regularly. Most communication with them occurs over the phone. I assist Gina with phone calls to her parents during the week and the nursing staff help her with these phone calls on the weekends.

Many people who have spastic quadriplegic CP have associated expressive language difficulties due to their inability to coordinate oral motor muscles and breath control. Gina is able to verbally express herself but her verbalizations are very difficult to understand for people who are not familiar with her speech patterns. In addition, due to attachment issues related to her separation from family, she uses her expressive language difficulty to engage therapy interns and volunteers in long-drawn-out interpretative sessions in order to prolong social interactions with them.

She has an expensive computerized voice communication device, a "Dynavox," funded by Medicaid for use in school, in her personal life at the RCF, or with her family. Although Gina is at the cognitive developmental level of a 3-year-old, she ascribes to adolescent social norms. Gina is very cognizant of her disabilities and strives for normality. She does not like the artificial voice that comes out of the Dynavox and refuses to use it. She also enjoys the lengthy social interactions with staff who try to figure out what she is trying to verbally express.

Gina's family also wishes she could speak normally and they do not understand why the therapists are not working more on her oral motor coordination. As a result, when she is with her family, she is not encouraged to use the device. They believe that if Gina becomes proficient at using the Dynavox, it would hamper her ability to improve her expressive language skills. Gina may be able to pick up on her parents' negativity and this seems to reinforce her reluctance to use her Dynavox. Additionally, when she remains difficult to understand, she can continue to engage in long-drawn-out interpretation sessions with volunteers and interns. See Figure 8.1 for Gina's ecomap.

Goals

A first step in achieving an adaptive coping response is to define and facilitate realistic (achievable) goals with IWDDs (Augoustinos, Walker, & Donaghue, 2014). If goals are unrealistic and are unable to be achieved, people feel incompetent; they may experience negative emotional responses such as anger, depression, or anxiety. As part of the initial assessment process, the interdisciplinary team and the parents work together to develop goals. Parents are invited to complete a Parent Input Form that becomes incorporated into the social work assessment. Every year thereafter, goals are re-addressed with the team and family and updated to reflect whether the goal was achieved, if it is an ongoing "continuing goal," or if the goal should be discontinued. For children in the school program, this reassessment typically occurs during the annual school district meeting to reevaluate the child's IEP.

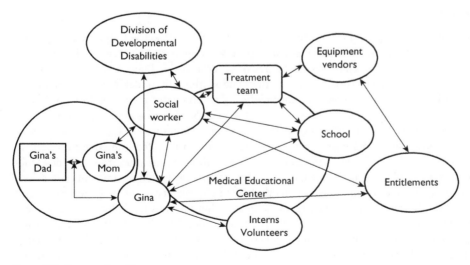

Figure 8.1 Ecomap for Gina

For Gina, family input was hampered by their inability to be physically present at the meetings and their lack of compliance in returning the Parent Input Form. In addition, Gina and her family were reluctant to express any feelings that were contrary to the recommendations of the treatment team. Her mother often said, "I trust the team and whatever they think is fine with me." She would sign off on the annual plan and the IEP that was developed in conjunction with Gina's school district without comment or dispute. When the proposal for Gina's training on the Dynavox voice communication system came up for discussion, all appeared to be in agreement.

Developing objectives and contracting

The family was not present at the initial meetings to discuss obtaining the equipment and training Gina how to use her communication device. This was an error on the part of the interdisciplinary team. Although she had tried a loaner device with her speech pathologist, Gina had never actually consented, nor was asked to consent, to its use. In addition, the adoption of the Dynavox was not presented to the family in the context of an interdisciplinary team meeting. Rather, the speech pathologist individually recommended to the family that Gina trial the device. Only when the team realized Gina was inconsistently using the equipment, or failing to use it at all, did the issue become a team discussion including the social worker and the family.

Meeting place

I met with Gina on a weekly basis in my private office. She arrived independently at our sessions via motorized wheelchair. I petitioned a private funding source to cover the purchase of a Star speaker phone system to enable students (and me) to communicate with their families. We would teleconference Gina's parents into our sessions by speaker phone.

Use of time

Over time, it became apparent that the device was not being effectively utilized. The team asked me to investigate the situation and intervene with Gina and her family. I spent time counseling Gina and her parents over the course of several weeks. I needed to spend substantial time with the parents in order to ensure they had sufficiently understood and integrated the information about the Dynavox. Additionally, I wanted them to feel free to identify and articulate their concerns. My priority was to meet the needs of Gina and her family. Even so, the treatment team was focused on their own perception of what was in Gina's best interest. Oftentimes, time constraints pressure professionals and families for immediate consent to new treatments. Yet families need the time to research, think about and formulate additional questions prior to a plan being enacted. Families are often intimidated by medical professionals and may acquiesce to care suggestions despite having reservations or concerns. Social workers must advocate with our care teams to ensure that families understand the treatment plan and have enough time to make an informed decision. Telephone communications are also problematic in that many important nonverbal communications are missed by not being able to attend to the person's body language and facial expressions. My contact with Gina's family was critical to our care of Gina.

Strategies and interventions

Despite the advantages of being able to communicate clearly with the voice communication device, Gina and her family were not convinced that the advantages outweighed their other needs/concerns. Gina refused to use the device and frequently broke or lost parts and this behavior seemed to be supported through implicit and explicit messages from her family. Clients and families are often reluctant to express their choices when they perceive that they are going against their treatment team's recommendations. IWDDs and their families may view themselves as lacking power and autonomy and feel compelled to accept the medical professionals' advice despite reservations they may hold.

It was incumbent upon my role as social worker to work with the family and Gina to uncover their unspoken concerns and fears. I used a variety of clinical techniques and, eventually, I was able to discover their core concerns. I met with Gina over the course of several weeks and used reflective discussion along with observation of behavioral cues and body language. In addition, I had established a history of trust and reasonable rapport with Gina and her family as I provided clinical and concrete interventions. I was able to create an environment for them where they felt free to express their concerns about Gina becoming dependent on the device and not ever becoming able to use her voice for communication.

Gina acknowledged her enjoyment in eliciting interactive conversations with unfamiliar staff as they worked to interpret her language. In addition, she admitted she was horrified by the artificial voice that emerged from the device. She felt alienated and excluded from social interactions when using the device. I engaged Gina in supportive counseling with a focus on developing other strategies for appropriate social interactions with peers and support staff. In addition, I enlisted ancillary team members to assuage the parents' concerns. Ultimately, the team agreed that focus would be placed on enhancing Gina's ability to verbally express herself rather than continue to move ahead with the AT device.

Stance of the social worker

The medical model situates families in a position lacking power and knowledge so they typically adhere to the recommendations of the medical team despite reservations they may hold regarding treatment options (Brashler, 2002). In addition, families and patients may not even be able to fully articulate their concerns. A crucial role for the social worker is to assist families to understand, identify, and articulate any issues that have not been fully fleshed out at the treatment team meetings.

As Gina's social worker, my directive is to facilitate client self-determination and to meet the client where he or she is. In this case, the "client" is both Gina and her family. Her family has tremendous influence on her decision-making. My social work role had profound impact as I helped create a communication bridge between Gina, her parents, and the interdisciplinary treatment team. Information needed to be broken down into basic language for the family and they needed appropriate time to digest and reflect on the various options the team identified.

A component of my work as the liaison between the interdisciplinary treatment team and the family was to serve as the family's advocate and represent their fears and concerns. In addition, I provided background information, insight into the family dynamics, and some problem-solving options for the team to consider. I educated the team about, and encouraged them to adopt the principles espoused by a person-centered planning perspective (or in this case: a family-centered perspective) (O'Brien & O'Brien, 2000). This perspective acts in concert with the principles of the Social Model of Disability to transfer power back to the IWDD and their family; they must decide which care options they prefer. As a result, we change the focus to what the person perceives as important to him/herself rather than focus solely on the preferences of the interdisciplinary treatment team.

Reassessment and evaluation

Gina's and her family's needs and concerns were not satisfactorily addressed earlier by the treatment team. If one is to obtain optimal outcomes and compliance, the client and family must be included in the decision-making process about AT (Schlosser, Sigafoos, Rothschild, Burke, & Palace, 2009). While the team obviously saw the benefits of using the device, Gina and her family had other objectives that were not being addressed. Once they felt safe enough to articulate their concerns and desires to the treatment team, the goals and objectives were modified to include their input and the Dynavox was withdrawn from the plan.

Ultimately, in this case there was a failure on the part of the interdisciplinary team to listen adequately to the family and client in the development of the treatment plan including the use of AT. A lot of valuable therapeutic time and resources were lost that could have been directed towards achieving more mutually accepted goals. Families need to be actively involved in the decision-making process for their children from the beginning (Parette & Brotherson, 2004). A family-centered approach may involve a systematic process comprising: (1) information gathering from the client's and family's perspectives, (2) matching the AT decision-making process with the family's cultural background(s), and (3) aligning specific characteristics of the child within the environments they navigate to the features of the device (Judge & Parette, 1998; Parette & Brotherson, 2004).

Transfer and termination

I followed Gina throughout her school years into the extended high school 12+++ program. Children with developmental disabilities are entitled to special education through age 21. Upon graduation, Gina transitioned into the RCF's adult day program and I transferred her to a social worker who works with adults in the RCF. Gina had an opportunity to meet jointly with her new worker and me over the course of several weeks to outline what we have been working on and her goals for the future in the Adult Services Program. These meetings took place months prior to her graduation. Her parents were included in the meetings when they were available by phone or in person. As Gina identified with her newly emerging adult status she was eager to move on and was motivated to transition to the new worker and the new program.

Case conclusion

Gina continued to eschew the use of AT until the advent of the iPad and the discovery of software that could be installed on the device and used effectively as a communication device. She perceived the iPad as "cool" and "hip" and so the stigma attached to using an artificial communication device diminished. Interestingly enough, despite her family's continued resistance to having her use the technology, Gina appeared to be "rebelling" and used the technology despite her family's reluctance. Although IWDDs may be functionally/cognitively delayed developmentally, they may still ascribe to age-appropriate developmental crises and norms, such as the rebellion Gina exhibited in true adolescent fashion. She was at a point where she was ready to assert her own wishes despite, or maybe even because of, her family's opposition.

Differential discussion

There were specific communication lapses on the part of the interdisciplinary team when considering Gina for an augmentative communication device. Honoring the client's self-determination in using AT is an important element in any treatment plan and the client/ guardians should be included in planning discussions. Excluding the client and family from team meetings and not paying attention to nonverbal communication such as behaviors and noncompliance with the device led to great frustration. My role as a communication bridge between Gina, her family, and the care team was crucial in interpreting the family's unspoken fears and concerns regarding the use of the device and relaying this information to the team.

A careful balance must be maintained in using AT, which can be viewed by IWDDs as both a help and a hindrance. For example, a voice communicator device can be an advantage in facilitating communication, but may also be perceived as ostracizing and alienating. Some devices have artificial voices which sound tinny, childlike, or robotic. Many young adults and adolescents dislike the sound of these devices and prefer not to use them. Some individuals prefer to use communication boards, switches, sign language, or their own vocalizations which may be difficult for others to understand, even when familiar others understand them. IWDDs' self-determination is a crucial element in determining whether an AT is the right option for an individual (Cook, 2009; van der Meer, Sigafoos, O'Reilly, & Lancioni, 2011). In addition, family, caregivers, and staff "buy-in" becomes a huge component in determining whether the individual is motivated, supported, or dissuaded from using the device (Hammel, 2003) as illustrated in Gina's case.

There are also ethical problems when AT devices require maintenance but insurance no longer covers the device. If the AT device is not upgraded regularly, or repaired when damaged, then it can be unsafe and of no use for the individual. In addition, failure to pay careful attention to maintenance issues can exacerbate social undesirability rather than increase their ability to engage in social interactions (Cook, 2009). For example, improper positioning in a wheelchair can impact an IWDD's posture, exacerbate drooling, impact their respiration (breathing), and hamper their ability to self-propel and negotiate environments effectively, safely, and independently. Each AT has benefits and drawbacks, and IWDDs and their supporters are continually required to assess the balance among them (Dorsten, Sifford, Bharucha, Mecca, & Wactlar, 2009). Guidelines need to be utilized in approaching the ethical concerns of utilizing AT. Typically, many agencies apply the following four ethical principles:

- Non-maleficence means "do no harm." We must ask whether we are doing the individual more harm than good. Could that piece of equipment lead to confusion and distress that overrides the advantages of its use?
- Beneficence: Is this AT of benefit to the person? For example, does it assist with the ability of the person to communicate needs?
- Autonomy means that each person has rights to self-determination, privacy, freedom, and choice. How does the AT enhance these rights?
- Justice refers to treating everyone fairly and respecting their rights. Are all individuals provided with equal access to technology available?

Ethical issues

In addition to the above principles, research suggests a scarcity of information about appropriate teaching practices for proper usage and orientation to AT devices (Campbell, Milbourne, Dugan, & Wilcox, 2006). This situation may have potential ethical implications as well as impacting successful engagement, performance, and improvement of individuals and families utilizing the technologies. Some specific ethical concerns surrounding the use of AT might include the following:

- Types that monitor individuals for safety purposes might also impinge on privacy rights. For example, video cameras for distance learning need to be carefully monitored to preserve an individual's privacy and dignity. While of great potential benefit for those who are bedridden and unable to attend classes or programs, caregivers need to be aware of the person's need for protection from exposure during intimate care activities. The IWDD's privacy must always be preserved. Covering the camera may also be necessary.
- AT might cut back on services and reduce human contact. This is a common concern among users of technology in general but also for IWDD in particular. Interpersonal interactions can be beneficial in and of themselves, especially if the IWDD tends to be isolated. While computer use and distance learning can certainly serve to meet gaps, use of these technologies should not completely substitute for the benefits that come from social and group class experiences.
- Concerns regarding AT supplanting the individual's ability to do an activity independently without the aid of such a device and fears that AT use may exacerbate problems in the long run. The cost/benefit ratio must be analyzed through the lens of "non-maleficence." At what cost do the benefits of utilizing the technology enhance quality of life parameters for the individual? Again, this problem requires a very individualized analysis of the particulars in the situation.
- Obtaining full consent of the family and assent of IWDD to utilize such devices. Not only does the treatment team need the family's approval and permission, but also the IWDD's (for those who are unable to consent on their own) assent. The IWDD needs to "buy into" the process. If this is not the case, the client can sabotage the efforts to effectively learn and utilize the equipment which can certainly waste time, resources, and energies of those involved, as depicted in the case of Gina and her Dynavox.
- Issues surrounding the maintenance and/or withdrawal of technology. This last issue has significant implications with regards to individuals and patients' human rights issues. Once an IWDD has the ability to independently navigate his or her environment (as an example), what are the ramifications of withdrawing or disengaging the equipment? Our facility views this as a human rights violation. Hence the ethical dilemma is posited: what happens if funds are withdrawn and an outdated or broken device cannot be replaced?

In summary, the flow of communications between Gina, her family, me (as their social worker), and the treatment team was flawed. While I had developed a rapport with the family, I was unaware that the treatment plan developed by the therapy team was to move ahead with providing a Dynavox for Gina. Maintaining regular communication with the team may help avoid this occurrence. In addition, this case underscores the importance of including all members of the treatment team, including the patient and family, in the initial planning and implementation of AT devices.

Discussion questions

1   How might you work with a family that is rejecting technologies that have the potential to ease their child's lives? How does your approach differ if the child him- or herself is not interested in the technology that medical staff believe is necessary?
2   What do you believe about the duty of governments/societies to provide expensive technologies to individuals with disabilities?
3   What new "cool" technologies might be leveraged to help IWDDs have more integration into typical communities?

References

Augoustinos, M., Walker, I., & Donaghue, N. (2014). *Social cognition: An integrated introduction*. Thousand Oaks, CA: Sage.

Brashler, R. (2002). Social work practice and disability issues. In S. Gehlert & T. Browne (Eds.), *Handbook of health social work* (pp. 219–236). Hoboken, NJ: John Wiley & Sons.

Brown, J. & Radford, J. (2007). Historical overview of intellectual and developmental disabilities. In I. Brown & M. Percy (Eds.), *A comprehensive guide to intellectual and developmental disabilities* (pp. 17–34). Baltimore, MD: Paul H. Brooks Publishing Co.

Burkhardt, T. (2004). Capabilities and disability: The capabilities framework and the social model of disability. *Disability & Society, 19*(7), 735–751. doi: 10.1080/0968759042000284213

Campbell, P., Milbourne, S., Dugan, L., & Wilcox, M. (2006). A review of the evidence on practices for teaching young children to use assistive technology devices. *Topics in Early Childhood Special Education, 26*(1), 3–13. doi: 10.1177/02711214060260010101

Cook, A. M. (2009). Ethical issues related to the use/non-use of assistive technologies. *Developmental Disabilities Bulletin, 37*(1, 2), 127–152.

Dorsten, A., Sifford, K. S., Bharucha, A., Mecca, L. P., & Wactlar, H. (2009). Ethical perspectives on emerging assistive technologies: Insights from focus groups with stakeholders in long-term care facilities. *Journal of Empirical Research on Human Research Ethics*, 25–36. doi: 10.1525/jer.2009.4.1.25

Hammel, J. (2003). Technology and the environment: supportive resource or barrier for people with developmental disabilities? *Nursing Clinics of North America, 38*(2), 331–349. doi: 10.1016/S0029-6465(02)00053-1

Judge, S. & Parette, H. (1998). Family centered assistive technology decision making. *Infant-Toddler Intervention, 8*(2), 185–206.

McNaughton, D. & Bryen, D. N. (2007). AAC technologies to enhance participation and access to meaningful societal roles for adolescents and adults with developmental disabilities who require AAC. *Augmentative and Alternative Communication, 23*(3), 217–229. doi: 10.1080/07434610701573856

O'Brien, C. L. & O'Brien, J. (2000). The origins of person-centered planning: A community of practice perspective. In S. Holburn & P. Vietze (Eds.), *Person-centered planning: research, practice, and future directions*. Baltimore, MD: Paul H. Brookes.

Parette, H. & Brotherson, M. (2004). Family centered and culturally responsive assistive technology decision making. *Infants and Young Children, 17*(4), 355–367.

Race, D., Boxall, K., & Carson, I. (2005). Towards a dialogue for practice: Reconciling social role valorization and the social model of disability. *Disability and Society, 20*(5), 507–521. doi: 10.1080/09687590500156196

Schlosser, R., Sigafoos, J., Rothschild, N., Burke, M., & Palace, L, (2009). Speech and language disorders. In I. Brown & M. Percy (Eds.), *A comprehensive guide to intellectual and developmental disabilities* (pp. 383–402). Baltimore, MD: Paul H. Brooks Publishing Co.

van der Meer, L., Sigafoos, J., O'Reilly, M. F., & Lancioni, G. E. (2011). Assessing preferences for AAC options in communication interventions for individuals with developmental disabilities: A review of the literature. *Research in Developmental Disabilities, 32,* 1422–1431. doi: 10.1016/j. ridd.2011.02.003

World Health Organization (2001). *International classification of functioning, disability and health.* Geneva, Switzerland: Author.

Chapter 9

Genetic testing following a pediatric cancer diagnosis

A role for direct practice social workers in helping families with Li–Fraumeni syndrome

Allison Werner-Lin and Shana L. Merrill

Context

Li–Fraumeni syndrome (LFS) is a rare autosomal dominant cancer syndrome characterized by multiple, early, and aggressive cancers. LFS is caused by germline mutations, either inherited or *de novo* (new to the bloodline), in the *TP53* gene. Nicknamed "guardian of the genome," *TP53* regulates cell division, repair, and apoptosis (cell death), and maintains the integrity and functionality of human DNA. A mutation to the *TP53* gene disables essential functions that protect cells from environmental exposures, leaving them susceptible to uncontrolled cell growth and, consequently, tumors. Approximately 50% of *TP53* mutation carriers will develop cancer by age 30, and lifetime risk reaches 70% in men and nearly 100% for women (McBride et al., 2014). Core cancers commonly diagnosed in individuals with LFS include: osteosarcoma (bone cancer), soft tissue sarcoma, breast cancer, brain cancer, and pediatric adrenal cortical carcinoma (Gonzalez et al., 2009). Increased risk of melanoma and acute leukemia, as well as cancers of the stomach, kidney, colon, pancreas, esophagus, lung, and embryonic tumors also characterize LFS. "Since its description by Li and Fraumeni over 40 years ago, Li–Fraumeni syndrome (LFS) remains one of the most striking familial cancer predisposition syndromes" (Kamihara, Rana, & Garber, 2014, p. 654).

LFS is distinguished from other more commonly recognized hereditary cancer syndromes, such as hereditary breast and ovarian cancer, by the high risk of developing tumors in childhood, the lack of a clear management strategy (Mai et al., 2012), the rarity and lack of visibility of families with LFS, and the significantly increased risk for a shortened lifespan even with aggressive preventative measures. Typically, LFS patients are short-lived and have a history of multiple cancer diagnoses and treatments. Each biological child of a mutation carrier has a 50% risk to inherit the syndrome, and children of individuals with LFS are often known to have a markedly increased risk for cancer shortly after birth.

Due to the broad range of potential cancer sites and the belief of little long-term survival benefit, historically, screening was limited to the breast for adult women (Lammens et al., 2010). Now, LFS management is more proactive (Kamihara et al., 2014). Screening is offered "from birth to grave." Protocols recommend 3–4 month screenings for children with LFS with either bloodwork or imaging (Villani et al., 2011). Thus, children with LFS experience numerous doctor's visits with frequent blood tests and more intrusive medical care than most individuals have in a lifetime. See Table 9.1 for suggested surveillance strategies for individuals with Li–Fraumeni.

Until recently, testing for *TP53* mutations in minors was discouraged unless a child was symptomatic and testing results could be utilized to make treatment-related decisions. Today,

Table 9.1 Suggested surveillance strategy for individuals with germline TP53 mutations

	Pediatric surveillance recommendations	Adult surveillance recommendations
Adrenocortical carcinoma	• Every 3–4 months: • Ultrasound of abdomen and pelvis • Complete urinalysis • Bloodwork	
Breast cancer		• Monthly breast self exam, starting age 18 years • Clinical breast exam every 6 months starting at age 20–25 years, or 5–10 years before the earliest known breast cancer in the family • Alternate mammogram and breast MRI every 6 months starting at age 20–25 years, or individualized based on earliest age of onset in family • Consider risk-reducing mastectomy
Brain tumor	• Annual brain MRI • Annual rapid total body MRI	• Annual brain MRI • Annual rapid total body MRI
Soft tissue and bone sarcoma		
Leukemia/lymphoma	• Bloodwork every 3–4 months	• Bloodwork every 3–4 months
Intra-abdominal tumor (e.g., sarcoma)		• Annual abdominal ultrasound
Colon cancer		• Colonoscopy every 6 months beginning at age 40 years, or 10 years before the earliest known colon cancer in the family
Melanoma		• Annual dermatology examination
All other cancers:	• Regular evaluation with family physician with close attention to any medical concerns or complaints • Organ targeted surveillance based on pattern of cancer observed in family	

Source: NCCN (2012); Villani et al. (2011).

pediatric genetic testing for LFS is initiated if an immediate family member is known to carry the *TP53* mutation in order to establish risk estimates, to plan surveillance, to enable early detection, to (eventually) inform family planning, and/or to provide relief from anxiety regarding cancer risk (if results are normal) (Alderfer et al., 2015).

Psychosocial overview

Although identification of a *TP53* mutation can increase a family's sense of control over their future (Peterson et al., 2008), a positive test result might trigger a variety of distress reactions among family members (Lammens et al., 2011). Decisions regarding testing, cancer risk management, and family communication around illness and loss impose great psychosocial burdens on families who are often grieving the loss of a close relative to cancer, coping with medical anxiety, and supporting family members who are undergoing similar struggles at the same time. Families may decline testing due to concern about the potential for unbearable anxiety in parents, fear of being a burden on children, a general disinterest in aggressive preventative medical care, concerns about discrimination, or effects on marriage and reproductive decisions. Adolescent and young adult (AYA) views regarding genetic testing and preventative medical care may diverge from their parents; often AYA patients experience extreme familial pressure to act according to their parents' wishes regarding testing and management decisions.

Policy

Private payer insurance and health care reform

In most circumstances, regular preventative screening is covered by U.S. insurers for children and adults with LFS. Due to the frequency and extensive nature of scans, as well as the fact that patients are often asymptomatic at the time of screening, expertise working with insurance companies may be required to secure coverage. High co-pays or deductibles may deplete family resources, particularly in families who have many members requiring annual screening. Fewer than 10 institutions in the United States currently offer rapid full-body MRI, often only under research protocols. Therefore, families in rural or underserved areas with limited resources may need to travel regularly to the National Institutes of Health or large academic research centers to participate in funded protocols associated with research studies on families with LFS.

Genetic Information Nondiscrimination Act

The Genetic Information Nondiscrimination Act (GINA), federal legislature passed in 2008, protects individuals from health insurance or employment discrimination based on genetic information (www.eeoc.gov/laws/statutes/gina.cfm). The protections of GINA are relevant to individuals with family histories of cancer because they allow healthy individuals to pursue genetic testing and engage in surveillance without concerns about discrimination. GINA does not extend to life insurance, short-term disability, or long-term care coverage (see Chapter 13 for more on GINA), nor does it apply to women and men in the military who, due to the recommendations for sophisticated screening, are usually restricted from active duty.

Technology

Detecting genetic mutations

Most individuals undergoing *TP53* testing have had counseling about LFS, yet the population of patients diagnosed with LFS has expanded to individuals who may not have a personal or known family history of cancer. This is largely due to the use of multi-gene panels and whole-exome sequencing, representing a genotype-first approach to risk assessment (Merrill & Guthrie, 2015), in addition to direct to consumer testing. In these cases, individuals and families may not understand the implications of the abnormal *TP53* result. Once a family's specific mutation is identified, those at risk to inherit the mutation can be tested for that specific genetic change to determine whether or not they also have an increased risk for cancer.

Increased detection of LFS also comes from genetic testing of pediatric tumor samples (somatic testing), which have the potential to suggest (although cannot confirm) that a patient has a germline *TP53* mutation. With aggressive screening protocols in place for children with LFS syndrome, the vast majority of experts currently support early testing to determine appropriate medical management strategies. Although most families pursue genetic testing for minors at risk for LFS (Alderfer et al., 2015), parents may exercise their right to decline such testing.

Prevention and medical management

Historically, LFS-involved families were counseled to have children avoid unnecessary radiation exposures or other carcinogens, encouraged to have a low threshold for seeking evaluation for medical complaints, and given general cancer prevention advice. Research on LFS is very limited because LFS is rare and family members are often quite sick or deceased, reducing subjects available for research. Anecdotally, providers and families often equate the capacity to test for a *TP53* mutation, and developments in screening, with the potential for reducing the risk of early and recurrent cancers, and early mortality. Yet, despite a shift towards more aggressive treatment (Langan et al., 2013), reduced mortality subsequent to screening is not yet proven. Available data suggests knowledge of a *TP53* mutation may lead families to believe disease can be managed with early detection (Lammens et al., 2010), yet this misconception may create a false sense of hope for cancer avoidance or long-term survival. Further, questions about the benefit of screening are raised by children's experiences of pain and treatment complications.

"Scanxiety" and surveillance fatigue

Knowledge of significantly increased risk for cancer can lead patients to avoid the use of tobacco products, maintain a healthy diet, and increase physical fitness. Still, frequent and comprehensive screening evaluations often provoke anxiety, or "scanxiety" (Feiler, 2011). Such worry is particularly salient for pediatric patients who may have limited understanding of the goals behind evaluations and for individuals with a history of cancer in themselves or a close family member. Patients (or the parents of young children) who feel they are "living scan to scan" may struggle to balance motivation for screening with distress about cancer risk.

Reprogenetic technologies

The early incidence of cancer in individuals with LFS affects the reproductive choices of young adults. Like other hereditary cancer conditions (Werner-Lin et al., 2012), families with LFS wish to avoid passing the mutation to biological children. Emerging reproductive technologies enable prospective parents to give birth to a child free of a familial condition using pre-implantation genetic diagnosis after *in vitro* fertilization. *In vitro* fertilization is invasive, can be emotionally taxing, expensive, and has no guarantee of a successful pregnancy. Nevertheless, some families are not informed about such options, either due to lack of provider knowledge or to providers' opinions regarding their appropriate use; in these cases couples may only learn of these options after they have completed their family, leading to resentment. However, these options may provoke ethical or social conflict among family members or those with religious or cultural beliefs regarding intervention in reproduction.

Genetic amniocentesis at approximately 18–20 weeks of pregnancy and chorionic villus sampling at approximately 11–13 weeks of pregnancy are other options for prenatal genetic diagnosis of pregnancies with *TP53* mutations. Institutions vary in willingness to perform prenatal testing for LFS (or terminate a pregnancy for LFS in the second or third trimester). Additionally, prospective parents may elect to use donor gametes (eggs or sperm) to avoid passing on the genetic material of an affected parent. Some individuals diagnosed with cancer and facing chemotherapy treatment regimens will freeze eggs or bank sperm to increase the length of their child-bearing years and/or to enable the use of a surrogate.

Organization

Community providers may care for families with LFS, especially in geographic areas with limited access to genetic services. Most care teams housed at major academic facilities include primary care, a variety of relevant sub-specialty physicians, genetic counselors, and psychosocial support staff. Having access to pediatric and adult hospital-based care is ideal for avoiding fragmentation of care. Such an arrangement is particularly useful as adolescents transition from resource-rich pediatric settings to adult-oriented centers.

Though social workers employed within our cancer center are available for consultation as needed for families affected by LFS (those with and without cancer or genetic diagnosis), the scope of their services is limited by the hospital setting. Typically, our oncology-based social workers provide services at the time of cancer diagnosis or when called upon to navigate care issues or crises; however, their services are time-limited and rarely ongoing. As a result, hospital social workers are often unable to provide long-term counseling and instead refer to private practitioners. Families with LFS may appear to providers, on cursory assessment, to handle cancer diagnoses better than other patients who have limited experience with cancer and cancer treatments. Therefore, they may be overlooked for referrals to social work services as they typically "know how to hold it together about cancer" on the surface.

Private or community-based social workers are able to provide ongoing services to families affected by cancer or chronic bereavement. The international Cancer Wellness community provides a host of services at no cost to individuals and families (https://cancerwellness.org/). Yet, these systems of support are often unprepared to address the psychosocial concerns of families with hereditary cancer syndromes such as LFS. Social workers in private practice, although costly, may be well positioned to support families to make sound medical decisions, cope with complicated grief, and balance ongoing cancer risk with the normative tasks of child and family development.

Typical clients and situations

Every person in the LFS family system is a significant stakeholder; some are connected through shared lineage/DNA, others through present, past, or anticipated caregiving, and all are linked together by anticipatory grief and loss. Family life is often characterized by concurrent diagnoses across the family system, and often across generations, as well as by cancer-related death. Parent loss during childhood is not uncommon. Families often struggle to balance normative development of well family members with hypervigilance about physical symptomology and medicalization during childhood and adolescence. Social work practice with LFS families may focus on coping and ongoing adjustment to grief and illness, support in medical decision-making, balancing family dynamics between normative development and the demands of the condition, and advocating for services and insurance coverage.

Decisions about practice

The number of experts who provide care to families with LFS is limited. As a result, providers typically care for all individuals within an entire family system, regardless of closeness of relationship and communication among family members. This requires providers to establish individual relationships with each family member, balancing a bird's eye view of the family's medical and psychosocial history with individual risk estimates and illness narratives. Providers must balance knowledge of a family member's genetic testing or cancer screening results, as well as prognostic or treatment information that might directly impact the care of a relative. Often, the intimacy of patient/provider relationships leads patients to disclose deceptions or secrets about family members regarding testing status, results, or even questions of paternity. Providers also share the burden of grief alongside families.

The clinical care team may identify a need for family members to seek private consultation with social workers, particularly in an environment that facilitates attention to the evolving needs of individual clients. The following case study exemplifies common scenarios as they apply to social work practice for families with LFS. In this case, the social worker at the hospital (SM) referred Jack to a social worker in private practice (AWL) in order to meet his individual and developmental needs and to permit a holistic approach to the stress generated by hereditary conditions in families.

Definition of the client

Jack was diagnosed at age 3 with an early-stage adrenal cortical carcinoma and successfully treated with surgical excision and close monitoring. He has very limited personal memory of that experience, with the exception of watching the model trains in the lobby of the children's hospital. At the age of 12, Jack was diagnosed and treated for spinal ependymoma, a rare tumor of the central nervous system. Jack completed surgery with subsequent radiation and a six-month course of chemotherapy. Despite a favorable prognosis, Jack's mother

Molly maintained a fatalistic view of his chances of survival. Jack completed an invasive and painful course of treatment, yet he remained thoroughly optimistic. Now at age 20, Jack has keen insight into the impact of his diagnosis and treatment of his spinal tumor on his identify formation, his relationship with his somewhat chaotic blended family, and his future career goals.

Jack's father, Leonard, was diagnosed with glioblastoma (brain tumor) at the age of 42 when Jack was 8 years old. Two decades prior, he had a sarcoma (bone cancer) in his leg that was caught early and resected without any additional treatment required. Leonard died 18 months after his diagnosis, just as Jack transitioned from elementary to middle school. During these 18 months, Leonard had aggressive radiation and chemotherapy treatment that left him physically scarred and exhausted. Metastases to the bones in his spine made him unable to walk due to intense and poorly managed pain. Leonard entered home hospice in the week before his death. By then, he was incontinent and unable to communicate. Jack's family had a positive experience with the local community-based psychosocial support organization for families affected by cancer and participated briefly in their bereavement program until the start of school in September drew the family's attention elsewhere.

Jack is regularly followed in the pediatric cancer survivorship clinic. His survivorship team is presently preparing to transition his care to adult oncology. In preparation for this change, Jack's pediatric oncologist referred him to medical genetics at the University Hospital for evaluation. Jack made an appointment with an experienced cancer geneticist and genetic counselor (SM). Jack attended the genetics appointment with Molly, who remains very active in his medical care. SM advised him to "consider formally looking into why he and his father had early tumors."

Jack has a sophisticated grasp of his medical history and a clear understanding of how to navigate medical systems. As a third-year pre-med student, he also has a good command of genetic processes and technologies. He told SM that he often wondered about whether his family had an hereditary cancer syndrome and whether he had a responsibility to his siblings and potential future children to discuss genetic testing. Molly has less familiarity and more skepticism with genetics; this created the need for simultaneous communication on different levels for mother and son regarding the diagnostic process, meaning and implications of results, reasons, risks, and benefits of testing.

Molly told SM about other siblings in Jack's paternal line, including his older half sister Amy, diagnosed with melanoma at age 16 years and with kidney cancer at age 22 years, his older half brother Mark, and his younger full brother Kevin. Although Molly felt general disdain towards Amy's mother, Leonard's first wife, she felt an obligation to foster continued bonds to Leonard's side of the family after his death. SM told the pair that Amy's diagnoses could be related to the genetic trait shared with their father, and, should a trait be identified, it could impact everyone in the family, including Amy's 4-year-old daughter Gillian and her son Avery. The cancer geneticist and SM suspected a *TP53* mutation, which was confirmed through gene-specific testing. SM suggested that Amy consider pursuing testing for the known familial *TP53* mutation.

Amy tested positive for the *TP53* mutation and immediately transferred her care from a regional hospital to University Hospital to enroll in a regular course of screening, and have her first rapid full-body MRI. At the time of her visit in genetics, Amy told SM that her 4-year-old daughter, Gillian, had recently started experiencing headaches and "sometimes goes cross-eyed." After urgent evaluation, Gillian was diagnosed with a brain tumor and underwent surgery. The surgery was successful and Gillian emerged with a moderate prognosis for long-term survival.

Amy's MRI results, which were positive for a substantial lesion in her chest, suspicious for metastatic cancer, came on the same day as her daughter Gillian's surgery. The family was aware the MRI results would be available and they requested them that day, despite the physician's hesitation. Amy and her husband, Oren, left messages with SM arguing that their medical experiences made them uniquely competent to receive their results at any time. The team met with the family over Gillian's post-surgical hospital bed to share the news that Amy had abnormal MRI results likely indicative of metastatic cancer that would require further evaluation. Oren felt he could not manage the imminent deaths of both his wife and his daughter. Amy reassured him they would both be fine, and she promised to pursue treatment as soon as her daughter recovered from surgery.

Gillian's headaches and vision trouble resolved following her initial surgery, yet she underwent a subsequent chemotherapy for an aggressive local recurrence of her tumor. She is closely monitored with imaging and not undergoing any treatment. Amy was subsequently diagnosed with metastatic thyroid cancer, requiring surgery and potentially additional therapies. Mark and Kevin remain cancer-free; both have a 50% chance of carrying the *TP53* mutation and both have declined genetic testing. Despite Kevin's rejection of genetic testing, Molly continues to contact SM about making appointments for Kevin. Amy initially wanted more children, but after consulting a reproductive endocrinologist, she and Oren decided against another pregnancy.

Use of time

Two weeks per month, Jack meets with a private practice social worker (AWL) with expertise in family therapy and familial disease. They use the time to discuss mourning Jack's father, as well as to process his ongoing relationships with Molly and Amy. Jack addresses his concerns about transitioning to adult oncology. Jack hopes his niece will be able to make the same transition one day, but he experiences pre-emptive survivor guilt that he has already lived much longer than she might. Molly refuses to visit the social worker on her own, yet she came in twice, at Jack's request, so Jack could learn more about Leonard's disease and death. Together, the two are working to rebalance the mother–son relationship to address Jack's wish for greater autonomy in his care. Jack suggested that Amy and her husband make an appointment with the same social worker to discuss changes in family structure, their fears about their daughter's cancer and recurrence, and Oren's fears about "being surrounded by cancer." To date, they scheduled and cancelled three separate meetings. See Figure 9.1 for Jack's genogram.

Strategies and interventions

The social worker who facilitates Jack's survivorship group uses supportive–expressive group psychotherapy. The group's aims are to provide a safe space to discuss cancer and survivorship as shared experiences, to normalize the trauma and growth that a pediatric cancer diagnosis predicates, and to share strategies for coping with survivorship concerns in a world with limited understanding of their struggles. On rare occasions, the group facilitator invites attendees to share meaningful music, create art, or to learn meditation through guided imagery.

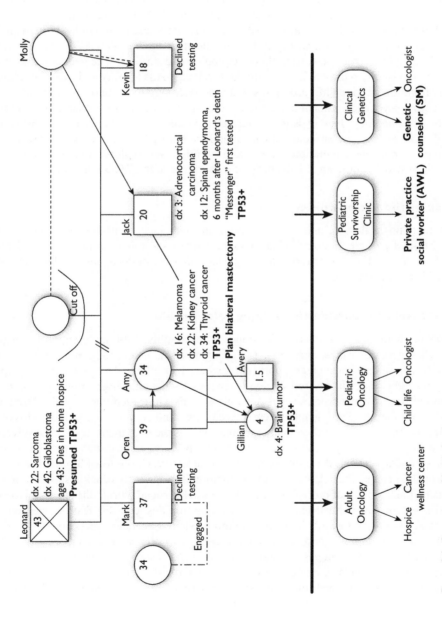

Figure 9.1 Genogram of Jack's family

AWL (the private practice social worker) operates from a narrative perspective, critical to work with hereditary cancer syndromes where generations of family members are affected, and technologies have substantially changed disease course, intervention strategies, and pathways towards the end of life (Werner-Lin & Gardner, 2009). Together, we (AWL and Jack) explore Jack's understanding of his family's history with cancer and death, the ways his diagnosis and survivorship fit into his family's story, and the places his plot diverges from that of his father and sister, in particular. We work to contextualize Jack's family dynamics in the family's shared history, to situate Jack within this context, and to see himself and his family as entities defined by processes greater than cancer and genetics. Finally, the narrative approach helps Jack connect to his deceased father beyond their shared genes.

Jack was familiar with his family's pedigree, a visual representation of his biological family to track cancer diagnoses, susceptibility, and death. Together with AWL, he constructed a genogram, shifting the focus from illness to coping and survival. The genogram gave Jack flexibility to visually represent those individuals critical to his identity and care, including his friends from the survivorship group, his pediatric oncology team, and his pre-med friends. AWL uses a psychoeducational approach to address Jack's concerns about transitioning his care to adult oncology. Jack feels guilt over his lingering desire to become a parent; he fears he will experience a new or recurrent cancer and die during his child's youth, or worse, that he will pass on the gene mutation to the next generation. We explored a variety of reproductive options which would enable the birth of a child free of the *TP53* mutation.

Stance of the social worker

AWL maintains a flexible and casual relationship with Jack. Together, we decide how to invite Molly's participation and what to address when she joins sessions. AWL identifies the soft limits of Molly's comfort zone and pushes on these limits to address Jack's need for family history information.

Use of resources outside the helping relationship

Alternating with such sessions, Jack attends a bi-monthly, 90-minute support group for young adult pediatric cancer survivors. The group meets in the evenings and is located at the community-based psychosocial support center where Jack attended a bereavement group following his father's death. At each session, attendees discuss challenges of integrating cancer into normative life cycle tasks, such as scheduling scans while attending school far from their primary care facility. Participants discuss "scanxiety" and surveillance fatigue (Hoskins & Greene, 2012) associated with regular screening. Jack is the only member of the survivorship group with an identified gene mutation, but the group shares concern about the risk of recurrent or secondary cancer. AWL also encouraged Jack to reach out to LFS organizations and social media groups. Participation in these communities augments Jack's support network, increasing the visibility of other families with LFS in his social world. She is careful to probe about the extent to which participation in these communities feeds his fears of recurrence or induces survivor guilt towards families with more extensive cancer expression.

AWL attends monthly case conference meetings in clinical oncology genetics at the University Hospital and attends international meetings on cancer and genetics to stay abreast of current developments in hereditary cancer care and risk management. In these settings, she adapts her style to match the professional environment of her genetics colleagues. She is becoming increasingly comfortable suggesting psychosocial referrals and educating the physicians and counselors about hospital and community resources, though she is careful not to advertise her services so she is not perceived to be "chasing ambulances." Participation in case conference enables AWL to help Jack separate risk estimates from beliefs about susceptibility based on his family history. This work allows Jack to explore where he has choice in his care and his life trajectory and where he feels limited agency.

Reassessment, evaluation, and termination

AWL checks in with Jack at the start of each session. She periodically assesses Jack for depression and anxiety. She does not conduct other formal psychosocial evaluation. She encourages Jack's attempts to bring Amy in for an evaluation and ongoing support, and she gives him language to address what he perceives to be Amy's ambivalence. She has also referred Amy to a colleague in the social work department where Gillian is receiving care to minimize additional burden on Amy's nuclear family unit.

As Jack approaches adulthood, living beyond his mother's prognostications, he is coming to understand his father's life and death from a mature perspective. He identifies with his father, but struggles morally with the decision to seek out a life partner (who he assumes will provide end of life care for him) and plan a family (which he assumes he will leave bereaved). Jack's ambivalence is complicated by Gillian's cancer diagnoses and ongoing risk. During school breaks, Jack spends time with his young niece and he finds her spirit refreshing, her suffering familiar and understandable, and their time together enjoyable.

Evaluation (ongoing)

Family evaluation is ongoing. AWL anticipates that Jack will go through periods where he does not need ongoing psychotherapy, and thus maintains an "open door" policy. The therapeutic alliance is strong and both of us recognize his ongoing need to adapt to the demands of LFS on his life and in his family context. Jack may exit and enter the therapeutic space during breaks in his academic calendar, he can schedule phone sessions, and he can check in by email as needed.

Medically, families seldom terminate care unless they have a grave prognosis or they decide to stop screening. Families typically terminate pediatric relationships and transfer care during late teenage years/early twenties unless their medical issues dictate a need to do so earlier. At some facilities, LFS care teams may straddle pediatric and adult contexts. This can present challenges if a young patient must be followed at an adult care center or vice versa. At-risk families wishing to decline all testing or screening for either themselves or their children pose a challenge to the genetic counselor or physician, as it is difficult to know if they are making informed decisions for reasons consistent with their personal values, if they have limited resources or information, or if decisions were based on misperceptions. If a patient relocates, the care team refers to an appropriate specialist at their new home and establishes ties with new providers for them.

Differential discussion

LFS requires a multi-disciplinary, multi-arm approach to the care of patients and families. Balancing Jack's needs with the needs of his family challenges the resources of any single service provider. Because Jack was the only member of his family to seek out and participate regularly in psychosocial care, he felt separate from his family's process and assumed responsibility for his mother's and sister's emotional experiences. He attempted to forge a closer relationship with his burdened brother-in-law and his healthy brothers but felt separate from these three men based on their LFS negative status. In retrospect, greater communication among social workers, particularly between AWL and the inpatient pediatric oncology social worker, would have facilitated a family-centered approach, consistent with the nature of, and needs of families affected by, LFS.

The capacity to test for and (to a certain extent) manage hereditary cancer syndromes is developing in parallel with an ethic towards intervention and medicalization. The ethical challenges of presymptomatic genetic testing, particularly of children, remain underexplored. Efforts to understand the psychosocial implications of genetic discovery on family life are evolving *after* technologies are disseminated into research and clinical settings. The management of LFS in family groups requires a resource-rich environment. Urban teaching and research hospitals with federal funding and protected time for providers and researchers can provide this. Less attention is given to families who cannot access these environments. Disparities in access to care are likely to grow as genetic technologies are scaled up and medical practitioners and individual families begin to utilize technologies in varied ways (Collins, Green, Guttmacher, & Guyer, 2003).

Discussion questions

1   Consider the roles the two authors have with regard to Jack and his extended family's care. Where can hospital and private practice social workers help their clients and each other and where might there be tensions? How does the Health Portabililty and Privacy Act affect such partnership?
2   Genetic information is generally given as a "risk" statement ("You have a 50% greater chance of developing breast cancer than a typical woman of the same age"). How does this fit your own style? Do you see this as risky or not risky?
3   When genetic conditions are life-threatening and yet have little treatment that is effective, what do you believe your responsibilities are to individuals and families as they are diagnosed?

References and resources

Alderfer, M. A., Zelley, K., Lindell, R. B., Novokmet, A., Mai, P. L., Garber, J. E., Nathan, D., et al. (2015). Parent decision-making around the genetic testing of children for germline *TP53* mutations. *Cancer, 121*(2), 286–293. doi: 10.1002/cncr.29027

Collins, F. S., Green, E. D., Guttmacher, A. E., & Guyer, M. S. (2003). A vision for the future of genomics research. *Nature, 422*, 835–847.

Feiler, B. (2011, June 2). Scanxiety. *Time*. Retrieved from http://content.time.com/time/specials/packages/article/0,28804,2075133_2075127_2075107,00.html

Gonzalez, K. D., Noltner, K. A., Buzin, C. H., Gu, D., Wen-Fong, C. Y., Nguyen, V. Q., et al. (2009). Beyond Li Fraumeni syndrome: Clinical characteristics of families with p53 germline mutations. *Journal of Clinical Oncology, 27*(8), 1250–1256. doi: 10.1200/JC0.2008.16.6959

Hoskins, L. M. & Greene, M. H. (2012). Anticipatory loss and early mastectomy for young female *BRCA1/2* mutation carriers. *Qualitative Health Research, 22*(12), 1633–1646. doi: 10.1177/1049732312458182

Kamihara, J., Rana, H. Q., & Garber, J. E. (2014). Germline TP53 mutations and the changing land-scape of Li–Fraumeni syndrome. *Human Mutation, 35*(6), 654–662. doi: 10.1002/humu.22559

Lammens, C. R., Aaronson, N. K., Wagner, A., Sijmons, R. H., Ausems, M. G., Vriends, A. H., et al. (2010). Genetic testing in Li-Fraumeni syndrome: Uptake and psychosocial consequences. *Journal of Clinical Oncology, 28*(18), 3008–3014. doi: 10.1200/JC0.2009.27.2112

Lammens, C. R. M., Blieker, E. M. A., Verhoef, S., Ausems, M. G., Majoor-Krakauer, D., Sijmons, R. H., et al. (2011). Distress in partners of individuals diagnosed with or at high risk of develop-ing tumors due to rare hereditary cancer syndromes. *Psycho-oncology, 20*, 631–638. doi: 10.1002/pon.1951

Langan, R. C., Lagisetty, K. H., Atay, S., Pandalai, P., Stojadinovic, A., Rudloff, U., & Avital, I. (2013). Surgery for Li-Fraumeni Syndrome: Pushing the limits of surgical oncology. *American Journal of Clinical Oncology, 38*(1), 98–102. doi: 10.1097/COC.0b013e3182880bc5

Mai, P. L., Malkin, D., Garber, J. E., Schiffman, J. D., Weitzel, J. N., Strong, L. C., et al. (2012). Li-Fraumeni syndrome: Report of a clinical research workshop and creation of a research consor-tium. *Cancer Genetics, 205*(10), 479–487. doi: 10.1016/j.cancergen.2012.06.008

McBride, K. A., Ballinger, M. L., Killick, E., Kirk, J., Tattersall, M. H., Eeles, R. A., et al. (2014). Li-Fraumeni syndrome: Cancer risk assessment and clinical management. *Nature Reviews Clinical Oncology, 11*, 260–271. doi: 10.1038/nrclinonc.2014.41

Merrill, S. L. & Guthrie, K. J. (2015). Is it time for genomic counseling? Retrofitting genetic counseling for the era of genomic medicine. *Current Genetic Medicine Reports,* E-pub ahead of print. doi: 10.1007/s40142-015-0068-8

NCCN (National Comprehensive Cancer Network) (2012). *The National Comprehensive Cancer Network clinical practice guidelines in oncology: Li–Fraumeni syndrome* (Version 1.2012). National Comprehensive Cancer Network, Inc., 2012.

Peterson, S. K., Pentz, R. D., Marani, S. K., Ward, P. A., Blanco, A. M., LaRue, D., et al. (2008). Psychological functioning in persons considering genetic counseling and testing for Li-Fraumeni syndrome. *Psycho-oncology, 17*, 783–789. doi: 10.1002/pon.1352

Villani, A., Tabori, U., Schiffman, J., Shlien, A., Beyene, J., Druker, H., et al. (2011). Biochemical and imaging surveillance in germline TP53 mutation carriers with Li-Fraumeni syndrome: A prospective observational study. *The Lancet Oncology, 12*(6), 559–567. doi: 10.1016/S1470-2045(11)70119-X

Werner-Lin, A. & Gardner, D. S. (2009). Family illness narratives of inherited cancer risk: Continuity and transformation. *Families, Systems and Health, 27*(3), 201–212. doi: 10.1037/a0016983

Werner-Lin, A., Rubin, L. R., Doyle, M. H., Rapp, R., Stern, R., Savin, K., et al. (2012). "My funky genetics": *BRCA1/2* mutation carriers' understanding of genetic inheritance and reproductive merger in the context of new repro-genetic technologies. *Families, Systems & Health, 30*(2), 166–180. doi: 10.1037/a0028434

Website resources

Cancer Wellness Centers, https://cancerwellness.org/

GeneReviews: Li-Fraumeni syndrome, www.ncbi.nlm.nih.gov/books/NBK1311/

Genetic Alliance, www.geneticalliance.org

Li-Fraumeni Syndrome Association, www.lfsassociation.org

National Cancer Institute, Division of Clinical Epidemiology and Genetics. Li-Fraumeni Family Study, http://lfs.cancer.gov/

Chapter 10

Family-focused care of an adolescent with a burn

A multi-disciplinary approach

Anne Hahn

Context

Description of the setting

The Johns Hopkins Burn Center is situated within the Johns Hopkins Bayview Medical Center, part of the Johns Hopkins Medical Institutions. Accredited by the American Burn Association, the burn center treats patients age 15 and over for all types of burn injuries and also treats other skin conditions requiring complex wound care. Here, a multi-disciplinary team of medical and psychosocial providers work together to comprehensively treat burn injury with all of its complexities.

Policy and reimbursement variables

Reimbursement issues are a major challenge for burn centers due to the high cost of acute care and the need for long-term follow-up. Survivors often need rehabilitation and multiple surgeries for reconstruction, and they and their families may need psychological follow-up for extended periods (Phillips, Fussell, & Rumsey, 2007). Limited insurance or lack of insurance present challenges to obtaining follow-up care.

The American Burn Association, National Burn Repository (2014) reports that uninsured burn patients have been decreasing due to an increase in patients insured by medical assistance and through the Affordable Care Act. For those who are insured, many insurance companies do not understand the complexity of wound care and healing. Reimbursement for acute hospital care varies from state to state, and social workers need to be aware of these variances.

Reimbursement: implications for social work

Because burn unit services are very costly, a major focus for me must be to ensure that the patient has coverage for care and hospital reimbursement so the initial assessment of the patient includes insurance coverage. I can assist with patient/family referral to the hospital's financial counseling office. A major reimbursement issue, consistent with national policy concerns, is that of undocumented immigrants (Martin & Burke, 2010) for whom only limited financial assistance is available. Emergency medical assistance can be authorized for the acute phase but does not cover additional care needs such as rehabilitation or reconstruction service (Young & Soleymani Lehman, 2014). Reimbursement for, and access to, follow-up mental health care is often a challenge, particularly in rural areas (Cukor, Wyka, Leahy, Yurt, & Difede, 2015).

Burn injury

A large burn is a major assault to the body and all its systems (Herndon, 2012). The human skin is a large organ whose major function is to act as a barrier to an inhospitable environment, maintain body fluids, and regulate body temperature. The loss of fluid and temperature control can cause other organs such as lungs and kidneys to malfunction. A combination of internal mediators and external treatments can cause a cascade of events that can lead to multi-system failure. The treatment of a large burn is not just focused on the burned skin but on all systems of the body.

Patients are first evaluated and stabilized in the emergency department where the source of the injury, and the depth and the size of the burn are determined. It is important to know the source of the burn in order to decide on treatment. For example, in a chemical burn, the exact chemical components must be obtained to properly treat the burn; grease and/or steam burns are often deeper than on initial presentation; and an electrical burn will have an entrance and exit wound.

The depth of the burn is assessed. If a burn involves all layers of the skin and destroys hair follicles, nerves, and sweat glands, it is determined to be a full-thickness burn or third-degree. Ironically this deep burn is not painful because nerve endings are destroyed. This burn requires surgical treatment. A second-degree burn or partial-thickness can generally heal without surgery in several weeks. These burns are very painful. A first-degree burn is similar to sunburn and does not destroy skin layers. Most large burns are usually a combination of all three burn depths. In calculating the size of the burn or total body surface area (TBSA) only full- or partial-thickness depth burns are considered.

Patients are also assessed for inhalation and trauma injuries. When the patient breathes significant amounts of smoke, irritants can cause swelling of the airway. If an inhalation injury is identified or suspected, an endotracheal tube is inserted. Any delay may result in the patient's airway swelling, thus precluding the placement of a breathing tube. If the burn injury involves any type of trauma, patients are evaluated for fractures, particularly spinal cord injuries.

The assessment phase also consists of a history. The team looks at age, existing medical conditions, such as neurological and cognitive impairments, cardiovascular diseases, renal failure, and other chronic conditions, such as diabetes, and alcohol/drug and psychiatric disorders. Any preexisting condition can complicate wound healing and the burn plan of care. Age is a major factor in prognosis. Generally, advancing age (>50 years) and a large burn (50% TBSA) are associated with increased mortality (American Burn Association, 2014).

Technology

The burn center is a specialized surgical intensive unit. Patients are monitored in ways that require lines and catheters to monitor internal functions. A feeding tube may be inserted to provide nutrition during the time the patient is in an induced coma. An important part of initial treatment of a large burn is fluid resuscitation. Patients lose fluid when skin is damaged or lost, yet care must be taken not to overload the patient with too much replacement fluid, which could result in respiratory or kidney failure.

The most important part of burn therapy is wound care. All patients are bathed daily in a specialized tub room. Patients are sedated and the wounds are washed, dead skin removed, and the wounds covered with creams and bandages. Advances in the types of dressings can now promote faster healing, and some wound care products can be left on for several days, thus avoiding wound care pain and facilitating earlier discharge.

Other specialists treat the patient as well. Physical therapy begins range-of-motion exercises to promote conditioning and prevent contractures. Occupational therapy works with upper extremities and may place splints to maintain positioning and minimize stiffening of arms and hands. The nutritionist initiates the proper diet for optimal wound healing. The bedside nurse assesses and treats pain. Other team members who assist include pharmacy, psychology, psychiatry, and palliative care. Pain rounds are conducted weekly and pain regimens updated as needed.

Infection is a constant threat and challenge. Patients' wounds are frequently cultured for any sign of infection and lines changed at specific intervals. Infectious disease specialists determine which antibiotics to prescribe. Hand washing is enforced and all staff and visitors gown and glove before entering a patient's room.

Burn patients are surgically treated by transplanting tissue from one part of the body to another – skin grafting. The grafting procedure requires viable skin on one part of the body (donor site) that can be used for graft tissue (autograft). If none is available, cadaver skin is used (allograft), but this is temporary until the patient's own skin can be used. Multiple grafting procedures may be necessary in large burns. A successful skin graft results in faster healing, shorter hospital stay, and better function and cosmetic effect.

Several advances assist in the success of a graft. One is the use of cell-cultured epithelial autograft (CEA), in which skin cells from the patient are grown in a laboratory that produces skin cell sheets. These sheets are applied as temporary coverage if the patient lacks enough donor sites. Unfortunately, these often do not take and are very expensive. Vacuum-assisted closures (VAC) are devices used to assist with closure of large wounds. The vacuum unit creates negative pressure through a system of foam, tubing, and bandages which seal the edges of the wound. It draws out excess blood and fluids that help to maintain cleanliness, reduce infection, promote the development of new blood supply, and increase the success of the wound graft.

Treatment and technology: implications for social work

I am often the first person whom families meet, and they are usually frightened and bewildered. They have no idea what to expect. Patients with a life-threatening burn injury can sometimes walk to the ambulance and talk to families in the emergency department. This can give families the false impression that the injury is minor and easily overcome. They do not realize that the critical nature of the injury will manifest itself in the first 24 hours. It is part of my responsibility to prepare the family for the realities of the injury; that is, the patient may become critically ill from respiratory or infection issues. Patients may be intubated and sedated and unable to communicate with them, or they may look very distorted – bloated from an infusion of fluids and attached to multiple lines and machinery. I educate families about the course of care and about the members of the multi-disciplinary team, the roles they play, and how to have access to them. Referral is provided to such agencies as the American Red Cross, financial counseling, and other community resources. At the same time, I am gathering important information about the patient that can affect the course of care. A careful history includes asking about previous medical and psychiatric illnesses, as well as the patient's and family's previous experience with crisis situations and how they dealt with them. This gives me an idea of how the family will cope and what kinds of assistance they will need.

Organization

The burn center consists of a 10-bed surgical intensive care unit, an intermediate care unit for patients who are recovering from critical burns or for those with less serious burns, and its own rehabilitation suite and tub room. The operating rooms are nearby. Our multi-disciplinary team has expanded over the last years to include intensivists and physician's assistants who specialize in critical care and are responsible for the day-to-day management of critically ill patients in the burn and surgical intensive care units. They work closely with the burn surgeons to improve the quality of care and reduce mortality.

Leadership is provided by two attending burn surgeons. Two burn fellows assist the surgeons and are key players in providing consistent care and tending to the technical aspects of burn care. The nurses are cross-trained to work in the acute critical care burn or surgical units as well as the intermediate unit to accommodate the fluid bed census. Physical and occupation therapists are assigned to the burn center but rotate through other services. I am assigned full-time to the center and am an integral part of the team, and I am part of a centralized Department of Social Work. Other team members include a psychologist and two fellows, a nurse case manager, and a nutritionist. There is continuity of staff, many of whom have worked in the burn center for years despite the emotional distress sometimes associated with this type of work (Kornhaber & Wilson, 2011). Newly hired nurses are mentored by a senior nurse who trains them and introduces them to the culture of the center. The team approach is supported through a variety of rounds that everyone attends.

The burn center is also a community of interdependent and equal professionals who could not accomplish their work without each other (Kerson, 2002). The sense of community has developed from a core group of individuals who were part of the center at its inception, and who have the sense of both its history and its future that is essential to a sense of community. There is a shared ethos of good patient care.

Organization: implications for social work

It is imperative that social workers analyze and understand the context of their practice to be effective (Kerson, 2002). A social worker who is isolated and cannot work effectively with the team will not be successful with patients. This requires that I understand my role, function, and place on the team as well as what other team members do. Mintzberg (2007) refers to this as an organization with operational fluidity and high collaboration. This requires mutual and reciprocal respect among disciplines.

I can assist the team in conflict resolution in relation to ethical issues (Jonsen, Siegler, & Winslade, 2015) by promoting communication and collaboration and minimizing confrontation. For example, burn surgeons may interpret "good patient care" as being as aggressive as possible to save a life while other team members may view "good patient care" as evaluating quality of life and/or providing comfort care. An ethics consult might be suggested as a way to unblock communication, remove blame, and energize the team to arrive at a decision.

Visibility is very important. Just as community organizers work within the community to promote change and meet needs, I must be a visible and viable member of the burn/critical care team to inspire and increase productivity, which in this case is good patient care (Cohen, 2013).

Decisions about practice

Description of the patient and injury

Charlie was a 15-year-old boy admitted to the burn center with burns to both legs. These burns covered 15% of the TBSA and were assessed as partial thickness or second degree. Skin grafting was not necessary, but debridement (removal of dead skin) and wound care were. Pain was a major issue for him because nerve endings were exposed. He was also confined to bed and non-ambulatory to promote healing to the lower extremities.

The injury occurred when Charlie and a friend set a fire with gasoline for "fun." He was burned when he tried to stomp out the fire with his feet. Charlie came from a rural part of the state. I met him on day three of his admission because he was in too much pain to talk with me earlier. Charlie was an attractive, smiling young man who looked older than his age and who did not appear to be in distress, though he had little to say. He did not have a good explanation for the accident and admitted it was "stupid." His injury was complicated by diabetes. He had been diagnosed with type 1 insulin-dependent diabetes at age 10, and it was never well controlled.

Definition of the client

After meeting Charlie, I spoke to his parents who provided background information and details about the accident and Charlie's non-adherence to his diabetic regimen. Charlie lived with his mother and younger brother, age 12. His mother's extended family (her parents and siblings) lived nearby. Charlie's parents had been divorced for 5 years, at the same time that Charlie was diagnosed with diabetes. His father lived in another state where the family had lived prior to the divorce. Following the divorce, his mother moved with her two sons to be closer to her family. Charlie's father and his parents remained involved in the boys' lives. His father came to the burn center as soon as he learned of his son's injury and visited his son for a week. Charlie's parents were amicable, taking care not to blame one another for what had occurred. They expressed their distress over the injury, and their primary concern was their son's healing from the burn and total recovery.

Both were very concerned about Charlie's behavior. Charlie was described as impulsive, rebellious, and non-adherent to his diabetic regimen. His parents' efforts to redirect his behavior were not successful. His behavior issues predated their divorce but had worsened since. Charlie had been in counseling, as well as family therapy, but it had not been effective. His school and pediatrician were all aware of the behavior issues and were trying to be helpful, but nothing seemed to be effective.

Charlie's mother described what she knew of the circumstances surrounding the injury. She was concerned that Charlie was socializing with friends who were not a good influence. They were older than Charlie but accepted him into their circle because he appears older. She also thought that he was using marijuana and occasionally drinking. He was with one of these friends when the injury occurred.

Charlie's parents and I discussed discharge issues. Since we knew that he would not be hospitalized long, we needed to establish plans for home care. Charlie's mother was prepared to take a leave of absence from her job to care for her son until he could return to school. His father was returning to his home and would not be available to assist. It became clear the aftercare for Charlie would fall to his mother who was concerned for her own job and finances. Charlie had good health coverage through his mother's employment.

We discussed referrals for diagnosis and treatment of Charlie's behavior issues. Both agreed that he needed some help but it was not clear how this could be arranged. His mother was pessimistic that Charlie would cooperate in counseling. She was familiar with outpatient psychiatric resources in her area because of her background as a social worker. She said that few resources were available. I told the parents that the burn center's psychologist would evaluate Charlie and that we would work together to find some resources and assist Charlie to accept the referral. Charlie's pediatrician also spoke to me about her concerns; she felt that Charlie's mother was not taking sufficient responsibility for the management of Charlie's diabetes. She had considered a referral to Child Protective Services because the mother missed pediatric appointments and did not follow through on the doctor's recommendations.

From my on-going assessment, I knew that the definition of the client was much more than just Charlie. Multiple strained relationships existed in Charlie's life. It became clear to me that assisting Charlie to heal physically, emotionally, and socially from his burn injury would require an interdependent endeavor.

Goals

Setting a goal for social work intervention is based upon the definition of the problem, which is often a moving target that can change over time and may be dependent upon one's perspective. In Charlie's case, the goal from the burn center's perspective was to heal his wounds and minimize permanent impairment. From my perspective as the social worker, the goal was to assist the family to address Charlie's diabetic management and behavior issues. From the pediatrician's standpoint, the goal was to change the mother's behavior. The mother's goal was to maintain her own equilibrium and deflect judgments about her as an uncaring mother while caring for her son. Charlie's goal seemed to be non-involvement with his issues, including family dynamics.

In order to adequately address the goals, we had to determine priorities. The first goal was related to the problem for which the patient and family sought help – burn treatment. The second goal – diabetic management – related to the first. Unless Charlie's diabetes could be managed, he would not heal properly from his burns. The burn occurred while the patient was participating in risky and impulsive behavior which, by history, was a pattern and not an isolated incident; therefore a third goal was acceptance of a referral for psychiatric diagnosis and treatment. My work was to facilitate the identification, acceptance, and completion of these goals by all involved: patient, family, and multi-disciplinary team.

Contract and objectives

Contracts, particularly in a hospital setting, are flexible and often informal, as the needs may change. After my initial meeting with Charlie and his family, I returned to discuss identified problems: Charlie's burn healing and aftercare, diabetic management, and mental health care. I explained how I could assist them with referrals to home care resources, consultations with a pediatric social worker about diabetic referrals, and assistance with identifying mental health care and follow-up. We agreed to work toward achieving the following objectives: discharge to home with follow-up appointments, information and referral for a pediatric endocrinologist and education resources, and referral for diagnosis and treatment of behavior issues.

While working with the family, I observed the mood, body language, and voice inflections. Charlie was outwardly cheerful and agreeable to all suggestions but he said very little.

His father was often angry and overbearing, criticizing Charlie for his reckless behavior. Although verbally supportive of the objectives, he provided no specific offers of how he would assist. Charlie's mother agreed with the objectives but brought up barriers to achieving them such as lack of resources in her rural area, long waiting lists for psychiatric care, and her own work schedule. I recognized everyone's frustration and acknowledged that the objectives might not all be achievable at once, but we could prioritize one. We agreed to work on locating resources for diabetic management.

Meeting place

Sessions with Charlie and his family were held in a number of places including the patient's room, my office, and the burn center conference room. This is typical of my work with patients and families.

Use of time

The percentage of TBSA involved in the injury usually corresponds to the number of days the patient spends in the hospital. Charlie received a 15% TBSA burn. His hospitalization in the burn center was 17 days. I saw the patient and his mother almost every day but not necessarily for a therapeutic intervention. Often it was a brief conversation to inquire how things were going. This is typical. Most of my interactions take place at the time of admission and at the time of discharge. The middle phase is often more task-related unless the family contracts with me for more intense and structured counseling.

Much can be accomplished in a short period of time if the intervention is clear and the family agrees. Families are usually in crisis and more open to admitting to underlying problems and accepting assistance due to the rising tension (Parad & Parad, 2006; Rainer & Brown, 2007). Inner resources can often be mobilized to seek long-needed help.

Strategies and interventions

Social workers in intensive care units participate in multiple activities (McCormick, Engelberg, & Curtis, 2007). Often patients are too ill to participate in the assessment and pre-discharge planning phases and, thus, interventions are often directed toward the families. Although the first intervention is assessment, this can also be therapeutic for families because it is not only about information gathering but also education about the burn center's organization and treatment protocols, and referrals to resources. Charlie's burn injury was a symptom of a bigger problem, an undiagnosed psychiatric disorder within the context of a fractured family. The mother was overwhelmed and felt blamed and judged by others, and the father was physically and emotionally absent. In addition, the intervention also had to address burn healing and management of a chronic illness.

My interventions are guided by a systems approach to integrating mental health and health care along with team collaboration (McDaniel, Hepworth, & Doherty, 2014). Recent evidence suggests that patients and families can experience post-traumatic stress, depression, and guilt (Bakker, Maertens, Van Son, & Loey, 2013; Dahl, Wickman, & Wengstrom, 2012; Klinge, Chamberlain, Redden, & King, 2009). Poor functioning prior to the burn injury can complicate coping and be a predictor of a longer adjustment period (Wibbenmeyer et al., 2014). The degree of distress can be associated with the size of the burn and how much it affects appearance (Maskell, Newcombe, Martin, & Kimble, 2013).

Families are usually willing to engage with the social worker during the assessment phase because they are in crisis. They may then shut down as they begin to experience feelings of loss, shame, or guilt (Bakker et al., 2013). These feelings may be heightened when other family members arrive to be supportive but may add to the tension if there is a history of poor family relationships. The assessment phase needs to be on-going as families' moods and behaviors can change from the initial evaluation.

Stance of the social worker

Charlie's case presented a challenge. I believed that focusing on the mother was important to meet the agreed upon objectives. The mother was the primary parent in Charlie's life. I sensed that as the hospitalization continued, the mother became less engaged and more superficial in her interactions with me. About the same time, I received a call from Charlie's pediatrician who wanted me to know of her concerns about Charlie and his mother. The pediatrician was concerned that the mother was not accepting responsibility for Charlie's diabetes management.

This was difficult for me because the mother was a professional social worker. I wondered if the mother might feel judged by me as an inadequate mother; perhaps I was embarrassed about confronting her with our concerns. We met several days before Charlie's impending discharge. The mother asked what the psychologist thought about Charlie. I suggested we all meet to discuss her concerns because I thought that an additional team member might promote communication. Prior to the meeting with the mother, the psychologist and I met. We went over the data we had gathered: Charlie's non-adherence and impulsive behavior, possible neglectful mother, absent father, concerned pediatrician, and lack of community resources, and we decided to take an open and non-judgmental approach. We wanted to hear the mother's assessment of the situation both as a parent and a professional social worker. This was successful. We met in a comfortable and private conference room. The mother opened up about her son's violent behavior, her attempts to deal with it, and the poor relationship she had with the children's father.

At one point, I asked her if it would help her if we made a referral to Child Protective Services. She did not want this because she felt that Charlie might get lost in the system and never receive the help he needed. She admitted to feeling very sad about her mothering and believed that her husband's family thought she was an inadequate parent. However, she felt that her children were better off with her than their father who lacked the emotional resources to deal with them. By the end of the session, the psychologist and I saw a caring mother who was overwhelmed by multiple stressors: an out-of-control adolescent with a serious health problem, another son to protect, minimal social support, and financial issues. We acknowledged that she was a caring mother who was doing the best she could but needed help and had the courage to ask for it.

Use of outside resources

Following the meeting the psychologist and I discussed how Charlie's wounds were almost healed and that the other equally important issues needed to be addressed. We could not accomplish this in our unit. We worked, with the help of the attending physician, to have Charlie transferred to the main hospital's pediatric unit. The psychologist spoke to Charlie about the plan and his agreement to participate. I followed up with Charlie and his mother to support the plan, discuss ambivalent feelings, and assist with the technical aspects of the transfer. Once Charlie was transferred, he was able to receive evaluation and treatment for his behavior and diabetic issues. He was diagnosed with a mood disorder and ADHD and referred to the adolescent psychiatric day program. From there he was transferred to a similar program closer to his home. He was stabilized on a diabetic regimen and appointments arranged for him with a community pediatric specialist and a nurse diabetes educator. Charlie's pediatrician was made aware of the referrals. I informed the pediatrician that the burn team did not feel that the mother was negligent but overwhelmed, and I explained that the mother could benefit from the pediatrician's support for Charlie's on-going care at these community resources.

Charlie did not need any other services for his burn injury. He and his mother returned to the burn clinic once for follow-up and he was discharged to the care of his pediatrician. Appearing happy and relaxed, they visited the inpatient burn center and thanked everyone for his care. Charlie was back at school, participating in outpatient psychiatry visits, and his mother had returned to work.

Evaluation and reassessment

The review of Charlie's case was positive in that all goals were met. Charlie's burns were treated, his diabetes better managed, his behavior and psychiatric issues assessed, and treatment had begun. Additionally, we were able to support his mother validating that she was a caring mother, and at the same time relieving her of the burden of finding the appropriate care for her son and trying to make him adhere to the plan. We advocated with the pediatrician so that she could be a source of on-going support. The pediatrician was also made aware of resources such as the Phoenix Society (www.phoenix-society.org), a national support organization for burn survivors.

Differential discussion

This case is representative of the types of burns and cases seen in our center. The burn injury often occurs in the context of preexisting poor functioning and chronic psychosocial problems. Admission to the burn center may have the effect of not only treating the burn but also addressing the underlying issues and providing assistance.

Burn units have the luxury of a multi-disciplinary team and more time to address issues because burn patients often have longer-than-usual acute stays. The burn team can be mobilized to assess and intervene with the patient and family, and the critical nature of the burn can mobilize the patient and family to address underlying conditions and accept assistance. The role of the social worker is twofold: assessment of the patient and family for underlying issues, and communication with the multi-disciplinary team. The positive outcome in Charlie's case was due to assessment, relationship building with the family, and in collaboration with the psychologist. The social worker must be able to quickly form relationships with patients and families while working with the team, and be willing to share the work with others with the goal of good patient care.

In reviewing Charlie's case, it is not clear if anything else could be done differently. It is likely that the timing of events was consistent with the mother's comfort level with me, as well as her anxiety as Charlie's discharge was approaching. The involvement of the pediatrician was key. Once she understood the pressures the mother was under and the mother's willingness to work with us, she became a willing support for the mother. Each case is different. The multi-disciplinary team is a vehicle to address complex medical and psychosocial problems and I contribute to the teamwork by remaining open and flexible in order to use myself as a resource for patients and families.

Discussion questions

1 How can a social worker assist the team to better understand family dynamics, address conflicts among the health care team, and work through ethical dilemmas?
2 What are strategies for dealing with your own discomfort in working with a patient and/ or family member who is also a professional social worker?
3 Burn care is extremely expensive due to long length of stay and the labor-intensive nature of wound care. Can you think of ways that burn care could be provided in a less expensive and perhaps more humane manner?

References

American Burn Association (2014). *National Burn Repository*. Retrieved January 28 2015 from www. Ameriburn.org/2014NBR AnnualReport.pdf

Bakker, A., Maertens, K.J., Van Son, M. J. M., & Loey, N. E. E. (2013). Psychological consequences of pediatric burns from a child and family perspective: A review of the empirical literature. *Clinical Psychology Review, 33*, 361–371. doi: org/10.1016/j.cpr.2012.12.006

Cohen, W. A. (2013). *The practical Drucker*: *Applying the wisdom of the world's greatest management thinker*. New York: Amacon Books.

Cukor, J., Wyka, K., Leahy, N., Yurt, R., & Difede, J. (2015). The treatment of posttraumatic stress disorder and related psychosocial consequences of burn injuries: A pilot study. *Journal of Burn Care & Research, 36*, 186–192. doi: 10.1097/BCR.0000000000000177

Dahl, O., Wickman, M., & Wengstrom. Y. (2012). Adapting to life after burn injury – reflections on care. *Journal of Burn Care and Research, 33*, 595–605. doi: 10.1097/BCR.0b013e31823d0a11

Herndon, D. N. (Ed.) (2012). *Total burn care*. Philadelphia, PA: W. B. Saunders.

Jonsen, A.R., Siegler, M., & Winslade, W. J. (2015). *Clinical ethics*: *A practical approach to ethical decisions in clinical medicine* (8th edn.). Philadelphia, PA: McGraw-Hill.

Kerson, T. S. (2002*). Boundary spanning. An ecological reinterpretation of social work practice in health and mental health systems*. New York: Columbia University Press.

Klinge, K., Chamberlain, D. J., Redden, M., & King, L. (2009). Psychological adjustments made by post burn injury patients: An integrative literature review. *Journal of Advanced Nursing, 65*, 2274–2292. doi: 10.1111/j.1365-2648.2009.05138x

Kornhaber, R. A. & Wilson, A. (2011). Psychosocial needs of burn nurses: A descriptive phenomenological inquiry. *Journal of Burn Care & Research, 32*, 286–293. doi: 10.1097/BCR.0b013e31820aaf37

Martin, E. & Burke, C. (2010). Health reform: What is the future for undocumented aliens? Retrieved from http://healthaffairs.org/blog/2010/10/15/health-reform-what-is-the-future-for undocumented-aliens/

Maskell, J., Newcombe, P., Martin, G., & Kimble, R. (2013). Psychosocial functioning differences in pediatric survivors compared with healthy norms. *Journal of Burn Care & Research, 34*, 465–476. doi: 10.1097/BCR.0b013e31827217a9

McCormick, A., Engelberg, R. & Curtis, J. R. (2007). Social workers in palliative care: Assessing activities and barriers in the intensive care unit. *Journal of Palliative Medicine, 10*, 929–937. doi: 10.1089/jpm.2006.0235

McDaniel, S. H., Hepworth, J., & Doherty, W. (2014). *Medical family therapy and integrated care* (2nd edn.). Washington, DC: American Psychological Association.

Mintzberg, H. (2007). *Tracking strategies*. New York: Oxford University Press.

Parad, H. J. & Parad, L. G. (2006). *Crisis intervention book 2*: *The practitioner's source book for brief therapy* (2nd edn.). New York: Fenestra Books.

Phillips, C., Fussell, A., & Rumsey, N. (2007). Considerations for psychosocial support following burn injury – a family perspective. *Burns, 33*(8), 986–994. doi: 10.1016/j.burns.2007.01.010

Rainer, J. & Brown, F. (2007). *Crisis counseling and therapy*. New York: Routledge.

Wibbenmeyer, L., Liao, J., Heard, J., Kealey, L., Kealey, G., & Oral, R. (2014). Factors related to child maltreatment in children presenting with burn injuries. *Journal of Burn Care & Research, 35*, 374–381. doi: 10.1097/BCR.0000000000000005

Young, M. J. & Soleymani Lehman, L. (2014). Undocumented injustice? Medical repatriation and the end of health care. *New England of Medicine, 370*, 669–673. doi: 10.1056/NEJMhle1311198

Chapter 11

The Young Women's Program

A health and wellness model to empower adolescents with physical disabilities in a hospital-based setting

Nancy Xenakis

Context

Policy

The Young Women's Program (YWP) is the only program of its kind in the region. Its purpose is to teach young women with physical disabilities, ages 14–21, how to lead a healthy lifestyle. This is accomplished by providing a planned curriculum with a variety of group classes and workshops, individual health and wellness planning, expert instruction, access to resources and a network of peers and mentors. Over the past four decades, the nation's health focus has shifted from acute care to long-term chronic care for persons with disabilities. The current emphasis on continuity of care is an outgrowth of a series of legislative initiatives, the most influential and widely known being the Americans with Disabilities Act of 1990 (ADA) which addressed the need and ability of persons with disabilities to function optimally in their environment. In 1999, the Supreme Court's decision in *Olmsted v. L. C.* outlined a remedy for states to achieve the ADA's goal of community care in the most integrated, public settings appropriate to an individual's needs by implementing reasonable accommodations. The decision accomplished a legal standard for measuring the adequacy of publicly funded health program design for persons with disabilities, most notably Medicaid, the largest public health care for persons with disabilities (Rosenbaum, 2000).

The Affordable Care Act (ACA) of 2010 aims to move the health care system towards a coordinated model delivering high-quality, low-cost care. Changing methods of payment and reforming health care delivery (creating high performing organizations will help to prevent and treat illness, improve access to care, patient safety and satisfaction, and coordinate services) is allowing new care coordination programs to be developed to serve people with disabilities.

Of the current 62 million Medicaid enrollees, 9.3 million are non-elderly persons with disabilities (Kaiser Commission on Medicaid and the Uninsured, 2013). Over time, Managed Care Organizations (MCOs) for the Medicaid program have proven more restrictive to people with disabilities incorporating younger people with disabilities into their managed care programs and attempting to limit spending and services, equipment, and supplies. Another component of the ACA expands Medicaid to cover millions of previously uninsured low-income adults and children, and to better meet the needs of its subpopulations (Kaiser Commission on Medicaid and the Uninsured, 2013). An example is Health Homes which were established to provide primary and acute physical health services, behavioral health and long-term community-based services and supports through a network of providers including hospitals and community-based organizations (Substance Abuse and Mental Health Services Administration, 2014).

Social workers have assumed a major role in advocating for clients with disabilities, assisting them to find appropriate managed care plans to meet their medical needs and to apply for exemptions when appropriate. Since funding for the YWP is provided by the Hospital's operating budget and foundation grants, the YWP itself is unaffected by managed care. Nevertheless, in discussion groups and planning sessions, participants discuss the restrictive measures of Medicaid managed care and efforts are made with involved parties to find resolutions. The young women are now asking questions about the ACA and enrolling in Health Homes.

Technology

People with physical disabilities should have equal access to telecommunications equipment and services that can improve their lifestyle, social interaction, security, and independence (Nguyen, Garrett, Downing, Walker, & Hobbs, 2007). Assistive devices for activities of daily living such as motorized wheelchairs and augmentative and alternative communication devices have allowed participants of the YWP to travel independently and communicate clearly. The Individuals with Disabilities Education Act (2004) requires public schools to make available to all children with disabilities a free appropriate public education in the least restrictive environment possible with an Individualized Education Program (IEP) developed for each child. This IEP describes each student's specific special educational needs including an assistive technology evaluation (United States Office of Special Education, 2014). This and general technology increase access and allow most participants to use smart phones and laptops as do their able bodied peers. Devices such as laptops, DVDs, videos, and digital cameras are utilized during the program and for community outreach. Devices also enabled YWP participants to make a CD of YWP songs, with their artwork and photographs used for the CD case.

A DVD highlighting different program sessions is also played during program outreach presentations to professionals, potential participants, and their parents (legal guardians), allowing audiences to visualize the program and fostering referrals and registration.

Organization

The YWP is a program within the Initiative for Women with Disabilities (IWD), a hospital-based center serving women across the life span with chronic physical illnesses and/or conditions. It offers accessible gynecology, primary care, physical therapy, nutrition consultations, exercise/fitness classes, wellness and social work services. The IWD is part of NYU Hospital for Joint Diseases (NYUHJD), and is part of a larger academic medical center, New York University Langone Medical Center, USA (NYULMC). NYUHJD maintains its identity with its areas of medical specialization, familiarity, and accessibility among physicians, staff, and patients, and contained space that is easily navigated. It also benefits from being part of NYULMC: with financial security, sharing of best practices and resources on the clinical, technological, and ancillary levels. The mission of NYULMC is the relief of human suffering caused by disease and disability through patient care, education, and research. This mission resonates throughout NYUHJD and the IWD. The IWD, a nationally known center that is about, for, and run by women, was established in response to the Office on Disability and Health's (ODH) selection of *Women with Disabilities* as a major area of emphasis. NYUHJD supports the mission and innovative programming of the IWD including the YWP. The team (director, program coordinator, primary care physician, gynecologist, social worker, physical therapist, nutritionist, wellness practitioners, nurse's aide, and administrative support staff) develops programming and provides services responsive to the needs of its patients.

Description of typical client situations

Young women with physical disabilities face barriers to leading healthy lifestyles. They often have difficulty developing healthy body images, and as they reach adolescence, they become aware of how different their bodies are when compared with their able-bodied peers. This awareness is often perpetuated by the perceived influence of the media, peers, and parents regarding the body ideal. These young women must also overcome myths that they are asexual or incapable of having sexual relationships (Piotrowski & Snell, 2007).

Also, young women with physical disabilities find practical barriers to socialization. For example, a need for special transportation reduces their ability to spontaneously participate in peer activities, or there are problems with physical access to a friend's home (Antle, 2004). Such barriers often affect their ability to find friends, mentors, and role models and can lead to problems with depression and isolation. Many adolescents with physical disabilities are more physically, behaviorally, and socially dependent on their parents than are adolescents without disabilities. This can be attributed to families sheltering young women with disabilities. As a result, these young women may not become independent in sync with other teenagers. Further, parents may be unaware of, or disinclined to seek, helpful resources.

Girls with disabilities have few options for learning about their changing health care needs and discussing maturation issues as they move from adolescence to adulthood. They often stay with their pediatricians well into adulthood, long after most young women have met with a gynecologist. As the stage is set in adolescence for many of the physical and emotional issues they will face as adults, barriers to health services and wellness activities can have an enormous impact on these young women's lives. Young women with disabilities should be active partners in choosing activities to promote wellness and well-being, such as exercise, physical activity, nutritional guidance, and stress management support groups (Piotrowski & Snell, 2007).

Obstacles to health care can be very practical. Women with disabilities have difficulty in locating physicians knowledgeable about their disability and the secondary conditions they are prone to, such as chronic urinary tract infections, heart disease, depression, and osteoporosis. The most common problem is getting onto a doctor's exam table. Physicians can also view these young women as asexual and infantilize them well into adulthood, though many have aspirations of marriage and motherhood (Chevarley, Thierry, Gill, Ryerson, & Nosek, 2006). Only in the last 25 years has our attention moved away from protective notions and towards assisting adolescents to strategize to promote their self-competence and functional capacity. Aligned with this philosophy, YWP promotes participants' self-determination by offering learning and empowering experiences in individual and group settings. We aim to increase their sense of self-competence, ability to achieve their personal goals and to form new relationships.

Decisions about practice

Definition of the client

YWP clients are adolescent females with physical disabilities, primarily in high school, ages 14–21, whose physical disabilities are congenital or acquired due to accident or illness. Some have secondary cognitive impairments and many struggle with mental health issues such as depression and anxiety. To be eligible, clients must be able to follow instructions, behave appropriately, and function within a group structure. A telephone screening with a parent (legal guardian) allows YWP to discuss the potential participant's functioning, accommodations, and interests, review program expectations and determine fit. Participants are either self-referred or referred by a health care or academic professional. Participants and their parents (legal guardians) complete registration paperwork including a consent form. Parents (legal guardians) can participate in an orientation to the program but afterwards are encouraged to allow the young women to participate independently. The YWP offers separate educational and wellness workshops for parents (legal guardians) as they have a vital and often complex role in the participants' development and can benefit from a support network.

Program participants are from diverse racial, ethnic, and socioeconomic backgrounds, and although they all have a physical disability their types of physical disability and level of functioning varies. The YWP staff are experienced in working with different cultural backgrounds; they believe that being culturally competent involves respect for difference, eagerness to learn, and a willingness to accept that there are many ways of viewing the world. Staff are sensitive to participants' various needs and are willing to explore differences to enhance the group's overall experience. The nutrition classes focus on healthy eating where the foods of different cultures represented by the participants are prepared and discussed. In the discussion groups issues relating to familial relationships and parental roles are explored. During the individual health and wellness planning sessions, participants develop their own personal goals; in the spiritual domain specifically, they often share their sociocultural and ethnic beliefs and practices.

Goals

The YWP's mission is to provide the opportunity for girls with physical disabilities to mature into young women, through age-appropriate health, social, and wellness activities. This is achieved by helping young women take charge of their health and wellness, and respect and honor their bodies. The program also serves as a bridge helping young women with disabilities meet the need for age-appropriate gynecological medical care and mental health services through referrals to the IWD. Most importantly, it provides young women an opportunity to socialize with their peers, develop friendships and share resources. Its main objectives are:

- to introduce girls with physical disabilities to concepts of health and wellness through classes and workshops in exercise/fitness, wellness, expressive arts, and discussion groups;
- to provide young women the opportunity to explore and develop friendships, share concerns and feelings with other young women with disabilities, discover new and rewarding goals for their future focused on independence; and
- to develop and utilize self-advocacy skills through experiencing mentorship through a partnership with young adult women with disabilities, introducing girls to available resources on health and wellness for persons with disabilities and helping participants learn how to access appropriate medical care, both primary and gynecological.

Each participant develops an individual health and wellness plan identifying achievable goals for the coming year. The purpose of this exercise is to apply the concepts that are learned in the group sessions to one's own life and develop meaningful, short-term goals in the five well-being domains: recreational, physical, emotional, educational/vocational, and spiritual. It is intended to improve one's feelings of self-worth and self-competence. Every six months, each participant reviews, evaluates, and updates her goals.

Developing objectives and contracting

Contracts are established with participants, staff, vendors, and funding sources. Written contracts are completed with companies that provide efficient transportation. The majority travel with a para transit company serving persons with disabilities. Participants who attend the same schools or reside in the same areas are scheduled on the same vehicles to enhance socialization and increase the comfort level of parents (legal guardians) to allow their daughters to travel independently. A transportation service brings a large group of participants who attend a high school outside of the para transit company's jurisdiction to the program.

Contracts between the YWP and program participants and their parents (legal guardians) stipulate policies and procedures including attendance and a consent to participate/liability form. This ensures that participants understand expectations and participate safely, and allows the hospital to be free from liability. Individual health and wellness plans developed by each young woman reflect short-term personal goals and serve as a contract between the participant and program coordinator. Each participant and the program coordinator review, sign, and keep a copy of the plan. Written contracts also exist with funders. When a grant is awarded, the grantor designates how funds are to be used and provides timelines and specifications for reporting funding use.

Meeting place and use of time

Group sessions of the YWP are held at IWD's own new fully accessible building a few blocks from NYUHJD. It includes multi-purpose rooms, medical exam and treatment rooms, and conference rooms as well as staff offices. YWP programming is offered seamlessly. The program consists of 10 consecutive 3-hour sessions offered weekly after school in the fall and spring. Specialized workshops (drama, beauty, rowing, track, and writing) are offered during weekends and school recess. Table 11.1 gives an overview of the after-school program structure.

Table 11.1 Table of activities: after-school program structure

Time period	Activity
4:00–5:00 p.m.	Homework/studying (tutoring available), review of resource table, socialization, healthy snacks
5:00–5:45 p.m.	Health and wellness class 1[a]
5:45–6:30 p.m.	Health and wellness class 2[a]
6:30–7:00 p.m	Healthy dinner, guest speaker on program/service, socialization

[a] Class categories are: exercise/fitness, expressive arts, wellness, discussion groups.

This structure permits a combination of organized class time and informal participant interaction. Classes are of a duration that engages participants and holds their interest. The 10 consecutive 3-hour sessions in one program season enable the young women to meet program objectives including learning new skills and developing friendships. Specialized workshops provide year-round program continuity and the opportunity to offer classes that require longer duration. One example is collaboration between YWP and The Visible Theatre, Inc. to develop a creative writing workshop called "A True Story Project: I am Heard" (TSP). TSP's experiential approach of connecting women with disabilities to each other and facilitators/mentors through the writing and sharing of stories in a safe and nurturing environment fosters self-expression and empowerment.

At the end of the fall and spring programs, each participant meets with the coordinator individually for an hour-long session to complete health and wellness planning. The long interval between sessions allows time for participants to address their short-term personal goals. During after-school program sessions, some ongoing discussion focuses on the young women's individual health and wellness plans and provides an opportunity for group sharing. The young women can be part of the program while they are 14–21 years old. After they age out, 100% transition to the IWD's Empowerment Program, which strengthens living skills and offers enrichment activities until 32 years old. Afterwards they can participate in other IWD programs and services for the rest of their lifetime.

Strategies and interventions

The YWP addresses transitional challenges concretely with classes, workshops, and experiences related to living arrangements, independent travel, school, career, health care, community life, socialization, sexuality, taking care of one's body, and financial management, and socially by creating bridges to adulthood through developing skills in advocacy, goal-setting, empowerment, independence, communication, negotiation, persistence (even when facing adversity), navigating/being resourceful, and sharing information with others with similar needs.

The literature on persons with disabilities has identified the many needs of this population, the existing gaps in services, and their societal perception. Research points to types of programming and services that would make life for persons with disabilities more fulfilling professionally and personally. Primarily suggested are empowering experiences that promote self-determination and self-competence including goal-setting, opportunities for socialization with peers and mentors, exposure to community resources, and developing skills to take care of their bodies and lead independent lives (Rimmer & Rowland, 2008; U.S. Department of Health and Human Services, 2005; van Campen & Iedema, 2007). This literature informs and reinforces the structure and goals of the YWP.

Adolescents with disabilities are significantly lower in both independence (the disposition to express one's own opinions and to resist the pressure of others to conform) and persistence (the disposition to persist at tasks or goals until they are completed, despite obstacles or difficulties). Interventions to address these areas include involving the teenager in decision-making and goal-setting, encouraging problem-solving and role-playing around problem situations, and reinforcing behaviors related to the acquisition of competence.

The individual health and wellness programming is an intervention designed to serve several purposes. First, it fosters open, candid communication about thoughts and feelings related to health and wellness. Second, it serves as a tool by which to identify perceived strengths and gaps related to various health and wellness domains and rate the level of importance of these areas to the participant. Finally, it allows the participants to develop short-term, achievable goals in identified areas. Overall, this portion of the program provides an opportunity for each participant to express herself independently and freely and feel empowered to create, attain and evaluate her own goals (van Campen & Iedema, 2007).

Stance of the social worker

The stance of the social worker is primarily as the coordinator of this program, a provider of linkages to community resources, an advocate for persons with disabilities, and a facilitator of transition to the IWD Empowerment Program. The social worker also conducts individual health and wellness planning that includes supportive counseling, health education, and care planning.

The program coordinator has found that focusing on ego strengths and weaknesses with the young women as a group and as individuals helps to assess and explore issues. Assisting the participants to identify their strengths as a group and individually has been effective in improving their self-confidence, developing a more positive sense of self, and having a more optimistic and goal-oriented attitude towards the future. No matter what they are facing, all people have the strength to better their lives. Establishing rapport by being a reflective listener reduces the level of threat and brings trust to the client/social worker relationship (Hepworth, Rooney, & Larsen, 2006). In the YWP, this is done with both parents (legal guardians) and participants during our group and individual sessions. Further, Antle (2004) states that in the social model of disability, social workers need to challenge dominant notions of life with disability as tragic, painful, and difficult, and to support parents (legal guardians) as influential players in the evolving self. The group sessions reflect this paradigm shift. They aim to help young women with physical disabilities build esteem-enhancing opportunities and broaden their supportive network beyond their family not only individually but on a larger systems level.

Use of resources outside of the helping relationship

According to the Surgeon General's report, *Call to action to improve the health and wellness of persons with disabilities*, an important strategy is to continue to develop community-based public–private partnerships to facilitate coordinated care and services (U.S. Department of Health and Human Services, 2005). The YWP partners with the community in several ways that mutually benefit the program, its participants, and the community: first, by organizing field trips to different recreation and learning institutions and organizations as a way for the young women to learn what each offers, which are fully accessible and how to navigate transportation; second, through collaboration with other programs which serve the disabled population and conducting cross-marketing and recruitment to maximize participation; and third, by offering joint workshops with programs that incorporate the mission and services of each. To heighten community awareness, we reach out to students, parents, teachers, therapists, and counselors at public and private accessible high schools, and present to professionals at medical centers and community-based organizations focused on health and social services for persons with disabilities. The program coordinator works with community partners on referrals and feedback regarding participants' performance.

Given the program's structure within the IWD, the young women have accessible gynecology and primary care services at the center. The program emphasizes the importance

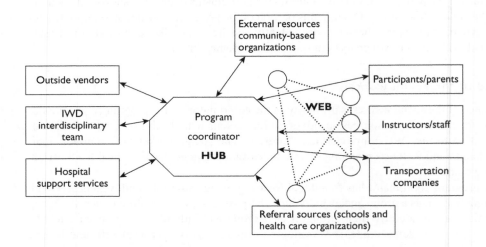

Figure 11.1 Young Women's Program organigraph – a hub with a web. Adapted from Mintzberg & Van der Heyden (1999)

of these medical services, introduces the practitioners, and facilitates the referral process. In addition to coordinating transportation discussed earlier, the coordinator collaborates with the IWD team members and program instructors on program design, curriculum, and individual participants as appropriate. Referrals are made for social work services where individual biopsychosocial assessments are completed and connections made for ongoing mental health services, if needed. The organigraph in Figure 11.1 illustrates the functionality of the program.

Reassessment and evaluation

Group sessions provide opportunities to discuss the unique challenges faced by young women with physical disabilities and yield many positive results. The participants engage in many forms of physical activity for the first time, brave new approaches to wellness, broaden their skills set through the instructors and their peers, discuss their feelings, and begin to connect to each other as friends. Participants initiate independence when parents (legal guardians) allow their daughters to travel and attend the YWP on their own. Participants who were once partially or fully dependent for eating and drinking are initiating autonomy and many young women are trying new activities that they were hesitant about (for example, acupuncture, rowing, drama). Many parents have noted positive changes in their daughters' behavior and attitude which are reflected in this feedback. One mother noted, for example,

> My daughter has really blossomed this year through her experiences at the IWD, especially the course on healthy eating. The transportation was fabulous, thanks for arranging that and it helped her learn to travel on her own. She really likes coming. Even when she is tired or has a lot of school work she always insists on coming. She always leaves happy.

Young women began to develop friendships by communicating with each other and sharing ideas and feelings about being adolescents with physical disabilities. They are empathic, and support one another on how to cope with stressors. They exchange valuable resources on summer internships and camps, attending events at accessible venues and obtaining extra help at school. We know that social support, particularly emotional support, plays an important role in enhancing health and quality of life in women with physical disabilities. This mutual support is expressed in these anecdotes: from a participant, "The program gets me out of the house, I learn new things and meet new people. It is important for my development as a person," and from a parent, "The program helps my daughter socialize and be with other young women with disabilities outside of school."

Community outreach has resulted in increased participation. Inquiries from professionals, primarily in health care and school-based settings, have grown exponentially. Participants' satisfaction has resulted in serving as ambassadors of the program and marketing it to their peers. Several have requested and volunteered to participate in formal presentations to community organizations. 75% of first-time attendees return to future sessions. The classes serve many purposes for the young women. First, 45 minutes seems to be the appropriate time length to teach a topic and hold their interest. Second, classes are diverse in subject matter and focused on experiential learning. Third, classes teach new skills and resources either through the expert instructors and the curriculum. Finally, they give participants the opportunity to learn from each other and socialize in a structured, safe environment.

These quotes offer a small window into the class experiences of the young women: "The exercise helps my body. The discussions teach me things." "I liked all of the classes. The talk we had on traveling with a physical disability is important; we need to know how to do that. I do yoga now at home that I learned at the program." "I liked learning about how to eat healthy, especially the healthy snacks . . . I plan to try those and hopefully with that and exercising I can get in better shape." "It (the program) gives me an outlet. I have freedom and a voice." Related to TSP, "I never knew that I could do this (write and share my writing). TSP pushed me to reach deep inside myself and pull out my feelings which I've always suppressed." "As I was reading my notebook after the workshop ended I realized what deep feelings I expressed. It (TSP) inspired me to enroll in a creative writing course at my college."

Exposure to the program's various health and wellness services through its classes and development of personal goals has resulted in many young women scheduling appointments for medical, wellness, and social work services at the IWD. Several of the young women now see the IWD gynecologist and primary care physician regularly for preventive care and many are seeking nutrition and physical therapy consultations and mental health services.

Program evaluations are completed at the end of each program season to inform future programming and have consistently yielded favorable results. Average results over the past 6 years demonstrate that 70% of participants were highly satisfied in the areas of goal accomplishment, classes and instructors, learning new skills and applying them to everyday situations, and improved overall quality of life in areas of independence, self-confidence and competence, self-advocacy and socialization. In the individual health and wellness planning, 87% responded that they thought the health and wellness planning was helpful in identifying and achieving their own personal goals. The distribution of a typed, signed plan provides something tangible that reinforces goals and provides something to which they can refer to throughout the year. Statements from some young women convey their thoughts about the health and wellness planning. "It gives me something to work towards. I've never really pushed myself like this before." "I like talking about and writing down my goals. It makes it real. Even though I didn't complete all of my goals, I feel a sense of achievement."

Transfer and termination

Conferences are held with participants and sometimes parents (legal guardians) regarding referrals and transitions to other IWD programming. If the participant is interested in pursuing other programs, the coordinator speaks with colleagues regarding the transfer and they connect with the participant for the transition. Participants' files including their demographic and medical background and individual health and wellness plans are forwarded to the appropriate personnel.

Differential discussion

Despite positive evaluations and verbal sentiments from the participants and the achievement of health and wellness goals, it is difficult to formally evaluate the YWP. Health and wellness planning with goal achievement should be measured including a large number of participants over several cycles. A longitudinal study following the YWP participants as they enter adulthood and measuring items such as high school and college graduation rates, employment, independent living, financial independence, and active participation in health care would strengthen our knowledge of program effectiveness. A research study by Stewart, Law, Rosenbaum, and Willms (2001) that examined the transition to adulthood for youth with disabilities reported that many of their youth recognized that their generation is the first of its kind surviving into adulthood and remaining in their communities. Given this fact, the YWP certainly serves a need. With 3,000 participants in the IWD, the Center wishes to expand its mission to study the services it provides for the disabled population, share empirical data, serve as a resource to other organizations specializing in this population, and heighten awareness among the general public. Funding must be secured for this research arm to be developed. The addition of other program components such as partnering participants with adult mentors and expansion of the current cadre of community partners including a linkage with high schools to improve academic performance will enhance future programming.

Discussion questions

1   As social workers, how can we empower the more resistant young women with physical disabilities to take steps towards their independence and provide them with the tools they need?
2   As social workers, how can we work with parents (legal guardians) of young women who are more protective (and often busy with work/other obligations) so they allow/ encourage their daughters to participate in opportunities that will lead towards their self-empowerment and independence?
3   Although passage of legislation and general and assistive technology advances have improved the quality of life for persons with disabilities, what limitations do you think still exist and why? What do you think social workers can do to address these limitations?

References

Antle, B. J. (2004). Factors associated with self-worth in young people with physical disabilities. *Health and Social Work, 29*(3), 167–173. doi: 10.1093/hsw/29.3.167

Chevarley, F., Thierry, J. M., Gill, C. J., Ryerson, A. B., & Nosek, M. A. (2006). Health, preventive health care and health care access among women with disabilities in the 1994–1995, National Health Interview Survey. *Women's Health Issues, 16*(6), 297–312. doi: 10.1016/j.whi.2006.10.002

Hepworth, D., Rooney, R., & Larsen, J. A. (2006). *Direct social work practice: theory and skills* (7th edn.). Pacific Grove, CA: Brooks/Cole.

Kaiser Commission on Medicaid and the Uninsured (2013). *Medicaid: A primer.* Henry J. Kaiser Family Foundation. Retrieved from http://kff.org/medicaid/issue-brief/medicaid-a-primer/

Mintzberg, H. & Van der Heyden, L. (1999). Organigraphs: Drawing how companies really work. *Harvard Business Review,* 87–94.

Nguyen, T., Garrett, R., Downing, A., Walker, L., & Hobbs, D. (2007). Research into telecommunications options for people with physical disabilities. *Assistive Technology, 19*(2),78–93. doi: 10.1080/10400435.2007.10131867

Piotrowski, K. & Snell, L. (2007). Health care needs of women with disabilities across the life span. *Journal of Obstetric, Gynecologic and Neonatal Nursing, 36*(1), 79–87. doi: 10.1111/j.1552-6909.2006.00120x

Rimmer, J.A. & Rowland, J. L. (2008). Physical activity for youth with disabilities: A critical need in an underserved population. *Developmental Neurorehabilitation, 11*(2), 141–148. doi: 10.1080/17518420701688649

Rosenbaum, S. (2000). The Olmstead decision: Implications for state health policy. *Health Affairs, 19*(5), 228–232. doi: 10.1377/hlthaff.19.5.228

Stewart, D., Law, M. C., Rosenbaum, P., & Willms, D. G. (2001). A qualitative study of the transition to adulthood for youth with physical disabilities. *Physical and Occupational Therapy in Pediatrics, 21*(4), 3–17. doi: 10.1080/J006v26n04_02

Substance Abuse and Mental Health Services Administration (2014). Health care and health systems integration. Retrieved from www.samhsa.gov

United States Office of Special Education: Family Center on Technology and Disability (2014). Retrieved from www.fctd.info

U.S. Department of Health and Human Services (2005). *The Surgeon General's call to action to improve the health and wellness of persons with disabilities.* Retrieved from www.surgeon general.gov/library/calls/

Van Campen, C., & Iedema, J. (2007). Are persons with physical disabilities who participate in society healthier and happier? Structural equation modeling of objective participation and subjective well-being. *Quality Life Research, 16,* 635–645. doi: 10.1007/s11136-006-9147.3

Additional web-based resources

Achilles Track Club, www.achillesinternational.org. "With chapters and members in 65 locations within the United States and abroad, Achilles provides athletes with training opportunities in a community of support to gain measurable physical strength and build confidence every day at parks, gyms, and tracks."

Assistive Technology, https://www.disability.gov/resource/disability-govs-guide-assistive-technology/. Assistive technology for persons with limited mobility, vision or dexterity; Computer/electronic accessibility program (CAP); Workplace personal assistance services and assistive technology; State assistive technology financial loan program; Using computer based tests with student with disabilities.

Center for Independence of the Disabled, New York (CIDNY), www.CIDNY.org. CIDNY is part of the Independent Living Centers movement – a national network of grassroots and community-based organizations that enhance opportunities for all people with disabilities to direct their own lives. CIDNY is the voice of persons with disabilities in New York City. It speaks for everyone who lives with a disability, whether it came at birth, by injury, disease, or during the process of aging. It educates the public and advocates for civil rights and a string safety net of benefits and services.

Center for Research on Women with Disabilities (CROWD), www.bcm.edu. CROWD's mission is to promote, develop, and disseminate information to improve the health and expand the life choices of women with disabilities. The faculty and staff accomplishes this by working with a consortium of local and national research collaborators, medical advisors and consumer advisors.

Centers for Disease Control and Prevention: Disability and Health, www.cdc.gov/ncbddd/disability andhealth. Basics; Healthy living; Data and statistics; Partners and programs; Specific groups; Articles; Resources and free materials; Emergency preparedness.

Disability Rights Advocates, www.dralegal.org. Founded in 1993, with offices in California and New York, Disability Rights Advocates (DRA) is one of the leading non-profit disability rights legal centers in the nation. Its mission is to advance equal rights and opportunity for people with all types of disabilities nationwide. DRA is run by people with disabilities for people with disabilities.

Girls Health, www.girlshealth.gov/disability. Information on body, fitness, nutrition, illness and disability, drugs, alcohol and smoking, your feelings, relationships, bullying, safety, your future.

Got Transition/Center for Health Care Transition, www.gottransition.org. An agreement between the Maternal and Child Health Bureau and the National Alliance to Advance Adolescent Health whose aim is to improve transition from pediatric to adult health care through new and innovative strategies for health professionals and youth and families.

Health Information Tool for Empowerment (HITE), www.hitesite.org. An online resource for social workers and other referral providers. HITE's comprehensive customizable directory helps the health and social services workforce provide fast, accurate linkages for uninsured and low-income individuals.

Initiative for Women with Disabilities (IWD), http://iwd.med.nyu.edu

United States Office on Special Education: Family Center on Technology and Disability, www.fctd.info.

The Visible Theatre, Inc., http://dsq-sds.org/article/view/3188/3078. Created opportunities where a diverse community of artists expresses their authentic voice through process and performance, with a belief that cultivating presence and celebrating our deepest humanity will empower and transform us.

YWP Summer Art Workshop Animation, https://www.youtube.com/watch?v=fwW8-OMowQc

YWP Videos on Facebook page: https://www.facebook.com/pages/Initiative-for-Women-with-Disabilities-Young-Womens-Program/145425442179457

Chapter 12

The role of the social worker in transgender health care

Russell Healy

Context

Transgender clients embody a paradox. Their lived experience tells them that they are not ill, but they somehow have found themselves living in a body whose assigned gender feels wrong. This produces a profound dysphoria that can best be addressed through medical intervention. Transgender clients want to experience authentic life without feeling alien in their bodies. In order to access the treatment they need, the transgender client must accept various psychiatric and medical diagnoses. For many trans*[1] persons, having to accede to being ill adds to their dysphoria.

This chapter will offer the social worker in health care a model for the assessment and treatment of young transgender clients and their families. The goal of intervention will be the reduction of gender dysphoria (GD) in the client by facilitating transition. The social worker who works with trans* clients will need specific medical knowledge and skills to interact and collaborate with medical professionals. Additionally, social workers who work with the trans* population must be able to use the *Diagnostic and Statistical Manual of Mental Disorders* (5th edn.) (*DSM-5*) (American Psychiatric Association [APA], 2013), and be able to accurately diagnose GD as well as any other co-occurring conditions. Working with the trans* client truly requires a biopsychosocial approach.

Gender is a complicated topic. Transgender prevalence rates vary because transgender clients or those who present for gender confirmation (surgical or medical procedures to bring bodily consistency with felt gender) are on the extreme ends of a spectrum that encompasses many expressions and experiences of gender. The *DSM-5* reports that 0.0005–0.014% of natal boys are transgender and that 0.0002–0.0003% of natal girls are transgender (APA, 2013, p. 454). Social workers who work with trans* clients will initially encounter the idea that gender is not a simple male–female binary. Rather, it exists on a fluid, multi-dimensional continuum that acknowledges and challenges social norms while also emphasizing how people relate to one another and understand their gender-self. Erin Markman writes that, "societal definition of gender as binary leaves no space for transgender experience to be considered normal" (Markman, 2011, p. 17). She believes that social work allies of the trans* community have an ethical obligation to work towards depathologization (Markman, 2011). Consistent with social work's person-in-environment perspective, trans* persons and their allies believe that the pathology exists in oppressive societal and cultural norms, not in the individual. It is also important to understand that for many trans* clients, issues such as gender fluidity may be meaningless. They have no problem with the notion of a gender binary. They simply believe that they are on the wrong side of the binary. As many trans* clients will tell us, they basically want to "pass" through life as the gender they know themselves to be.[2]

The *DSM-5* relies mostly on client report to diagnose GD in adolescents and adults. The diagnosis of GD may be made when "a marked incongruence between one's experienced/ expressed gender and assigned gender, of at least six months' duration" is manifested by at least two of six criteria. Adolescents and adults may experience or express marked incongruence with primary and/or secondary sex characteristics in addition to GD regarding their bodies. The *DSM* states that the client may express a "strong desire" to be rid of their genitals or secondary sex characteristics such as breasts, or to be the other gender or to be treated as the other gender. There may also be a "strong conviction" that the client has the feelings and reactions of the other gender. Some clients assert that they are "other gendered," one that is neither male nor female but contains elements of both. Finally, the client's condition must be "associated with clinically significant distress or impairment in social, occupational, or other important areas of functioning" (APA, 2013, pp. 452–453).

Words such as "discomfort," "distress," and "incongruence" are used in the *DSM* to describe GD. According to the *New Oxford American Dictionary*, the term dysphoria derives from the mid-nineteenth century Greek *dusphoria* or "hard to bear." Its antonym is euphoria. In my clinical experience, the language of the *DSM* minimizes the lived experience of GD. For example, many trans* youth will avoid mirrors because they do not want to see their faces or their bodies. When they do catch a reflection of their appearance, they describe a feeling of panic, horror, and helplessness. I believe that when they are aware, or are reminded, that they are living in the wrong body, they feel something akin to what people with post-traumatic stress disorder feel, except that these young trans* clients are not having flashbacks. They are re-experiencing trauma every time realizations of the wrongness of their bodies enter their minds.

Many transgender adolescents experience a crisis at the onset of puberty, when their vague feelings of "otherness" become clear, and their bodies begin to develop secondary sex characteristics. The *DSM-5* refers to these clients as late-onset types. In retrospect, some of these clients acknowledge that they always felt "different" but they never consciously thought about gender. Early-onset types are always children, some as young as 2 years old. In such cases the dysphoria is manifested behaviorally through a willful insistence on cross-dressing or cross-gender play and playmates. If they verbalize their feelings they simply state that they *are* the gender they experience themselves as (APA, 2013, pp. 453–456; Gregor, Davidson, & Hingley-Jones, 2014).

Both the World Professional Association for Transgender Health (WPATH) and the APA hold that gender non-conforming behavior and GD are different phenomena (APA, 2013; Coleman et al., 2012). Both organizations attempt to address the depathologization movement by acknowledging that gender expression is personal but constrained by social roles and cultural values. The trans* community refers to persons whose biologically assigned gender matches their experience as *cisgender*. The term is not hierarchical and does not imply normal and abnormal. In chemistry, the prefix *cis* means that molecule groups lie on the same side (of a carbon center) rather than *trans* where they are on opposite sides. Functionally, through their presence in our lives, trans* people are asking us to expand our view of gender and consider that gender exists in the self and the mind, not in anatomy.

In the past decade, health care providers have noticed a measurable and substantial increase in the referrals of children and adolescence with GD. A recent study has found that when the first multi-disciplinary gender clinic, the Gender Management Service (GeMS) in Boston, was established in the United States in 2007, the rate of referrals of children and adolescents increased fourfold (Spack et al., 2012). Similar results were found in the Netherlands when a gender clinic expanded (de Vries & Cohen-Kettinis, 2012). Very little explains this trend. Some wonder if social media and improvements in information technology (faster internet connection speeds and newer algorithms for retrieving data) have created opportunities for young people to gather information about their dysphoria and learn about treatment options earlier than ever before. Consequently, GD may become more pronounced and persistent. This is when parents may seek help for their child or adolescent.

Recently, there have been media reports linking trans* youth and the risk of self-injury or suicide. The research on the topic varies greatly, with some studies reporting that 45% of trans* youth have experienced suicidal ideation and as many as 26% have attempted suicide or engaged in "life-threatening behaviors" (Grossman & D'Augelli, 2007, p. 532). Research also identifies protective factors. According to social worker Caitlyn Ryan of the Family Acceptance Project, the risk of suicide for trans* youth decreases as the strength of family acceptance increases (Ryan, Russell, Huebner, Diaz, & Sanchez, 2010). It is important for social workers to understand the role of parental acceptance and to work with parents if they are struggling to accept their child. Other studies have suggested that in addition to suicide prevention, "parents of transgender youth may have a crucial opportunity to offset the mental health impact of societal harassment and discrimination their children receive" (Simons, Schrager, Clark, Belzer, & Olson, 2013, p. 793).

Policy

No established social or medical policy exists in the United States specific to trans* persons. From a legal perspective, trans* rights vary state by state and within federal statutes. A good deal of controversy exists regarding whether or not trans* individuals (especially children) ought to receive a psychiatric diagnosis in the first place. Understandably, many in the trans* community oppose the use of psychiatric diagnosis. Some advocate for the depathologization of transgenderism (Suess, Espineira, & Walters, 2014), arguing that the act of diagnosis contributes to the oppression they already experience. Others, more concerned with seeking medical assistance, accept that they have to adhere to the medical model in order to receive help. The root of the debate is the fact that research money and resources for treatment are tied directly to the existence of a diagnosis.

Outside of the United States the International Classification of Disorders (ICD) is used for all diagnosis (Eisfeld, 2014). While the ICD shares the same controversy as the *DSM*, specifically, coding transgenderism as pathology, some believe that the medical focus of the ICD can be an alternative to diagnosing trans* persons as having both a mental disorder and a medical disorder (Lev, 2013).

Full gender reassignment is expensive. In the United States, the system of private health care covers the medical needs of trans* patients on a policy-by-policy basis. Some procedures are covered, such as hormone replacement therapy (HRT) or surgical procedures such as mastectomies and hysterectomies. Insurance companies frequently challenge genital reconstruction surgeries. Medicare has begun covering some trans*-specific procedures, but at the time of this writing it is unclear exactly how such treatment will be administered. The social worker will need to learn, on a plan-by-plan basis, how different procedures are covered, and how to document for medical necessity.

In the absence of clear social or political policies, medical standards of care are recognized by most nations. A *Standards of Care* manual is frequently updated by WPATH reporting treatment technology and research advances. The current version also addresses ethical and social justice concerns. Therefore, WPATH's SOC v7 informs much of this chapter (Coleman et al., 2012).

Technology

Medical intervention for the trans* client falls into three categories: reversible, partially reversible, and irreversible. Reversible treatments are generally used with children with GD. Referred to as the "Dutch Approach" (de Vries & Cohen-Kettinis, 2012), puberty-delaying medications such as gonadotropin-releasing hormone analogs (GnRHa), luteinizing hormone-releasing hormone agonists (LHRH), or medroxyprogesterone are administered to suspend the development of puberty (Coolhart, Baker, Farmer, Malaney, & Shipman, 2013). This allows children who experience GD a window of about 2 years to discover whether or not their dysphoria will desist or continue to persist, without the added stress of the physical changes associated with puberty. It also allows them to experiment living as their experienced gender in at least one sphere of their life. Endocrinologists and WPATH recommend that the puberty-blocking treatment needs to begin at the onset of puberty, around Tanner stage 2.[3] At this stage there is *some* breast and *some* testicular development. This stage can occur as young as age 9 but more likely around age 12 (Coleman et al., 2012; Olson, Forbes & Belzer, 2011).

If, after a trial of puberty-suppressing treatment, it is clear that an adolescent requires gender-confirming treatment, then partially reversible HRT can commence. Fundamentally, HRT induces a second, more congruent puberty. The Dutch protocols also allow for HRT to begin while the adolescent is in puberty, thereby replacing an incongruent puberty with one that substantially reduces dysphoria. The belief is that if transitioning begins as early as is medically sound, the physical outcome will be greatly improved, which, in turn, improves the emotional and social well-being of the client (de Vries & Cohen-Kettinis, 2012).

Dr. Norman Spack of GeMS found that many of the children and adolescents referred to his clinic have significant psychiatric histories (44.3%) that include instances of self-harm (21.6%). He speculated that "psychological functioning improves with medical intervention . . . psychiatric symptoms might be secondary to a medical incongruence between mind and body, not primarily psychiatric" (pp. 422–423). I have seen the use of puberty-blocking medication or hormones work so well that psychiatric medications can be reduced or eliminated altogether.

The transition from female to male (FTM) may be seen as an easier one than transitioning from male to female (MTF). For FTMs, testosterone does a lot of the work: the voice gets lower in register, hair grows, and fat migrates to masculinize the body. Because of the effects of testosterone, FTMs can use exercise to amplify masculinization. Once testosterone is discontinued, the voice will not return nor will the hair go away. Some of the likely potential risks associated with testosterone replacement therapy are: acne, weight gain, polycythemia, balding, and sleep apnea. Possible and less likely risks include type 2 diabetes, hypertension, and cardiovascular problems. However, certain co-factors need to exist for these problems to manifest. Those are the main irreversible aspects of testosterone therapy for FTM clients. Some studies have suggested that ovarian, uterine, or breast cancer may be associated with testosterone treatment, but WPATH states that the data are so inconclusive that there may be no increased risk (Coleman et al., 2012, p. 40).

Estrogen therapy does not affect an MTF's voice, so voice training may be required. Estrogen can cause weight gain, so MTFs may need to change their diets and add exercise to their lifestyle. The irreversible effects of HRT on MTF clients include permanent breast development. Some of the potential risks of HRT for MTFs include the increased possibility of venous thromboembolic disease (if estrogen is administered orally rather than transdermally), elevated liver enzymes, gallstones, and weight gain. With the presence of additional risk factors, such as obesity or family history, there is a chance of developing hypertension and type 2 diabetes. As with testosterone treatment, WPATH states that the risk of certain cancers is inconclusive enough to speculate that there may be no increased risk (Coleman et al., 2012, p. 40). These risks justify having an endocrinologist monitor HRT, not outright rejection of HRT.

The irreversible treatments for trans* clients involve surgery. For FTM clients, double mastectomies, otherwise known as "top surgery," are the first and perhaps most essential procedure. Frequently, breast removal initiates a significant reduction in GD. If that continues, many FTMs elect not to proceed further. If they are using testosterone effectively, eating well, and exercising regularly, they pass easily as men. If they wish to pursue a full gender transition, then a hysterectomy and an oophorectomy are recommended. Once these procedures occur, the trans* man must remain on testosterone for life. The next step would then be genital reconstruction surgery. There are several procedures from which to choose, but success often depends on the degree to which testosterone has enlarged the clitoris. For FTM persons, their biggest concern, beyond passing and eliminating GD, is the maintenance of sensation in the nipples and genitals. For top surgery, the symmetric appearance of the nipples is highly valued.

Surgical procedures for MTF clients generally involve an orchiectomy, the removal of the testes, and a penectomy, the removal of the penis. After the genitals are removed, genital reconstructive surgeries such as vaginoplasty, clitoroplasty, and vulvoplasty may occur. According to WPATH, "sex reassignment surgery is effective and medically necessary" (Coleman et al., 2012, p. 54). A full description of the various procedures may be found in the WPATH SOC v7, in addition to the ethical reasons for such procedures and why they are not simple cosmetic surgeries (Coleman et al., 2012), an important rationale when advocating for a client's insurance coverage of procedures.

Young MTF clients have reproductive issues to address. Many choose to have sperm samples frozen and stored for later use should they want to have biological offspring, especially if they forecast partnering with women. In addition, MTF transwomen may require cosmetic procedures in order to feminize their appearance effectively. These include trachea shaves as well as extensive hair removal through electrolysis or by laser. If HRT does not promote the development of breasts to the client's satisfaction, breast augmentation procedures may be necessary.

Information technology comes into play because gender transitions are social and legal as well as medical. Legal transitioning refers to name changes and changes in gender markers on identification such as driver's licenses, passports, and birth certificates. Most documents clients will need are available online. Moreover, social transitioning is enhanced through the use of information technology. Many young trans* clients use the internet for social support or even social life. Online, trans* persons can be who they truly are through names, avatars, and narrative.

Organization

Trans* clients may be encountered in mental health as well as health care settings. The social worker's role can be multi-faceted. Licensed clinical social workers may be required to function as both primary counselor and gatekeeper. They may also function as case managers in gender clinics or hospitals, providing counseling, assessments, resources, and support. Another important social work function is advocacy. We may be called on to provide education for the various systems in the trans* client's life. We may also be asked to train colleagues in various realms of health care.

Historically there has been distrust between trans* patients and their providers. Social work specialists in trans*-specific care frequently believe that advocacy and assessment should be "trans-affirmative." Because the gatekeeping function of the clinician can create a power differential between trans* clients and social workers, the trans* affirmative approach helps to build a trusting alliance that respects the gender language the client prefers (Collazo, Austin, & Craig, 2013). Whether practicing independently or on a gender team, social work with trans* clients requires that we use our full range of assessment, engagement, and relationship-building skills.

In Canada and Western Europe, gender clinics provide trans* persons with one-stop shopping. In the United States, there are limited gender clinics (usually affiliated with universities or hospitals), such as the GeMS in Boston. In cities with large lesbian, gay, bisexual, or trans* populations (LGBT), quality transgender care is offered by centers that serve the LGBT community, for example, the Mazzoni Center in Philadelphia.

I work as a solo practitioner in a metropolitan area. Clients are referred to me through various sources including physicians, other clinicians, school systems, youth centers, and parent support groups such as Parents and Friends of Lesbians and Gays (PFLAG). The biggest challenge for the independent provider is maintaining a network of medical professionals with whom the social worker can collaborate. Such professionals include pediatric and general endocrinologists, primary care physicians, plastic surgeons, and psychiatrists. Many trans* clients prefer to research surgeons on their own, and are willing to travel out of State for the surgeon with whom they are most comfortable. Others prefer one-stop shopping and are willing to travel to a nearby city with a gender clinic.

Decisions about practice

One of the most unnerving things that can happen to an FTM adolescent is the menses cycle. Horrified by their periods, some FTM teenagers will induce anorexia in an attempt to stop the menses cycle. As I will illustrate in the case example that follows, there are better ways to address the dysphoria FTM adolescents experience as a result of unwanted menstruation.

Description of the client

Jack, 15, was a natal female who recalls having felt "like a boy" since early childhood. Because he appeared to be a tomboy, his family never took notice of his gender non-conforming behavior. Shortly after turning 13, Jack began to isolate himself when he was not at school or playing sports. He spent a lot of time alone in his room playing interactive, online games during which he passed himself off as a boy to the other players. Eventually, Jack made a few online friends and revealed that he was an FTM transboy. His new friends suggested several online trans* youth forums where Jack learned that anorexic girls often lose their periods as a consequence of not eating. He managed to keep up his grades, so, again, his parents were not concerned about how much time he was spending alone. He began losing weight, which his parents attributed to his athleticism and puberty.

Jack successfully managed to eliminate his period for two months, but his emaciated appearance alarmed his parents. They took him to a pediatrician who had him admitted to an inpatient program for adolescents with eating disorders. While there, Jack revealed to a psychiatrist that he developed anorexia to avoid having periods. This was as close as he could get to revealing to an adult that he was trans*. No one recognized this disclosure's import and meaning, so Jack withdrew into himself again.

Jack was discharged to an intensive outpatient program for adolescent girls with eating disorders (ED). He hated the all female milieu. From early childhood, he had always related better with boys. He resisted the eating plan imposed on him by the program's nutritionist. In less than a year, Jack went from being a friendly and cooperative teen into an oppositional and sullen adolescent. His parents were understandably alarmed. One evening during the usual power struggle over eating dinner, his mother lost her composure and asked Jack directly "why" he was "doing this." Jack locked himself in the upstairs bathroom, burst into tears, and took a handful of pills. His parents called the mobile crisis response unit and Jack was evaluated and treated at the local emergency unit. Feeling tired and hopeless, Jack told the crisis worker his secret.

Goals, objectives, and contracting

The crisis screener referred Jack to me but I insisted that he remain in the ED program while he and his family were seeing me concurrently. Anorexia is a compulsive and potentially fatal condition; I needed to be certain that Jack was sufficiently in remission before he could discontinue ED-specific therapy. The WPATH SOC states that all "co-existing mental health concerns need to be optimally managed prior to, or concurrent with, treatment of gender dysphoria" (Coleman et al., 2012, p. 25). Fortunately the ED treatment team was happy to collaborate. All parties involved wished that Jack had revealed his true self to us, but his tendency to withdraw inwardly is a common method of coping for trans* adolescents. They do not expect to be believed and are afraid of the rejection they might face. Their thinking becomes constricted until they break through or act out.

I met first with Jack's parents. They were unconditionally supportive but struggled to accept that their daughter was now their son. Understandably, his suicidal gesture alarmed them as well. I talked with them about what is known about suicide risk and prevention, and how their acceptance and support could mitigate future instances of self-harm. At this stage of counseling, there are two concerns. First is what needs to be done in the family to begin to reduce an adolescent's GD. Second is what can be done medically to alleviate any distressing physical symptoms, such as Jack's periods. Priority is based on what is most pressing for the trans* client. In Jack's case it was his menses cycle.

Jack was too old to begin puberty-blocking therapy. Besides, at 15, Jack's GD had not desisted. That meant that he would continue to experience GD until he could begin to transition to male. I was comfortable recommending HRT, but I was concerned that his parents would find this to be a radical move so early in the treatment. To help Jack, I needed the trust of his parents. I knew that I had a small window of opportunity to recommend a treatment that could help yet be reversible.

Strategies and interventions

In cases like Jack's, the administration of long-term birth control (continuous oral contraception) may be used to disrupt an FTM trans* client's menstrual cycle. This seemed like the best recommendation, one that could relieve Jack's distress and would appear reasonable to his parents. To his immense relief, Jack's parents agreed to use continuous oral conception. I referred them to a pediatric endocrinologist who could also begin HRT when Jack was ready.

After this intervention, individual sessions with Jack had more utility. One measurement of trust in the social worker is if a trans* client will reveal what is most often on their mind: their bodies. Trans* youth are especially preoccupied with how they appear. They worry about their hips, the size of their hands or feet, facial structure, facial hair (or lack thereof), and all manner of physical presentation. Jack was almost disarmingly open with me when discussing his body. He would show me his stomach and ask me if I saw abs or flex his arm and ask me if they were "girl's arms or boy's arms." He had begun to eat normally and gained enough weight to be discharged from the ED program in three months. In preparation for HRT he began a sensible exercise program. He wanted to acquire the habit of exercise so that he could take full advantage of HRT.

Stance of the social worker

Should the social worker take a position regarding HRT or even surgery for a minor? That is a matter of professional preference and cumulative experience. Cisgender social workers can assume a professional stance, an ally stance, or even an activist stance. Our primary role is to reduce persistent GD. My stance is that of an ally with professional social work skills that allow me to advocate for my clients, work with family and community, and help navigate the world of complex information and medical systems.

Jack had exceptionally supportive parents, and that made my work easier because they initiated the vital medical interventions proactively. When Jack turned 16 they felt he was ready to begin HRT and asked me for a referral letter, thereby eliminating the issue of informed consent. They were open to non-medical interventions from the beginning. For example, Jack disclosed that he had been wrapping ace bandages around his chest to make it look flat. I took out my laptop and showed him a website where he could purchase "binders" made for FTM adolescents. I recommended family tasks regarding proper pronoun use such as "he" and not "she." For every pronoun error two quarters would be placed in a jar. For every proper pronoun use a quarter could be removed. Although such paternalistic interventions are sometimes uncomfortable, this family accepted the guidance.

Working with trans* youth may require that the social worker function as a consultant to the various stakeholders and systems in the social life of the client. In Jack's case and at his request, I met with key administrators, faculty, and staff at his high school to explain why Jack needed access to a single bathroom and to be allowed to dress for gym in a private area. Jack preferred to go "stealth" (pass as a tomboy) in every other aspect of his social transition at school, so pronoun use at school was not a concern. If safety were an issue, then I would have taken a stance that the school should institute policies and procedures around issues such as bullying. I would offer to provide in-service training for all faculty and staff. Such interventions would have to be done without violating Jack's confidentiality. In other contexts one could argue that the social worker would have a dual role if they were providing an in-service seminar that is essentially about a client. One resolution to this ethical dilemma would be to recommend another resource. But, if one does not exist, the social worker would have to navigate those waters skillfully and personally.

Termination and conclusion

My work with Jack and his parents ended when he turned 19. He decided to take a year off between high school and college. He underwent top surgery the summer after high school ended and used the rest of the year to work on transitioning socially and legally. He changed his name legally and was able to get the gender marker on his driver's license changed to male. With some difficulty he was able to get the gender marker on his birth certificate changed to male. The problems he encountered were bureaucratic, and they triggered a temporary increase in GD symptoms. His parents offered to hire an attorney to handle the birth certificate issue. Jack, to his credit, insisted on doing it himself. He researched colleges that would be trans* accommodating and friendly. He was accepted at the school of his choice. At his last visit Jack appeared happy.

What would I expect if Jack were to return for more care? The issues would likely revolve around genital and bottom surgeries. The duty of the clinician is not to help the client decide whether or not to undergo surgery. Clients have to decide for themselves, or, most likely, they already have. The social work clinician's primary task is to determine readiness and eligibility, and assess informed consent. If Jack wanted a full gender transition he would likely require three surgical procedures: a hysterectomy, an oophorectomy, and genital reconstruction surgery. The latter surgery may involve multiple procedures and a relatively lengthy period of recovery. I believe the best way to assess informed consent is if the client does their own research and comes to sessions informed. If he had not already, I would ask Jack to do his research and bring his findings to a session. Our conversations would focus on four factors: the benefits and drawbacks of surgery and the benefits and drawbacks of not having surgery. This is not to suggest that supportive counseling would not be required. Trans* clients live in a cisgender world. Essentially, they are always transitioning. The counseling function of social work can be helpful; however, it is important to keep in mind that transgender-specific counseling is not psychotherapy for a mental disorder. It is about helping trans* clients adjust to and live in a world that can be inhospitable towards them.

Differential discussion

Jack's case could have gone very differently if Jack was less responsive or if his parents were unaccepting. If Jack continued to withhold or did not respond to the ED treatment program, I would have either terminated trans*-specific treatment or muddled through on my own. The latter would be risky because at the time I had very little training in working with ED. Had his parents been unable to shift their perspective to one of active and loving acceptance of their former daughter, now a son, Jack's GD most certainly would have persisted and increased. Moreover, if Jack's high school was resistant to the recommendations, his oppositional and defiant behavior likely would have continued.

Instead, what I experienced reflected the finding that parental support, and by extension, community support, are powerful protective factors for trans* youth. As I continue to work with this population I am struck by how attached trans* youth are to their accepting parents and to what lengths those parents will go to protect and help their child. Interestingly, most trans* youth from accepting families I have seen do not go through a rebellious phase. Jack's oppositional and defiant behavior ended when his parents agreed to the use of continuous birth control.

There is one thing I would have done differently. I would have collaborated more closely with the ED program Jack attended. Social work's person-in-environment perspective suggests that treatment ought to be holistic and not split off into pieces. I was correct to trust them; they ran a great program, but a little more communication from me might have helped Jack to overcome his ED more quickly.

If the trend continues, trans* clients will present for services during childhood or adolescence. Social work, as a profession, is in a unique position to assist and advocate for this client population. Some social workers will undoubtedly feel uncomfortable with the idea that a young person's gender can be reassigned by medical technology. Perhaps it seems technology is advancing faster than our ability to acquire a moral grasp. History contains many examples of useful technology that initially appeared to outpace our social development. Having worked with clients with GD for a number of years, I have witnessed first hand how much trans* people suffer. Regardless of the area of practice a social worker chooses, it is a matter of justice to do whatever we can to alleviate suffering in the lives of persons, according to our individual capacities, our personal beliefs, and our values as professional social workers.

Discussion questions

1   How comfortable are you as a clinician viewing gender as a continuum rather than a binary? What arguments support either view?
2   How might you approach Jack, recognizing that he needs his parents support, yet also is of an age where he needs to rebel developmentally?
3   What creative ways might you suggest to reach the peer groups of trans* youth to educate them and advocate for acceptance while avoiding ostracizing any individual trans* youth?

Notes

1 The asterisk is part of trans* culture. It is used to acknowledge the wide and fluid range of gender experience, gender expression, and gender identity (Tompkins, 2014). Although in current use, preferred usage changes rapidly and this reflects preferred usage in 2015 when this chapter was written.
2 For purposes of this chapter, the focus will be on the transgender client who is seeking gender confirmation, previously called reassignment. There are many expressions and experiences of gender on the fluid spectrum. They deserve their own consideration.
3 The Tanner stage model (Coleman, et al., 2012, p. 18) offers endocrinologists and pediatricians a method of determining an adolescent's stage of puberty.

References

APA (American Psychiatric Association) (2013). *Diagnostic and statistical manual of mental health disorders* (5th edn.). Arlington, VA: American Psychiatric Publishing.

Coleman, E., Bockting, W., Botzer, M., Cohen-Kettenis, P., DeCuypere, G., Feldman, J., & Zucker, K. (2012). *Standards of care for the health of transsexual, transgender, and gender-nonconforming people, version 7*. World Professional Association for Transgender Health (WPATH). Retrieved from www.wpath.org/site_page.cfm?pk_association_webpage_menu=1351

Collazo, A., Austin, A., & Craig, S. L. (2013). Facilitating transition among transgender clients: components of effective clinical practice. *Clinical Social Work Journal, 41*(3), 228–237. doi: 10.1007/s10615-013-0463-3

Coolhart, D., Baker, A., Farmer, S., Malaney, M., & Shipman, D. (2013). Therapy with transsexual youth and their families: A clinical tool for assessing youth's readiness for gender transition. *Journal of Marital and Family Therapy, 39*(2), 223–243. doi: 10.1111/j.1752-0606.2011.00283.x de Vries, A. L., & Cohen-Kettenis, P. T. (2012). Clinical management of gender dysphoria in children and adolescents: The Dutch approach. *Journal of Homosexuality, 59*(3), 301–320. doi: 10.1080/00918369.2012.653300

Eisfeld, J. (2014). International statistical classification of diseases and related health problems. *TSQ: Transgender Studies Quarterly, 1*(1–2), 107–110. doi: 10.1215/23289252-2399740

Gregor, C., Davidson, S., & Hingley-Jones, H. (2014). The experience of gender dysphoria for pre-pubescent children and their families: A review of the literature. *Child & Family Social Work.* doi: 10.1111/cfs.12150

Grossman, A. H. & D'Augelli, A. R. (2007). Transgender youth and life-threatening behaviors. *Suicide and Life-Threatening Behavior, 37*(5), 527–537. doi: 10.1521/suli.2007.37.5.527

Lev, A. I. (2013). Gender dysphoria: Two steps forward, one step back. *Clinical Social Work Journal, 41*(3), 288–296. doi: 10.1007/s10615-013-0447-0

Markman, E. R. (2011). Gender identity disorder, the gender binary, and transgender oppression: Implications for ethical social work. *Smith College Studies in Social Work, 81*(4), 314–327. doi: 10.1080/00377317.2011.616839

Olson, J., Forbes, C., & Belzer, M. (2011). Management of the transgender adolescent. *Archives of Pediatrics & Adolescent Medicine, 165*(2), 171–176. doi: 10.1001/archpediatrics.2010.275

Ryan, C., Russell, S. T., Huebner, D., Diaz, R., & Sanchez, J. (2010). Family acceptance in adolescence and the health of LGBT young adults. *Journal of Child and Adolescent Psychiatric Nursing, 23*(4), 205–213. doi: 10.1111/j.1744-6171.2010.00246.x

Simons, L., Schrager, S. M., Clark, L. F., Belzer, M., & Olson, J. (2013). Parental support and mental health among transgender adolescents. *Journal of Adolescent Health, 53*(6), 791–793. doi: 10.1016/j.jadohealth.2013.07.019

Spack, N. P., Edwards-Leeper, L., Feldman, H. A., Leibowitz, S., Mandel, F., Diamond, D. A., & Vance, S. R. (2012). Children and adolescents with gender identity disorder referred to a pediatric medical center. *Pediatrics, 129*(3), 418–425. doi: 10.1542/peds.2011-0907

Suess, A., Espineira, K., & Walters, P. (2014). Depathologization. *TSQ: Transgender Studies Quarterly, 1*(1–2), 73–77. doi: 10.1215/232895252-2399497

Tompkins, A. (2014). Asterisk. *TSQ: Transgender Studies Quarterly, 1*(1–2), 26–27. doi: 10.1215/23289252-2399497

Resources

Laura's Playground, www.lauras-playground.com. A useful blog site for trans* clients.
twinfools, https://www.youtube.com/user/twinfools. A young transman chronicles his transition.
World Professional Association for Transgender Health (WPATH), www.wpath.org

Adults

Chapter 13

The social worker on the genetic counseling team

A new role in social work oncology

Susan Scarvalone, Julianne S. Oktay, Jessica Scott, and Kathy Helzlsouer

Context

In 1994, the highly penetrant genetic mutations *BRCA1* and *BRCA2* (Friedman et al., 1994; Wooster et al., 1995) that result in a high risk of breast and fallopian/ovarian cancer were discovered. This gave women with a strong family history of cancer the opportunity to clarify and manage their risk through genetic counseling, testing, and preventive care. Subsequently, additional genetic mutations associated with an increased risk of cancer have been identified, expanding the role of genetic counseling and testing for cancer patients (Minion et al., 2015). *BRCA1* and *BRCA2* explain the majority of genetic breast and ovarian cancer cases. Approximately 10% of women with breast cancer have a strong genetic predisposition to cancer and about half of these women carry mutation in *BRCA1* or *BRCA2* (Weltzel, Blazer, MacDonald, Culver, & Offit, 2011).

Description of the setting

The Prevention and Research Center provides cancer risk assessment and genetic counseling services for women at high risk for cancer based on their family history of cancer. The cancer risk assessment was designed as a multi-disciplinary team including a physician, genetic counselor, social worker, and nurse practitioner. The social worker is the primary clinician to address the social and emotional needs of patients in the Center. In addition to the cancer risk assessments, the social worker participates in program design, facilitates a variety of group support programs for patients and their family members, provides short-term counseling, and participates in a multi-disciplinary cancer survivorship clinic.

Policy

Several policy issues affect the provision of genetic counseling, including costs of testing, insurance coverage, confidentiality, and potential for discrimination (McEwen, 2006). Following the discovery of the genes *BRCA1* and *BRCA2*, the testing was only available through one laboratory. In 2013, the Supreme Court ruled that human genes could not be patented (Liptak, 2013) and now multiple laboratories offer genetic testing. Genetic tests use DNA isolated from blood or saliva samples and the genes are sequenced, looking for mutations (alterations) in the genetic sequence. If a mutation is present, the laboratory determines if that gene change leads to an increased risk of cancer. The cost for genetic testing varies by the type of test and the laboratory but can range from a few hundred dollars when testing for a specific gene mutation to several thousand dollars for full genetic sequencing for multiple genes.

The cost of genetic counseling and testing is usually paid by a patient's private or public health insurance. Although the passage and implementation (2010–14) of the Patient Protection and Affordable Care Act (ACA, 2010) reduced the number of Americans who do not have health insurance (ObamaCare Facts, n.d.), lack of adequate health insurance continues to be problematic in the United States, especially for those states that did not opt for Medicaid expansion.

While genetic services are covered by most health insurance programs, the coverage varies from program to program, as do deductibles and co-pays. Medicare, the primary coverage for individuals over age 65 or living with disability, covers the cost of genetic testing only if the person has a personal history of cancer and meets certain family history criteria. Other insurers cover those at risk of developing cancer, with some variation about the necessity of family history of cancer. In short, social workers must be aware of many individual and public variations in coverage. Cancer genetic testing costs are discussed as part of the genetic counseling process. If a mutation is found, additional costs related to preventive surgery, medications, and increased surveillance may be incurred.

Patients may worry about the potential for discrimination based on genetic testing. When genetic information first became available, discrimination in employment and insurance coverage, including health, long-term care, disability, and life insurances began to occur (Oktay, 1998). Since then, several federal and state legislative initiatives have been passed prohibiting discrimination based on genetic testing, such as the Americans with Disabilities Act of 1990 (ADA, 1990–2015), Health Insurance Portability and Accountability Act of 1996 (HIPAA) (U.S. Department of Health and Human Services, 2005), and the Genetic Information Nondiscrimination Act (GINA) (NCHPEG, 2010). However, GINA does not cover disability, life, or long-term care insurance policies and genetic test results may impact the insurability of patients with respect to these policies (Werner-Lin, 2015). Some states enacted genetic nondiscrimination laws and the ACA prohibits health insurance providers from denying coverage based on "pre-existing conditions," another protection for those who use genetic testing.

Social workers interested in genetic services should be familiar with insurance and workplace discrimination issues. Social workers can educate patients about the protections available to them and can also help patients weigh concerns about genetic testing against the fact that genetic test results can provide important clinical information for their health care providers. Social workers can also help patients to decide with whom, and how, to share their results.

Technology

Clinical genetic testing for *BRCA1* and *BRCA2* mutations became available shortly after the discovery of the gene in 1994. *BRCA1* and *BRCA2* genes are incompletely penetrant, meaning that not everyone who carries a mutation will develop breast cancer. For example, for women who carry a mutation in one of the *BRCA* genes, the lifetime risk of developing breast cancer can vary from 80% to 85% (Patenaude, 2005). The risk for fallopian/ovarian cancer may be 20–40%, compared to a less than 2% lifetime risk for the general population (Ford et al., 1998). Men who carry mutations in *BRCA1* or *BRCA2* are also at increased risk of cancer, including breast cancer, but the rates of cancer are lower than among women who carry mutations. Both men and women inherit these mutations in an autosomal dominant pattern, meaning that a child of a person with a mutation in one of these two genes has a 50% chance of inheriting the mutation.

Education and counseling before and after testing is critically important. Counseling includes assessment of the family history of cancer, determination of the most appropriate genetic test to order, discussion of the potential results and limitation of testing, discussion of the potential treatment options based on test results, and review of the impact of the test results more generally for the patient and his or her family. In-depth education about the test results, as well as limitations of testing, influences individuals' decisions about using genetic tests (Biesecker et al., 2000).

Organization

The program is based in an academically affiliated urban community hospital with a founding mission to provide high-quality care to the poor and underserved inner-city population. The patient population is diverse socioeconomically, racially, and culturally. The hospital is a full-service community hospital and includes an American College of Surgeons accredited cancer center with a strong focus on women's health. The cancer genetic counseling services are located in the same building as the Cancer Institute, which includes medical, surgical, and radiation oncology, and the Women's Health Center, which houses the Breast Center and the Gynecology Oncology Center.

Description of typical clients

Two primary groups of women seek genetic testing for hereditary breast cancer syndromes: women diagnosed with breast or ovarian cancer and women unaffected but who have a family history of cancer. Women diagnosed with cancer may be referred for genetic testing by their physician because the treatment plans may be tailored to specific genetic mutations. Characteristics that make a genetic mutation more likely include: having early-onset breast cancer (with diagnosis before age 50 years), having bilateral breast cancer, having a history of both breast and ovarian cancers, and having multiple similarly affected family members. Genetic testing may also be sought by women with a family history of cancer or a relative identified as a carrier of a genetic mutation. Some may seek genetic testing based on their ethnic background: there is high prevalence of genetic mutation in individuals of Ashkenazi Jewish ancestry (about 2.5%) (Manchanda et al., 2015).

The ideal process for genetic testing is to first test someone in the family who has had cancer in order to determine if the family history can be attributed to a mutation in *BRCA1* or *BRCA2*, or other genes. If a genetic mutation is identified, then subsequent testing of family members is conducted, testing only for that specific mutation. The targeted test costs less than full sequencing.

There are four possible results from the *BRCA1* and *BRCA2* genetic testing (Miller et al., 2006). The result can be "positive," meaning that a patient has a deleterious mutation that is known to cause increased risk for cancer development. A second result is "true negative," meaning that the patient is determined not to carry a previously found familial mutation. Two other types of results can occur. In families where there is a history of cancer but the carrier status of the family member with cancer is not known or a genetic mutation is not identified, the absence of genetic mutation in the person tested may be interpreted as "indeterminate."

The fourth possibility, a genetic variant of "uncertain significance," occurs when a gene change is found, but little is known about whether the change causes a problem.

A variety of management options including screening, chemoprevention, and risk-reducing surgical options are available for women who are found to carry a *BRCA1/2* mutation. Heightened breast cancer screening with breast MRI (magnetic resonance imaging), ultrasound, and mammography improve early detection of cancers. Unfortunately, there are no proven effective methods for early detection of fallopian/ovarian cancer, limiting the available screening options. Another option is to have risk-reducing surgery, removing the breasts (mastectomies) or ovaries and fallopian tubes (with or without hysterectomy), which greatly reduces, but does not eliminate, the chances of developing cancer. A third option is chemoprevention with tamoxifen, raloxifene, or aromatase inhibitors, but their effectiveness varies according to which gene is mutated. The physician or other health provider details all of these options, including their benefits and harms. For women of child-bearing age, discussion includes reviewing the risk of children inheriting a mutation and the availability of pre-implantation genetic diagnosis (PGD).

In the case of a "true negative" test result, where the individual tests negative for a known family mutation, the individual's risk for cancer is not zero but is similar to the risk for the general population. These individuals are instructed to follow general population screening and prevention guidelines. Although one might think that a woman receiving a negative result would be relieved, the reality is more complex; some feel "survivor's guilt," especially if family members have tested positive.

An indeterminate test means that the risk of cancer cannot be clarified based on the test results. Here, the risk is estimated based on the family history and personal risk factors, and a management plan is based on the degree of risk. This is difficult psychologically because there is a lack of information from the genetic test to more clearly determine degree of risk.

The assessment of risk and the results of genetic testing can lead to psychological consequences, such as depression, anxiety (Hallowell, Foster, Eeles, Ardern-Jones, & Watson, 2004), and family problems (Seymour, Addington-Hall, Lucassen, & Foster, 2010; Wiseman, Dancyger, & Michie, 2010). The social worker helps patients and families sort through the factors affecting their decision-making, consider the repercussions of the decisions, weigh the costs and benefits of genetic testing, and deal with the practical, medical, and emotional implications. These may include life-changing decisions affecting future fertility, body image, and sexuality. Patients seeking testing must consider with whom to share the results. Will she tell others in the family who may be at risk? Will they share their results with her children? If so, when? If they are not married, will they share the results with a future husband, wife, or partner? What if they have a sister who does not want to know the results, or a mother who does not want them to get tested? A social worker can help patients process these difficult decisions, their complex emotional reactions, and help the family to cope with the test results.

Decisions about practice

Definition of the client

Carla referred herself for genetic counseling when her sister was diagnosed with breast cancer and found to be positive for a *BRCA1* mutation. Carla and her husband are both employed full time and have been married for just over a year and have no children. The primary client in genetic counseling and testing is the individual seeking genetic services, but genetics by definition is a family matter. Therefore, the "family" includes not only the patient's siblings, parents, and children, but also the extended family.

Meeting place

The setting for genetic counseling services includes space for the client and family members. A small conference room, rather than an examination room, is used for the consultation. The setting is private and quiet.

Use of time

The consultation service includes an oncologist, a genetic counselor, and a social worker who meet with the client/family for one or two sessions. Obtaining family history and medical information before the consultation allows the patient more time to gather accurate information and means the session can be focused on education and counseling rather than on information gathering. For the initial consultation, the patient (and any accompanying family members) meets with the genetic counselor and social worker in the consultation room. After explaining the service, answering questions, and reviewing the family history, the genetic counselor leaves the room to discuss the medical information and family history with the oncologist. While the genetic counselor is with the oncologist, the social worker continues to process the psychosocial implications of testing, assessing whether additional counseling is required. The oncologist and genetic counselor return to the consultation room to discuss the results of their analysis and to make recommendations about genetic testing. If a patient decides to have genetic testing, a blood sample is taken and sent to the lab. The genetic counselor explains that she will contact the patient by phone with the results. If the patient tests positive, then a follow-up session is scheduled with the genetic counselor and oncologist to discuss management options and implications of results for family members. Indeterminate results may also be followed with a second in-person session.

Goals

There are six goals for genetic risk counseling:

1   Comprehension of genetic risk information to enable an adaptive decision and to determine whether family history suggests an inherited pattern;
2   Effective decision making regarding whether to undergo genetic testing;
3   Adjustment and minimization of the negative impact of genetic testing;
4   Adherence to surveillance recommendations;
5   Follow-up decision making regarding prevention options; and
6   Communication of test results to family members.

(Miller et al., 2006, p. 281)

The social work role in genetic counseling is to help ensure that the individual understands the implications for making the decision whether to be tested for potential risk for cancer, to identify the pertinent issues that may affect the patient and family, and to help the patient and family to consider the effect this information will have, and to determine if there are others in the family who may need additional intervention. In the first consultation session, I address the social and emotional implications of cancer risk screening and assess how the relationship between family members may affect their choices and decisions regarding cancer risk and prevention. I seek ways to support the decisions of the patient and to help them appreciate the complexity of their decision. I am also attentive to any barriers, both practical and psychological, that may affect the patient facing this decision. In the second session, I focus on how each individual faces living with the new information.

Contracting and developing objectives

At the initial visit, I clearly define my role as part of the consultation team, explaining that I help with the practical, social, and emotional aspects of genetic testing. Because the involvement of a social worker is provided as part of holistic care for the patient, there is no explicit contracting for social work services during the initial consultation. If additional counseling sessions are indicated, we contract about frequency and decide whether these will be provided in person or through telephone counseling. If further counseling beyond the cancer risk consultation service is needed, referrals are arranged.

Intervention

At the first session, Carla explained that her sister Sylvia, age 34, was recently diagnosed with breast cancer and undergoing treatment. Sylvia had genetic testing that confirmed a *BRCA1* mutation. Carla came prepared with written questions and took notes as the genetic counselor gave her an overview of genetics and genetic risk assessment, described the risk assessment process, and explained the very complicated medical implications and options. She answered Carla's questions and assessed her understanding. She then took a comprehensive history of Carla's family, with a focus on which relatives had a cancer diagnosis, when they were diagnosed, with which cancers, and other pertinent information (e.g., age at diagnosis) about these relatives.

The family history allows the genetic counselor and oncologist to assess any pattern of cancers related to a possible *BRCA1* or *BRCA2* mutation. Carla's parents are both alive and healthy and have never been diagnosed with cancer. Carla has two full siblings, her sister Sylvia, and a brother, age 22, who is healthy. Her maternal grandmother is alive at age 88, and does not have cancer. Her maternal grandfather died at age 89 with kidney cancer. Her paternal grandmother did not have cancer, but her paternal grandfather died of prostate cancer at age 62. She has three paternal great-uncles who all had cancer, but Carla did not know the types of cancer or ages when they were diagnosed. Carla's family originates from Eastern Europe, of Ashkenazi Jewish heritage, a higher risk group for *BRCA* mutations.

Carla raised some questions about insurance, confidentiality, and about how the test results might affect her plans to have children if she were to test positive. The genetic counselor reassured Carla that GINA protects patients from discrimination based on genetic test results. Once all of Carla's questions and concerns were discussed, the genetic counselor left the consultation room to meet with the oncologist.

I talked with Carla about what it was like for her to consider breast cancer risk testing and about her distress about Sylvia's breast cancer diagnosis. She knew of the increased risk for Ashkenazi Jews. When Sylvia's *BRCA1* results came back positive, she said "I knew I had to do something right away." She described herself as "not the type of person to hide from events" and said that her way of coping is "to face it head first." Sylvia had confided her *BRCA1* testing result to Carla alone and had not told her parents for fear of their response.

Although Sylvia's genetic counselor advised her to share the information, Sylvia was not ready. Carla understands that Sylvia does not want to disclose her genetic status to her parents and wonders how her parents, especially her father, will react.

Carla completed the distress screening tool prior to the consultation and rated her distress a "6" (10 being most distressed, 0 being least distressed), identifying family issues as causing the most concern. She was worried about Sylvia and her treatment, and she worried about her brother too. I explored with Carla how testing positive might affect her and her husband, and their plans for having children. I suggested that she contemplate what she would do if there was a positive, negative, or indeterminate finding, prior to deciding about testing. She offered different scenarios of how she would approach each of these possibilities. I have found that this technique helps patients explore their feelings about testing, being at risk for cancer, and the emotional impact not only on themselves, but also on their family members. In this case, we focused primarily on how Carla felt her husband was dealing with the uncertainty of her risk for developing cancer.

Timing of testing is an important focus for social work assessment. Genetic testing is not to be undertaken impulsively. Carla's sister's cancer diagnosis and testing positive for *BRCA1* were very recent. She and other family members were still in shock. Although Carla responded by moving quickly to determine her risk, I saw that Carla had given a lot of thought to the decision. She had explored information on the internet, talked to family, and was very knowledgeable about her options. Carla described a loving and close relationship with her husband. If testing was recommended, she was very determined to go ahead. Driving her decision to move quickly was her plan to have children someday. They had planned to wait for 4 or more years while they concentrated on their careers and saved money, but she realized that this plan might have to change. I believed that Carla was able to make an informed decision. She had a solid understanding of the implications of the test. Carla tended to "intellectualize," and her coping style is to seek knowledge to handle her anxiety. It was my assessment that she was in a position to deal responsibly with her potential risk.

When the oncologist and genetic counselor returned, they reviewed the pattern of cancer in Carla's family. Although the cancers noted in Carla's mother's family – kidney cancer and liver cancer – are not related to breast cancer risk, the prostate cancer of her paternal grandfather and cancers of her paternal uncles could indicate *BRCA* mutations. They explained that *BRCA1* and *BRCA2* mutations can be inherited through the paternal line. The fact that her sister was diagnosed at a young age and tested positive for the *BRCA1* gene, combined with the Ashkenazi Jewish family background, suggest that Carla has a 50% chance of being a carrier of this same mutation. They concluded that it would be prudent for Carla to complete the testing. She called her husband and he supported her decision to have the genetic testing. Her blood was taken immediately following the initial consultation.

Because a specific *BRCA1* mutation had already been identified in her family, Carla's blood was only tested for this known genetic mutation. The genetic testing results came back two weeks later. Unfortunately, Carla tested positive. The genetic counselor contacted Carla to give her the results and set up a second appointment. Carla and her husband arrived together for the second appointment. The genetic counselor reviewed the complex medical information, and the oncologist reviewed her recommendations for increased monitoring for breast and ovarian cancer. She mentioned that prophylactic surgery or hormonal medication were options that the couple might want to consider at some point in the future. She did not recommend an immediate oophorectomy due to the risks of premature menopause (medical and psychosocial). They discussed family planning and she supported the idea that they might have children sooner rather than later. The genetic counselor noted that future children had a 50% risk of inheriting the mutation and that they could obtain pre-implantation genetic diagnosis (PGD) if Carla conceived via *in vitro* fertilization. Before leaving, the oncologist arranged for Carla to begin ongoing follow-up and surveillance at the Breast Center.

After the genetic counselor and oncologist left, I stayed with the young couple. My goals were to assure that they understood the meaning of the test results, to help them deal with the emotional impact, to assist with decision-making about future surveillance and/or prevention, and to consider how this news changed their child-bearing plans and their relationship. The threat of a potentially life-threatening illness, and the uncertainty of whether one will even develop that illness, leaves the patient with the task of living their life as if all was well, yet knowing that there is always the real possibility that cancer can intrude at any time (Rolland, 2006). Carla and her husband were determined to carry on "as normal" while also acknowledging the sense that they can no longer take anything for granted. The news definitely changed their priorities. Carla's husband said, "I wanted to wait at least until we were 30 before having children, but I know I can figure out a way to financially change that."

We talked briefly about the surgical preventative measures that were discussed with the oncologist, including having a bilateral mastectomy or oophorectomy. Carla did not think she needed to consider this immediately and intended to consider these options after they had children. In my experience, the decision to have preventative surgery is more common after women complete their families. Carla and her husband were also concerned about how to communicate the news that she had tested positive to her family. Carla knows she needs to talk more with her sister about how to convey this information to the family, and this could raise ethical issues if Sylvia is not ready to share the information about her positive *BRCA1* mutation with her parents.

We also discussed how this would affect her younger brother. Carla talked about how complicated it would be for him if he tested positive as he is only just starting his career; he is single and this would now be part of his future life too. Carla was especially concerned about how her father would feel about the news and whether she would tell him that the oncologist recommended that he be tested to determine (confirm) that the *BRCA1* mutation originated on his side of the family. The benefit of this would be to identify others (e.g., cousins) who could be at risk. She worried that he would feel responsible for his children's genetic mutations and their ramifications. We also discussed disclosing the results to future children, but they were not concerned about this, certain that by the time their children were old enough to be told, advances in technology would create an entirely different set of circumstances. As a young couple, facing the knowledge that Carla is at a higher risk for developing cancer creates an experience that differs from other couples their age; with few who share similar circumstances, the isolation and difference may create social distance. The social work assessment includes identifying areas of potential distress, in this case increased pressure to start a family, and also areas of strength, such as the close and supportive relationship between Carla and her husband. Carla's pedigree is depicted in Figure 13.1.

Stance of the social worker

The multi-disciplinary team uses a "biopsychosocial" model of practice, as the intersection between biological (genetic, cancer in patient, and family), psychological and social

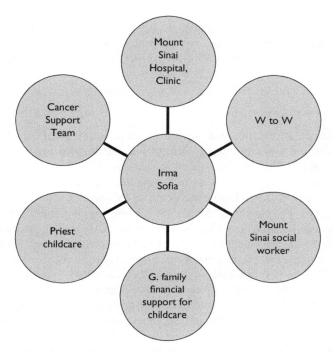

Figure 13.1 Pedigree for Carla's family

(including family) aspects of genetic testing are central to the intervention. I have a solid understanding about the state of knowledge of genetic testing for cancer risk, particularly for the *BRCA1* and *BRCA2* genes. I also have a background in oncology social work, so I am familiar with cancer treatment and the impact of cancer on the family. Equally important is the knowledge I bring about the complicated dynamics for the patient and family in evaluating cancer risk. I am familiar with practical resources, insurance, and financial considerations and I keep a comprehensive referral source database if additional services are needed. Because this is a very specialized service, with at most two sessions, the intervention I provide is psychoeducational. The focus is on informed decision-making. I also provide socioemotional support throughout the process, and assess emotional impact and family strengths and weaknesses. Because the service is limited, if I find a need for individual or family therapy, I make a referral to an appropriate setting.

Use of outside resources

There are few services for "previvors." There is no support group locally for those who are considering testing, but we do offer a monthly support group for individuals who have tested positive for a mutation or who have a strong family history of cancer. I also refer people to the FORCE organization (Facing Our Risk of Cancer Empowered), where patients and family members can connect with others, hear stories, and ask questions. Another important resource is Sharsheret, a national non-profit organization that supports young women of all Jewish backgrounds who are facing breast cancer or are at increased genetic risk.

Case conclusion

Our consultation model does not give us the opportunity to follow individuals or families over time. This means that our interactions generally end after the testing and plans for risk management are complete. This is sometimes frustrating on the personal level as we wonder about the outcomes.

Differential discussion

Carla was provided with adequate information and support to make an informed decision to engage in genetic testing, and she was supported as she and her husband dealt with their initial response to the testing results. This service is ideal for patients who have the ability to understand the genetic information and have access to the medical resources needed for long-term management. Like Carla, patients/families who utilize this service tend to have good economic and social support. The consultation does not provide any ongoing services for those who may need additional help, so screening for referral needs is a critical component of the service. Genetic testing has the potential to exacerbate family problems, and if not handled well, to create psychological symptoms (anxiety and depression) in those who are tested. There is a lack of funding for psychosocial services in the U.S. health system more broadly and it is difficult to find genetic support services that have ongoing availability.

It is important to recognize that all aspects of cancer prevention and genetic counseling are undergoing rapid change: the technology of genetic testing, our knowledge of its meaning, social policies about human genetics, and the structure of the health care system, including the payment system for health care services, keep evolving. It is our hope that with the increased recognition of the value of psychosocial services, social workers will not have to struggle to "fit" a person who is at risk for an illness into a "medical model" that steers funding to those already diagnosed. As our understanding of the genetics of cancer improves, we hope we will eventually be able to prevent cancer in those at risk through new technologies, such as "gene therapy." As the technology continues to develop rapidly, it is likely that policy in this area will lag behind the technology for the foreseeable future.

Discussion questions

1   What social justice issues arise as a result of genetic testing? How might a social worker advocate for more access to genetic testing for all who might benefit from it?
2   How do you envision counseling needs might differ between clients who have high levels of health literacy and those who do not? How comfortable are you personally with understanding the complexity of genetic risk?
3   What ethical issues do you identify when your patient wants to inform her family of her positive results, but other family members do not want to know about their own level of risk? How might you help to resolve such issues?

References

ACA (2010). Patient Protection and Affordable Care Act, 42 U.S.C. § 18001 et seq. (2010). Retrieved from www.obamacarefacts.com
ADA (1990–2015). Americans with Disabilities Act. Retrieved from www.ada.gov/

Biesecker, B. B., Ishibe, N., Hadley, D. W., Giambarresi, T. R., Kase, R. G., Lerman, C. & Streu-wing, J. S. (2000). Psychosocial factors predicting BRCA1/BRCA2 testing decisions in members of hereditary breast and ovarian cancer families. *American Journal of Medical Genetics, Part A, 93*(4), 257–263. PMID: 10946349

Ford, D., Easton, D. F., Stratton, M., Narod, S., Goldgar, D., Devilee, P., et al. and the Breast Cancer Link-age Consortium (1998). Genetic heterogeneity and penetrance analysis of the BRCA1 and BRCA2 genes in breast cancer families. *American Journal of Human Genetics, 62*, 676–689.

Friedman, L. S., Ostermeyer, E. A., Szabo, C. I., Dowd, P., Lynch, E. D., Rowell, S. E., & King, M. C. (1994). Confirmation of BRCA1 by analysis of germline mutations linked to breast and ovarian cancer in ten families. *Nature Genetics, 8*(4), 399–404. PMID: 7894493

Hallowell, N., Foster, C., Eeles, R., Ardern-Jones, A., & Watson, M. (2004). Accommodating risk: Responses to *BRCA1/2* testing of women who have had cancer. *Social Science & Medicine, 59*(3), 553–565. doi: 10.1016/j.socscimed.2003.11.025

Liptak, A. (2013, June 13) Justices, 9-0, bar patenting human genes. *The New York Times.* Retrieved from www.nytimes.com/2013/06/14/us/supreme-court-rules-human-genes-may-not-be-patented.html?_r=0

Manchanda, R., Legood, R., Burnell, M., McGuire, A., Raikou, M., Loggenberg, K., et al. (2015). Cost-effectiveness of population screening for BRCA mutations in Ashkenazi Jewish women compared with family history-based testing. *Journal of the National Cancer Institute, 107*, 380. doi: 10.1093/jnci/dju380

McEwen, J. (2006). Genetic testing: Legal and policy issues for individuals and their families. In S. M. Miller, S. H. McDaniel, J. S. Rolland, & S. L. Feetham (Eds.), *Individuals, families and the new era of genetics: Biopsychosocial perspectives* (pp. 506–529). New York: WW Norton.

Miller, S. M., Daly, M. B., Sherman, K. A., Fleisher, L., Buzaglo, J. S., Stanton, L., Godwin, A. K., & Scarpato, J. (2006). Psychosocial processes in genetic risk assessment for breast cancer. In S. M. Miller, S. H. McDaniel, J. S. Rolland, & S. L. Feetham (Eds.), *Individuals, families and the new era of genetics: Biopsychosocial perspectives* (pp. 274–319). New York: WW Norton.

Minion, L. E., Dolinsky, J. S., Chase, D. M., Dunlop, C. L., Chao, E. C. & Monk, B. J. (2015) Hereditary predisposition to ovarian cancer, looking beyond *BRCA1/BRCA2. Gynecologic Cancer 137*(1), 86–92. doi: 10.1016/j.ygyn0.2015.01.537

NCHPEG (National Coalition of Health Professional Education in Genetics) (2010). The Genetic Nondiscrimination Act (GINA). Retrieved from www.nchpeg.org

ObamaCare Facts (n.d.). Retrieved from http://obamacarefacts.com/

Oktay, J. S. (1998). Genetics cultural lag: What can social workers do to help? *Health & Social Work, 23*(4), 310–315.

Patenaude, A. F. (2005). *Genetic testing for cancer: Psychological approaches for helping patients and families.* Washington, D.C.: American Psychological Association.

Rolland, J. S. (2006). Living with anticipatory loss in the new era of genetics: A life cycle perspective. In S. M. Miller, S. H. McDaniel, J. S. Rolland, & S. L. Feetham (Eds.), *Individuals, families and the new era of genetics: Biopsychosocial perspectives* (pp. 139–172). New York: WW Norton.

Seymour, K. C., Addington-Hall, J., Lucassen, A. M., & Foster, C. (2010). What facilitates or impedes family communication following genetic testing for cancer risk? A systematic review and meta-synthesis of primary qualitative research. *Journal of Genetic Counseling, 19*, 330–342. doi: 10.1007/s10897-010-9296-y

U.S. Department of Health and Human Services (2005). Understanding HIPAA. Retrieved from www.hhs.gov/ocr/privacy/hipaa/understanding/summary/index.html

Weltzel, J., Blazer, K., MacDonald, D., Culver, J., & Offit, K. (2011). Genetics, genomics and cancer risk assessment. *CA: A Cancer Journal for Clinicians, 61*(5), 327–359. doi: 10.3322/caac.20128

Werner-Lin, A. (2015). The oncology social worker and genomics. In G. Christ, C. Messner, & L. Behar (Eds.), *Handbook of oncology social work: Psychosocial care for people with cancer.* New York: Oxford.

Wiseman, M., Dancyger, C., & Michie, S. (2010). Communicating genetic risk information within families: A review. *Familial Cancer, 9*, 691–703. doi: 10.1007/s10689-010-9380-3

Wooster, R., Bignell, G., Lancaster, J., Swift, S., Seal, S., Mangione, J., et al. (1995). Identification of the breast-cancer susceptibility gene BRCA2. *Nature, 378*, 789–792. PMID: 8524414

Resources

American Cancer Association, www.cancer.org

Facing Our Risk of Cancer Empowered, www.facingourrisk.org/index.php

Genetic Alliance, www.geneticalliance.org

National Cancer Institute, www.cancer.gov/

Sharsheret, www.sharsheret.org/

Chapter 14

Woman to Woman

A hospital-based support program for women with gynecologic cancer and their families

Arden Moulton

Context

Description of the setting

Woman to Woman (WtoW), the Gynecologic Oncology Support Program at the Mount Sinai Medical Center in New York City, was instituted in 2003 by a survivor of ovarian cancer. Feeling a lack of emotional support and access to information throughout her cancer experience inspired her to initiate a collaboration between the Mount Sinai Department of Social Work and the Division of Gynecologic Oncology in the Department of Obstetrics, Gynecology and Reproductive Science to create a dedicated psychosocial support program for women diagnosed with gynecologic cancer and their families. This partnership led to the creation of WtoW, an adjunctive social work program that provides peer-to-peer mentoring to women in treatment for ovarian, uterine, cervical, vaginal, and vulvar cancer.

I coordinate the program and in that role, in collaboration with each woman's physician, I identify volunteers, and train and support them throughout the process (see Fitzpatrick, Edgar, Remmer, & Leimantis, 2013 about the importance of training volunteers). Thus, throughout treatment and post treatment, women receive support, information, and advocacy training from volunteer survivors of gynecologic cancer, a model found to work well (Levine & Silver, 2007; Meyer, Coroiu, & Korner, 2014; Moulton et al., 2013). WtoW also provides support to the partners of women in treatment through an information guide (Moulton, 2012). Volunteers work with women in all inpatient and outpatient treatment areas. Survivor volunteers have monthly processing and continuing education meetings with me as program coordinator.

The role of program coordinator was originally part-time but as a result of both a growing number of women referred to Mount Sinai for medical care and the success of the WtoW program, the role was expanded to full-time and has allowed for an enriched partnership between the gynecologic oncology social worker, program staff, and volunteers. From the inception of the program in 2003 to the present, WtoW volunteers have provided support and information to over 1,000 women in treatment for gynecologic cancer. In 2012, the Ovarian Cancer Research Fund (OCRF) expanded its mission to include support for women in treatment for gynecologic cancer and their families using WtoW as the model for the expansion, hospitals apply for a US$50,000 one-year grant to start the program at their facilities. As a result, WtoW is available to women at 16 hospitals including Yale-Smilow, Stanford, Duke, University of Chicago, and Moffitt Cancer Center. I serve as a consultant to the OCRF and the hospitals that receive grants on all issues related to the expansion of WtoW.

The Mount Sinai Medical Center is an academic organization comprising a large tertiary hospital, the Mount Sinai Hospital (MSH), and a medical school, the Mount Sinai School of Medicine. Both are located between East Harlem, a very poor, culturally diverse area with a high proportion of immigrants, and the Upper East Side, one of the wealthiest areas in Manhattan and, perhaps, in the country. The Division of Gynecologic Oncology treats the largest number of women diagnosed with gynecologic cancer in the northeastern United States. In 2013, for example, over 500 women were treated at MSH and 1,000 more received care at its affiliate hospitals. In the United States in 2014, an estimated 12,300 women were diagnosed with cervical cancer, 52,630 with uterine cancer, and 21,980 with ovarian cancer. That year, an estimated 28,790 women died from gynecologic cancer (American Cancer Society, 2014). In New York State, 870 women were diagnosed with cervical cancer, 3,593 with uterine cancer, and 1,858 with ovarian cancer, and there were 1,870 gynecologic cancer deaths (New York State Department of Health, 2014).

Policy

WtoW is funded through a grant and private donations. In New York City, most women receiving Medicaid are enrolled in a managed care plan (New York State Department of Health, 2014). Women must be enrolled in a managed care plan accepted by Mount Sinai in order to receive care at our Gynecologic Oncology Clinic (GOClinic). While the goal of this policy is to provide comprehensive health care services to women, long waits, lack of consistent translation services, rotating medical personnel, and the financial impact of treatment for cancer negatively impact quality of life for these women. The consistent caring presence of our program attempts to assuage the effects of long waits and changing personnel. While our volunteers cannot affect system changes in entitlement policies or hospital admissions, they reduce some stress for women in treatment through hospital visits and phone calls. Knowing that a valued peer, one who speaks the same language, will provide emotional support consistently throughout treatment can help ameliorate the often difficult reality of hospital protocols (Macvean, White, & Sanson-Fisher, 2008). We also have a patient fund that provides financial support to women in treatment. Need is established at the time of diagnosis through intake interviews with the gynecologic oncology health care team. The fund has provided money to pay electric bills, transportation costs, and rent for a woman at risk for eviction.

Technology

Cervical, endometrial, and ovarian cancers characterize 95% of gynecologic cancers, and rank fourth in both incidence and mortality in cancers diagnosed in women (American Cancer Society, 2014). Although these cancers all originate in the female reproductive organs, they differ in diagnosis, treatment, and prognosis. While a diagnostic tool (the PAP) exists for cervical cancer and uterine cancer is typically detected early enough to treat successfully, ovarian cancer, the leading cause of death from gynecologic cancer in the United States, is most often diagnosed at stage III or IV, indicating spread of the disease to other organs. No reliable diagnostic tool exists for ovarian cancer. Women with gynecologic cancer are monitored throughout their lives with check-ups starting at three months following end of treatment. CAT scans, PET scans, blood monitoring (CA 125 test), and "second look" surgery for ovarian cancer are typical options (Connor & Langford, 2003).

The 15 WtoW volunteers are survivors of at least one of the most common gynecologic cancers: 11 of ovarian cancer, two of uterine cancer, one of cervical cancer. Three of the volunteers are survivors of both ovarian and endometrial cancers. The difficult treatment protocols and often grim prognosis for women diagnosed with stage III or IV ovarian cancer resulted in a multi-disciplinary decision to prioritize support for women diagnosed with the disease. Having 12 ovarian cancer survivor volunteers guarantees there will be consistent, ongoing support to newly diagnosed peers. The high recurrence rate (75%) is a difficult issue. If a woman successfully completes treatment, the longer she is categorized as NED or "no evidence of disease," the better her chance of a cure. Women are required to wait 2 years after the end of treatment to apply to be a volunteer, decreasing their odds of recurrence. Even so, the fact that cancer has recurred for three of the original five volunteers and all have died has profound implications for the volunteers and for the women they mentor.

Treatment for these cancers is determined by type and stage of the disease, along with consideration of the age and health of the patient. Women diagnosed in early stages typically have surgery and may not require chemotherapy or radiation. Cervical cancer is typically treated with surgery, chemotherapy, and/or radiation. Endometrial cancer is treated with surgery, usually a radical hysterectomy including removal of the cervix, uterus, ovaries, and fallopian tubes, followed by chemotherapy and/or radiation. Ovarian cancer is treated with surgery including a radical hysterectomy, debulking (removal of cancer cells visible in the peritoneal cavity), and chemotherapy. All the WtoW volunteers have experienced one or all of the above treatments. Their personal experiences with treatment and management of side effects are shared, if asked, with the patients they mentor. Receiving practical advice from a woman who has had a similar experience can be comforting and reassuring.

Organization

Highly regarded in the field and with a 100-year history, the Mount Sinai Department of Social Work has over 300 social workers who are an integral and necessary part of the functioning of the hospital and are accepted, valued members of multi-disciplinary teams. The WtoW program coordinator role is both clinical and administrative. The full time gynecologic oncology inpatient and outpatient social workers are responsible for assessment of patients, discharge planning, and clinical support throughout treatment. I provide clinical support to survivor volunteers through monthly meetings and individual sessions. I maintain relationships with patients in order to follow their progress medically and psychosocially, to monitor the relationship between volunteer and patient, and to assess the efficacy of the WtoW program. As coordinator, I manage volunteer schedules, fundraising (including grant writing and organizing benefits), write training and support materials, attend and sponsor education conferences, and do community outreach.

Description of typical clients

The women receiving support from the program are seen in the GOClinic, inpatient service, and Cancer Treatment Center. They are all in treatment for ovarian, uterine, cervical, vaginal, or vulvar cancer. All are in need of the peer-to-peer mentoring to women that WtoW provides. As program coordinator, I match women who are going through the treatment process with the volunteers, all survivors of ovarian, uterine, and or cervical cancer. I determine appropriateness of the referral (I do not match volunteers to women who have been diagnosed with dementia or serious mental disorders; volunteers are not mental health professionals). If the patient requests a referral and is appropriate, I match the patient with a volunteer of similar diagnosis and age. For example, a pre-menopausal 40-year-old woman newly diagnosed with ovarian cancer has likely been diagnosed at a late stage, lowering her chance of survival. She also faces loss of fertility following the standard of care treatment, radical hysterectomy, and premature menopause; the symptoms of menopause – hot flashes, mood swings, and vaginal dryness – are typically more severe than in natural menopause. I would typically match this woman with a volunteer who has had similar experiences with the psychosocial issues around diagnosis and treatment. I also consider cultural similarities, language, and family issues, as research suggests one should (Patten & Kammer, 2006). The specific concerns expressed by a patient are always considered.

Decisions about practice

Description of the client

Irma Fuentes, now 39 years old, was diagnosed with ovarian cancer in 2006 and has received various kinds of support from three volunteers in different settings during her cancer experience. Having emigrated from El Salvador in 1998, Irma is bilingual and is in the United States on a work visa. Irma's mother and 8 of her 11 siblings live in El Salvador. Her father died of a stroke in 2003. Irma and three of her brothers live in Yonkers, approximately 25 miles north of New York City. From 1998 to 2004, she worked in a factory, augmenting her income with a part-time job at her church. In 2004, Irma lost two fingers in a factory accident and has been on long-term disability (US$350 a week) since then. From 2000 to 2006, Irma lived with her boyfriend, and in 2006 she delivered a baby, Sofia, by cesarian section. On returning home, Irma experienced shortness of breath and was diagnosed with a blood clot in her lung. The next day her obstetrician told Irma that she had stage III ovarian cancer. Due to her complicated medical needs, Irma was transferred to MSH, had a radical hysterectomy for removal of all reproductive organs and debulking or removal of all visible cancer cells. Doctors also implanted a Greenfield filter in Irma's thigh to reduce the possibility of further blood clots. As a result of the hysterectomy, Irma is infertile and experiences symptoms of menopause. Following her diagnosis, Irma's boyfriend left their home, telling her that he was unable to manage the emotional and practical problems associated with fatherhood and her illness.

I meet with all women who express interest in WtoW. After consultation with my social work colleague and the health care team, I determined Irma's appropriateness for referral during our initial meeting and discussed the benefits of WtoW. While she was interested in meeting a peer, her principal concern was her financial situation. Her boyfriend's disappearance meant the loss of much needed income. Also, Irma did not have medical insurance and was concerned about the cost of care for Sofia throughout her treatment. Irma sued the factory where she was working when she lost her fingers, but the factory closed, making financial restitution unlikely. When diagnosed with ovarian cancer, Irma received an additional US$130 a week from Social Security.

Definition of the client

Irma became our client and both she and Sofia benefited from our support. Because Irma needed emotional, practical, and financial help, I referred her to three volunteers in two settings during her treatment. Bultz and Holland (2006) suggest that emotional distress is "the sixth vital sign" and support must be provided as well as medical care for oncology patients.

Goals

During our initial meeting, Irma identified her financial situation and its impact on her baby as her primary concern. While she was profoundly affected by the emotional turmoil of giving birth, facing a life-threatening clot, and being diagnosed with ovarian cancer in the space of one month, Irma's fear that her sudden financial instability would affect her ability to care for Sofia overwhelmed her ability to cope. Acknowledging this, I referred Irma to WtoW volunteer Valerie, a survivor of ovarian cancer and founder of WtoW. Valerie's status as a member of the Mount Sinai Auxiliary Board, a philanthropic organization that funds innovative programs within the hospital, helped her to raise the seed money to start WtoW. Her passion and dedication to helping women has contributed to the sustained success of the program. Valerie, at 71 years old, lives on the Upper Eastside, has been married for over 40 years to a successful lawyer and real estate entrepreneur, and is the mother of three adult children. While Irma and Valerie differ dramatically both culturally and demographically, Valerie's "founder" status and history of philanthropy became the most important qualities for an initial match with the financially devastated Irma. Sharing a diagnosis of ovarian cancer was another important criterion for the match and addressed the second goal, normalizing Irma's response to her diagnosis. Valerie's long-term survival would give hope to Irma and provide her with an advocate throughout treatment. Valerie met with Irma and her kindness, empathy, and unique understanding of Irma's medical situation and sharing of her own history helped Irma begin to acknowledge the overwhelming fear she felt about her diagnosis and its impact on her and her daughter's future. After consultation with Irma's doctors, we determined that support from the WtoW Patient Fund was warranted. WtoW covered two months of childcare. After two months, continued support was provided by Valerie and her husband through their personal foundation.

The third goal, Irma's need for advocacy, was identified during chemotherapy treatment. Being insured through emergency Medicaid meant she would be hospitalized for 48 hours three times a month for eight months. Every week, between treatments, Irma came to the GOClinic to monitor her blood chemistry levels. There, volunteers Jane, a 12-year survivor of uterine cancer, and Joyce, a survivor of breast, uterine, and ovarian cancer, developed a relationship with Irma. Their advocacy efforts included informal translating, serving as liaisons with the health care staff, helping with paperwork, and providing practical information about managing chemotherapy side effects. The volunteers provided Irma with a wig when she lost her hair, made sure she understood the doctor's words, provided her with snacks while she waited, and served as consistent support throughout treatment. When Irma's emergency Medicaid ran out, the volunteers acted as liaisons with the gynecologic oncology social worker to insure her treatments would not be delayed. The supports provided by the volunteers, including emotional and financial guidance and advocacy, helped Irma regain her equilibrium and learn new coping strategies.

Use of contract

A contract between volunteer and patient is established following a woman's initial agreement to be part of WtoW. First contact with a woman is made by the gynecologic oncology social worker, who ascertains the woman's interest in the program. The fear and confusion experienced by most women at the time of diagnosis results in a majority of women agreeing to participate in the program. Very few women refuse the program, and those who do are offered the program again during chemotherapy. Women uninterested in meeting with a volunteer immediately following surgery may not be physically or emotionally prepared for anything other than recovery from surgery and pain management. Irma agreed to join the program and I met with her 4 days after her hysterectomy and debulking and established a verbal contract agreeing to a visit from a survivor volunteer. I then discussed the referral with the team. Carefully reading her medical chart provided me with information necessary to determine her support needs; I gathered demographic information, medical status data, and information on Irma's family and social supports. Our verbal contract was backed up with chart notes from both the social worker and the program coordinator. A second, less formal contract was formed between Irma and the survivor volunteers. The relationship formed between Irma and the volunteer survivors included agreeing to share their stories, providing consistent availability, and educating Irma on techniques for coping with gynecologic cancer, and financial support.

Meeting place

Our team of professionals and volunteers works in all Mount Sinai treatment venues. Initial contact is made on the inpatient floor designated for women with gynecologic cancer. There are 16 beds, 13 of which are semi private, and volunteers meet with women in their rooms, join them for walks around the floor, or visit in the family waiting room. Irma first met with Valerie in her semi private room 5 days after surgery and 1 day before discharge. Irma had a roommate at the time of each visit, but the unusually large size of the room allowed Irma and Valerie to speak privately and did not impede their interactions. Irma discussed her main fear, that she would die and leave Sofia without a mother. As time went on, especially during post treatment, this fear receded and Irma began to feel hopeful about survival.

Irma met with Jane and Joyce weekly at the GOClinic, a large, crowded, uncomfortable space located in the basement of the inpatient building. Due to the Joint Commission: Accreditation, Health Care, Certification (JCAHO – or "Joint Commission") safety evacuation requirements, there is no access to private space in the clinic; all interactions must take place in the general waiting area. At times Irma requested help from Jane, who is able to speak some Spanish, to help her better understand her doctor's recommendations and treatment plans. These meetings took place in the examination rooms. The lack of privacy may have impeded Irma's willingness to share personal information with Jane and Joyce, but she continued to reach out to them.

Use of time

My initial meeting with women in treatment takes approximately 15 minutes. This usually takes place during post-surgical recovery, impacting duration of the intervention. Follow-up visits in treatment areas and the GOClinic are usually shorter, no more than 5 minutes. Most interventions involve WtoW volunteers who see patients in all treatment areas areas in the Hospital. Some volunteers meet with women outside the hospital and on the phone, and the time structure for these interactions is open ended and determined by volunteer and patient.

Use of time for hospital visits is determined by a number of factors. The most important consideration is always the patient's physical condition and availability. Women recovering from surgery may be unable to sustain conversations of any duration due to pain management and recovery from anesthesia. The volunteers ascertain availability by speaking to a woman's nurse to determine if she is in her room and if she is amenable to visits. Length of stay is determined by the volunteer and the patient but seldom exceeds 15 minutes. When a woman is receiving chemotherapy treatments, some of which are 5 hours in duration, visit times vary from a brief greeting to half hour discussions between volunteer and patient. Again, visit times are determined by both volunteer and patient.

Valerie's initial meeting with Irma was at her bedside following Irma's surgery for ovarian cancer. Irma's physical weakness and her emotional lability limited the duration of their visit. Valerie introduced herself, explained her role, and informed Irma of the financial support she would receive from WtoW. This visit lasted about 10 minutes. Longer, deeper discussions took place between Irma and GOClinic volunteers, Jane and Joyce. Irma had recovered physically at the time of these visits. She had begun to cope emotionally; her reduced anxiety allowed for longer interactions. Irma came to Mount Sinai for treatment every three weeks and was seen by a volunteer during each admission for chemotherapy. These visits varied according to issues discussed and volunteer availability.

Interventions

Interventions used by the volunteers include crisis intervention and social support, while group work techniques are used to help the volunteers themselves. The timing of the initial meeting between a survivor volunteer and the patient, and the nature of the peer model, results in a natural use of crisis intervention. Volunteers are trained in active listening and empathic interviewing but are not professionally trained in crisis theory (France, 2014). The interaction between peers includes sharing experiences in a manner that normalizes a confusing, stressful environment for patients. Volunteers' active listening encourages patients to tell their cancer story, helping them to process and understand their crisis.

Social support, in the form of providing information, emotional buttressing, and advocacy assistance in group and individual settings, is acknowledged to have a positive influence on health outcomes (Campbell, Phaneuf, & Deane, 2003). The WtoW model offers women in treatment for gynecologic cancer social support from peers who have had similar experiences. Women newly diagnosed with cancer often feel anxious, fearful, and out of control. The information that WtoW volunteers give to peers increases their knowledge of their illness, producing a sense of mastery and increasing feelings of control. The emotional empathy inherent in interactions between peers creates an interpersonal bond that encourages a hopeful outcome and models positive behavior. Encouraging self-advocacy through teaching and modeling helps women navigate the health care system, increasing their self-esteem and making the treatment experience more manageable. Meeting Valerie, Joyce, and Jane at the time of her diagnosis gave Irma hope that she could also expect a positive outcome. The practical information they provided encouraged Irma to advocate for herself with her health care team, the insurance system, and her community.

Group techniques are used for the volunteers. Established originally to process work with patients and further educate survivors on issues pertinent to their work, we now incorporate learning about cultural competency and teaching of additional mentoring skills; the monthly survivor volunteer group supports the powerful connection between members. Their common effort to cope with and find meaning in their illness, and the practical need to problem-solve around their work with patients, has resulted in personal growth and group cohesiveness. Most of the volunteers seek out membership in WtoW with the goal of helping others in similar situations. The volunteers all report improvement in their own lives through their work. They are often inspired and energized by the efforts of their group peers. The group has produced significant interpersonal relationships between members, a result of their common bond of survivorship and mentoring of others. The altruism they exhibit through their work with women extends to their relationships within the group further increasing group cohesiveness.

Stance of the social worker

My role as program coordinator of WtoW includes completing a brief psychosocial assessment of women in treatment who have asked for a referral to the program and who have been deemed appropriate by the gynecologic oncology social worker and the woman's doctor.

The demographic, diagnostic, and personal information I gather from my 15-minute interview helps me determine what needs should be addressed immediately and influences the match between patient and survivor volunteer. After meeting with Irma following her ovarian cancer surgery, I determined that her immediate need for practical support to pay for childcare for Sofia was her primary concern. Introducing her to Valerie at this time facilitated a donation from the WtoW Patient Fund, alleviating Irma's anxiety and allowing her to address other issues arising from her diagnosis. Irma's fear that her diagnosis would result in her death was partly addressed by meeting Valerie, a woman with a similar diagnosis who was doing well physically and emotionally. Her fear that all people with cancer die of the disease was further diminished after meeting Joyce and Jane, both of whom have survived their cancers and are living active, productive lives. Meeting Jane, who is bilingual, each week at the Mount Sinai GOClinic, gave Irma the opportunity to discuss her emotional and practical concerns in Spanish, her first language.

I continued to assess Irma's changing needs throughout her treatment through brief one-to-one contacts either in person or on the phone. I consulted with the three volunteers who worked with Irma as this was critical to my assessments, along with monthly discussions with Irma's health care team. Through our ongoing interactions, we determined that Irma's lack of knowledge about both her illness and the MSH system limited her ability to self-advocate. Jane and Joyce discussed their own treatment stories with Irma, teaching her about ovarian cancer through listening and example. They also discussed Irma's need for information with her doctors, who then took more time answering her questions and concerns. They encouraged Irma to write down her questions before meeting with her doctors, and Jane translated at times to ensure that Irma understood the medical information she received.

A challenge for me in my role as program coordinator and social worker is a tendency to micro-manage the work of the volunteers, over-involving myself in their interventions. Becoming too clinical and over-thinking each interaction could reduce the spontaneity between Irma and the volunteers and interfere with their natural bond, a bond I do not share because I have not had cancer. Irma trusted the volunteers because of the commonalities of their experiences and because they were lay persons who could remove the distance that can arise between staff and patient. Respecting the volunteers' unique and important role in Irma's recovery became a challenge for me that demanded constant monitoring of my thoughts and actions. Their support, while critical to Irma's success, augmented the medical and psychosocial support provided by the Gynecologic Oncology Interdisciplinary Team.

In my role as social work counselor to the volunteers, I lead monthly group meetings with the volunteers and meet individually with each volunteer every six months to determine her emotional wellness and discuss issues that arise from the often difficult work we do with patients in treatment. At that time, I reassess the appropriateness of that woman continuing as a volunteer. The group meetings are organized around the work the volunteers do with women, providing both ongoing education and training, and an opportunity to process the emotional issues that inevitably arise through the intimate relationships the program creates. Volunteers may see a woman once or they may develop a long-term relationship. It is a real possibility that a woman with whom they have developed a relationship does not respond to treatment and dies; they need to be able to process feelings of profound sadness and helplessness. My stance as social worker necessitates that I maintain a professional role as mediator and emotional support for the volunteers, but my own feelings of sadness have overwhelmed me. The death of a volunteer or her return to treatment is especially difficult for me. I like and admire these remarkable women. When the volunteers talk about their work "protecting" them from further illness, I empathize with their "magical thinking," and I become angry and sad when these brave women succumb to their disease.

The volunteers also strongly identify with some women, seeing themselves back in the role of patient, fearing recurrence that is never far from their consciousness. I have used the meetings to educate the volunteers about counter-transference and to normalize their feelings of anxiety and concern about their health. A strong mutual support group has evolved among the volunteers as a result of their work and the often difficult realities of their shared experiences. Volunteers have supported each other through the death of three of the volunteers, personal life events, and other health concerns. One of my challenges as group leader has been re-learning group dynamics to create a safe, effective environment encouraging group attendance and cohesiveness. The changes in the size and make-up of the group throughout the program's existence has been also been challenging, but the work the volunteers do bonds them quickly and overcomes initial reticence. Demographic differences among volunteers could present barriers, but mutual support of their shared experience as patients and as mentors emphasizes similarities more than differences.

Group discussion of the volunteers' work with Irma emphasized their various roles in providing her with practical help, emotional support, and advocacy training. We discussed her excellent medical prognosis and Sofia's thriving childhood. The volunteers expressed satisfaction about their role as mentors and we talked about their need to find meaning in their own illnesses through their work supporting Irma and other women.

Use of outside resources

When Irma requested information about support groups for women with ovarian cancer, the volunteers and I referred Irma to the Cancer Support Team, a support and information organization near her home. Irma also received counseling from her local priest. Childcare for Sofia, paid in part by the WtoW Patient Fund and Valerie's philanthropic trust fund, was provided by a relative in her home. The ecomap shown in Figure 14.1 reflects the various support systems offered to Irma throughout her treatment for ovarian cancer.

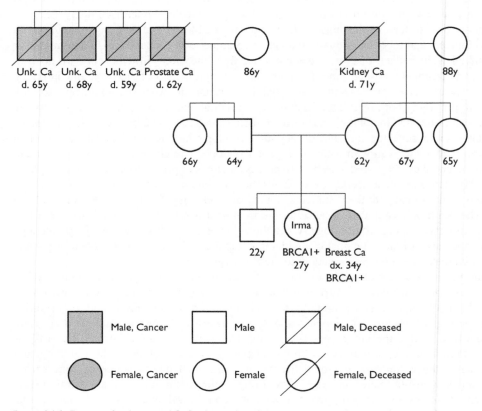

Figure 14.1 Ecomap for Irma and Sofia during Irma's cancer treatment

Reassessment and evaluation

Meeting with Irma at various times during her treatment allowed me to assess the effectiveness of the interventions of the volunteers and to make changes where necessary. At the same time, the volunteers discussed their work with Irma, its effectiveness, and their own response to working with her at our monthly processing meetings.

At the beginning of her treatment, Irma stated that practical issues, specifically financial concerns, were of critical importance as they involved the physical well-being of her daughter. The funds provided gave Irma immediate relief, allowing her to focus on her treatment and recovery. At my first meeting with Irma, she was grateful and relieved as a result of the financial support and more hopeful after meeting the survivor volunteers who helped her to know that she might survive her illness, advocate for herself and live to raise Sofia. Irma reported feeling secure in her knowledge of ovarian cancer and her ability to manage her appointments and interactions with her doctors. Her anxiety and fear decreased over time and she attributed feeling less anxious to a combination of gradual adjustment to her illness, the support of her family and the volunteers, and her love for Sofia, her "little miracle." Her insurance issues were a continuing problem and source of anxiety. Emergency Medicaid did not pay for her outpatient visits. The volunteers and I referred Irma to a social worker who manages insurance problems.

The volunteers discussed their work with Irma during our monthly meetings. Valerie was pleased to have helped, and Jane and Joyce both felt their limited interactions with Irma had a positive effect on her functioning. They were frustrated by the impact of Medicaid on Irma's care.

Case conclusion

Irma's cancer is currently in remission. The WtoW volunteers continue to see Irma every six months at her follow-up appointments. At her last appointment, Irma reluctantly told Joyce and Jane that she was experiencing ongoing financial problems related to her inability to find work. WtoW and the family who help financially support WtoW provided Irma with additional financial support, enabling her to pay for childcare for Sofia during her job search. The WtoW volunteers and I will continue to provide Irma with emotional and practical support.

The WtoW volunteer group will continue to meet consistently to support its members, encourage cohesiveness and sharing, and further educate the volunteers. The group allows me to monitor progress and current functioning of group members to identify individual distress resulting from work with patients.

Differential discussion

At the time of our initial meeting with Irma, our bilingual survivor volunteer, Nancy, had not yet joined WtoW. Spanish is not Jane's first language and while competent, she is not fluent. After Nancy's training, Irma was still receiving treatment and, on reflection, I think it would have augmented Irma's WtoW experience to talk with a survivor in Spanish, her first language. Nancy is also closer in age to Irma and might have engaged her in discussions about fertility and sexuality, issues of particular interest to younger women in treatment. Learning more about Irma's cultural heritage, including her extended family in El Salvador, her spiritual beliefs, and her values about healing would have better informed our work and given us greater sensitivity to the context in which her illness occurred.

Discussion questions

1   WtoW at Mount Sinai has received an unusual amount of financial support, mostly from various personal connections. Most medical centers provide no financial support to such programs. Is it morally and ethically appropriate to use the funds we raise for a demographically small population of patients? Should our mission be expanded to include other cancers? Do you think WtoW would be effective in an institution with a smaller census and fewer resources?
2   One of the central tenets of WtoW is to provide hope to women newly diagnosed so that they will have the same positive outcome as our volunteers. Knowing the survival rate of the volunteers is higher than the national statistics for most gynecologic cancers, is it ethical to promote hope for survival as a WtoW value?
3   How important are the criteria for matching survivors with women in treatment? Is the common factor of a diagnosis adequate to insure a meaningful and lasting relationship or are cultural and demographic issues equally important?

References

American Cancer Society (2014). *Cancer facts and figures*. Atlanta, GA: American Cancer Society.

Bultz, B. & Holland, J. (2006). Emotional distress in patients with cancer: The sixth vital sign. *Community Oncology, 3*, 311–314.

Campbell, H. S., Phaneuf, M., & Deane, K. (2003). Cancer peer support programs – do they work? *Patient Education and Counseling, 55*, 3–15.

Connor, K. & Langford, L. (2003). *Ovarian cancer: Your guide to taking control.* Sebastopol, CA: O'Reilly.

Fitzpatrick, T., Edgar, L., Remmer, J., & Leimantis, M. (2013). Job satisfaction among volunteers with personal cancer care experience. *Journal of Social Science Research, 30*(3), 203–305.

France, K. (2014). *Crisis Intervention: A handbook of immediate person to person help* (6th edn.). Springfield, IL: Charles C. Thomas.

Levine, E. & Silver, B. (2007). A pilot study: Evaluation of a psychosocial program for women with gynecologic cancers. *Journal of Psychosocial Oncology, 25*, 75–98. doi: 10.1300/J077v25n03_05

Macvean, M. L., White, V. M., & Sanson-Fisher, R. (2008). One-to-one volunteer support programs for people with cancer: A review of the literature. *Patient Education and Counseling, 70*(1), 10–24.

Meyer, A., Coroiu, A., & Korner, A. (2014). One-to-one peer support in cancer care: A review of scholarship published between 2001 and 2014. *European Journal of Cancer Care, 24*(3), 299–312. doi: 10.1111/ecc.12273

Moulton, A. (2012). *Woman to Woman information guide for partners.* New York: Mount Sinai Hospital.

Moulton, A., Balbierez, A., Eisenman, S., Neustein, E., Walther, V., & Epstein, I. (2013). Woman to Woman: A peer to peer support program for woman with gynecologic cancer. *Social Work in Healthcare, 52*, 913–929. doi: 10.1080/00981389.2013.834031

New York State Department of Health (2014). *Medicaid program information.* Albany, NY: Author.

New York State Department of Health (2014). *State Cancer Registry, statistics.* Albany, NY: Author.

Patten, Jr., C. & Kammer, R. (2006). Better communication with minority patients: Seven strategies for achieving cultural competency. *Community Oncology, 3*(5), 295–302.

Chapter 15

Liver Transplant 2015

Regina Miller and Senayish Addis

Context

The Liver Transplant Unit (LTP), a division of the Penn Medicine Transplant Institute (PMTI), is located at the Hospital of the University of Pennsylvania, USA, a 790-bed, university-affiliated teaching hospital. We are one of 137 liver transplant centers in the United States caring for candidates over age 18. Our center is one of a few in the nation performing multi-organ transplantation with a history of long-standing success.

Currently, 15,323 people in the United States await liver transplants, and in our region, the waitlist is 2,423. Since 1988, the LTP has carried out 2,337 transplants (OPTN, 2015). The 1-year survival rates for deceased donor grafts falls within the nationally estimated expected probability of survival at 89.36% at 1 year and 79.85% at 3 years. For the same time frame, the 1-year survival rates for the 19 living donor grafts reaches 100%, with recipients receiving living donations demonstrating best health outcomes overall. An individual's need for liver transplantation is defined by the model for end-stage liver disease (MELD) score and is unique to liver transplant candidates. A MELD >10 is a useful predictor for referral to a transplant center and also helps to rank candidates on the waitlist (Neuberger, Ferguson, & Newsome, 2013).

Our region's transplant centers collaborate to increase organ donation awareness though education and outreach, but there is still a dire need for organs, with 1,700 people dying of end-stage liver disease (ESLD) in 2011. The efficacy and outcomes of liver transplants will continue to improve, but the demand for liver allografts will exceed supply by a growing margin (Gedaly et al., 2008; O'Mahony & Gross, 2012). It is also important to note that patients with conditions such as severe hepatitis or severe alcoholic hepatitis might benefit from liver transplantation. They may be added selectively to waitlists; however, before adding them, a team must carefully and ethically weigh the consequences both in terms of the patient's benefit and in relation to global outcomes (Lucidi, Thierry, Moreno, & Donckier, 2015).

Policy

The Department of Health and Human Services oversees the Health Resources and Services Administration which gives direction to the Office of Special Programs which controls the Department of Transplantation, which, in turn, regulates the Scientific Registry of Transplant Recipients along with the Organ Procurement Transplant Network (OPTN). The OPTN operates the national network for organ procurement and allocation, and promotes organ donation through education and sound policy. Its role was created by the National Organ Transplantation Act of 1984 (NOTA, 1984) and it provides oversight that includes: organ match and placement; policies and procedures for organ recovery, distribution, and transportation; collection and management and dissemination of data; professional and public education; management of waitlists; oversight of transplant centers; and oversight of organ procurement organizations.

While public debate about ethical dilemmas related to organ transplant continues, collegiality and trust among the decision-makers, along with the presence of the United Network for Organ Sharing (UNOS), helps support a high level of professional and governmental oversight of the enterprise. For example, in 2006, a swift response by the Centers for Medicare and Medicaid Services (CMS) to specific questions surrounding organ allocation, questionable program statistics, and death rates for those on a transplant list resulted in active monitoring of heart, liver, lung, and intestine transplant programs. In 2007, new regulations established a single set of requirements and periodic reviews for all Medicare-approved transplant programs (Government Accountability Office, 2008).

All organ transplant programs must be located in a hospital with a Medicare provider agreement and must comply with both transplant and hospital Conditions of Participation (specified in 42 CFR 482.1 through 482.57) (CMS, 2015). CMS can visit any transplant center, without notice, to assure that standards are being met. Mandated reporting includes: changes in key staff members, decreases in the number of transplants performed or a program's survival rates, the termination of an agreement between the hospital and the organ procurement organization, and inactivation of the transplant program (Government Accountability Office, 2008).

In 2014, the OPTN/UNOS Committee published and circulated a concept paper for the entire transplant community and the public to encourage feedback and insight into an apparent trend of disparity noted within the liver and intestinal organ transplant population (OPTN/UNOS Liver and Intestinal Organ Transplantation Committee, 2014). Institutional bias or inequities based on geography of the distribution and allocation of solid organs was recognized with a commitment to change this trend through a formalized approach. The potential policy proposal was circulated for public comment in spring 2015.

Policies related to costs and reimbursement

Transplantation is unaffordable for most recipients without adequate insurance. A rough estimate places liver transplant, without complications, in the hundreds of thousands of dollars. Post-operatively, the non-reimbursed cost of a one-month supply of medicine can reach over US$4,000 (Milliman Research Report, 2014) and immunosuppression alone costs between US$13,000 and US$25,000 annually (Axelrod, Milliman, & Abecassis, 2010a, 2010b). Liver transplant recipients can expect to take immunosuppressant medications for life. If a candidate is underinsured due to a cap or a cost-sharing percentage, then obtaining transplant medications may be difficult. In theory, the improper use of immunosuppressant medications could result in poor outcomes, although, for various reasons, a direct correlation has not been shown between non-adherence and compromised graft or patient survival rates (Rodriguez, Nelson, Hanto, Reed, & Curry, 2013). Regardless, staff are concerned about mismanaged immunosuppression medication and fear rejection of a solid organ. The inability to obtain immunosuppressant medications following solid organ transplantation should be addressed with hypervigilance.

Liver transplantation is covered by Medicare, Medicaid, and private insurance. Medicare National Coverage Determination (NCD) began liver transplantation payment in 1991. Solid organ transplant costs encompass both medical and non-medical services and goods, and coverage varies according to the carrier. For example, private insurance may provide a stipend for short-term relocation, although Medicare does not reimburse for lodging, transportation, or meals. Medicare recipients tap into federal benefits and thus are eligible to access any National Center of Excellence for purposes of transplant; in theory, they are afforded increased access compared to private insurance. The caveat is that distance to centers and multiple listings at multiple centers present unique programmatic and individual resource challenges. In addition to Medicare A and B, supplemental insurance is necessary to cover the out-of-pocket expenses not reimbursed by Medicare B. Medicare A and B are limited in scope because 20% of the total costs are not covered, which includes doctors' visits, rehabilitation, pulmonary therapies, labs, radiologic testing, home IV nursing services, and pharmaceuticals. Medicare reimbursement policy sets the standard that private insurance companies consistently follow. Medicare A is an entitlement based on age or disability and work credits. Medicare B, Medicare D, and gap or supplemental insurance all come with a price which can be offset depending upon income and eligibility for Social Security Extra Help. Social Security Extra Help, also known as the Low-Income Subsidy (LIS), closes the Medicare Part D "donut hole," the name the United States gives to the gap between the time medications are covered by insurance (up to a certain dollar threshold) and when they become the consumer's responsibility until they reach "catastrophic "proportions (National Committee to Protect Social Security and Medicare, 2015). In 2015, beneficiaries with income below 135% of the poverty line are eligible for the LIS, which helps pay for all or part of the monthly premium, annual deductible, and drug co-payments (CMS, 2015).

The on-par contracts between transplant centers, programs, and insurers transfer high dollar amounts. Health Cost Guidelines place an average U.S. liver transplant cost above the half-million dollar mark. The total cost in this average includes 30 days pre-transplant care, procurement, hospital admissions, physicians' care during transplant, 180 days post-transplant discharge, and outpatient immunosuppressant therapy, for a total of US$739,100 (Milliman Research Report, 2014). The Penn Transplant Institute reviews billing and contracts annually with private insurance companies. At Penn Medicine, financial counselors meet with all potential recipients pre-transplant to determine coverage. While at some centers, social workers also act as financial counselors, at Penn Medicine, the roles are separate, but collaborative. Social workers take leadership roles in cases with financial and insurance barriers and work closely with recipients and families to identify plans or solutions.

Transplant recipients are expected to be affiliated with a transplant center throughout the continuum of care in order to ensure quality care and prevent complications. Transplant care can be formally transferred with the recipient's request after one year. Generally, procedures are planned, and surgery is interpreted as life-saving, not emergent. This so-called elective surgery risks a denial by insurers unless protocol is followed and authorization secured. The health care team is frustrated when a candidate's health care is jeopardized for economic reasons, and all involved turn to the social worker for direction and support. At times, Penn Medicine social workers have fielded calls from lawyers, government officials, and various other public and private agencies advocating for potential transplant recipients to identify problems and collaborate on solutions to insurance barriers and transplant costs.

The Affordable Care Act (ACA, 2010) increases access to those with ESLD because it has created the state health insurance exchanges that increase coverage and has eliminated the lifetime insurance capitation and pre-existing condition clauses that insurers previously imposed. In fact, improved access for this more recently covered population may even the playing field between those with Medicaid and those with private insurance in terms of earlier intervention and better outcomes. Social workers are highly attuned to such trends and advocate for uninsured and underinsured individuals deemed appropriate for transplant care.

In 2012, the federal government mandated that transplant centers develop, implement, and maintain a written, comprehensive, data-driven program designed to monitor and evaluate performance of services provided. In response, a dynamic, hospital-funded analytical center was created and a researcher hired whose purpose is to create and maintain a database. The goals here are proactive planning, improvements in transplant quality, and prompt responses to changes in regulations.

The care of donors is especially scrutinized by CMS; one adverse effect with a donor jeopardizes the donor program, and one donor death leaves the program shut down until a full investigation is completed. Living liver donor candidates are a unique cohort of healthy individuals opting for elective surgery to remove a lobe of the liver. Social workers play an essential role in assessing a living donor for psychosocial barriers and addressing ethical considerations, including the nature of the relationship and motivation to donate. The National Living Donor Assistance Center provides resources beyond the coverage paid by the recipients' insurance plan, or non-covered costs, which could include annual physicals, transportation, child care services, and lodging. Social workers can work with a recipient or donor, but not both; thus, each team must have more than one social worker.

In addition to the social workers, living donors are assigned advocates who hold a mandated role that is filled by physicians, nurses, community leaders, or social workers, depending upon the center. At PMTI, the leadership requests a social worker hold this highly valued position. The team includes three highly experienced licensed clinical social workers who can assess and act on behalf of a donor candidate. Social workers help to determine whether to move forward with surgery, and are available to advocate for the donor throughout the process, including a follow-up schedule of up to 3 years post donation (Hays et al., 2015).

Liver recipients can access Social Security Disability Insurance (SSDI) and Social Security Insurance (SSI) if they are deemed disabled by the medical provider and the federal government. SSDI requires predetermined work credits based upon a candidate's age, whereas SSI is based on both a disability and the income of the applicant. At times, a person can be both eligible for SSDI and SSI; for example, if someone has been working for low wages, the SSDI award will be low because the amount is based on the salary, thus potentially gaining access to additional income to supplement, or SSI income is allotted. In addition, candidates can be eligible for both Medicare and Medicaid, in which case Medicare is the primary insurance for similar reasons. If SSDI is approved, the candidate is entitled to Medicare 24 months after the first SSDI payment, or upon turning age 65. If SSDI is denied due to work credit shortage or a higher functional status, appeals may be possible. In some cases, help from a Social Security lawyer or legal clinic for the disabled may be necessary.

Technology

The first successful liver transplant occurred in the United States in 1963, and in the 1980s the discovery of the immunosuppressant cyclosporine started to boost outcomes. This orthotopic surgery, where the native liver is removed and replaced with a deceased donor's liver or the lobe of a living donor, remains a formidable procedure (Rustad, Stern, Prabhakar, &

Musselman, 2015). The length of hospital stay depends on the functional status and co-morbidities of the candidate, with many recipients requiring another level of care prior to discharge home. The greatest limitation continues to be the organ shortage. Gaps persist between donor organ availability and organs needed to supply the waitlist. Educational campaigns, policy changes, and creative strategies to increase donations have not closed the gap.

Organization

OPTN defines seven categories as liver transplant causes, and includes non-cholestatic cirrhosis, cholestatic liver disease/cirrhosis, biliary atresia, acute hepatic necrosis, metabolic disease, malignant neoplasms, and other (OPTN, 2015). A multi-disciplinary team is mandated with added consulting services, as needed. The primary liver team includes: administrators, transplant surgeons, transplant hepatologists, psychiatrist, nurse practitioners, nurse coordinators, pharmacist, nutritionist, medical assistants, and social workers. UNOS delineates all team roles and services, and requires that each solid organ transplant team hire a master's prepared social worker. UNOS broadly defines the mental health provider services as offering psychosocial evaluation of potential living donors and recipients, substance abuse evaluation, treatment, referral, monitoring, counseling and crisis intervention, support groups and newsletters, patient care conferences, advocacy; patient and family education, referral to community services such as vocational rehabilitation, housing; knowledge of available social services, regulations; and death, dying, and bereavement counseling, team building, running department meetings such as process improvement, participation in organ donation awareness initiatives, and community advocacy efforts (OPTN, 2015).

During the evaluation, it is first determined if the patient is medically and psychosocially healthy enough to be considered. Next, the team decides whether the person is ready for listing, must meet additional goals, or is ruled out. Patients hear the results in a follow-up appointment. If the person is ready, he or she is listed on the National Living Transplant Waiting List. The MELD score combines multiple variables, and the team observes this number to predict the best time to move the candidate up on the list (Wong, Gish, & Ahmed, 2014).

The post-operative phase lasts 5–7 days in hospital with social work being engaged in all aspects of care: rounding with the team on the floors, preparing for discharge, communicating with the team, making referrals, and providing psychosocial support throughout admission to best prepare the recipient and family for the post-op phase. Because recipients are being referred later for listing and transplanted more quickly, leaving less preparation time, the post-operative phase presents more acute challenges for all team members. The social worker works with all patients throughout the continuum of care, regardless of the phase of transplant.

Quality Assessment and Performance Improvement (QAPI) regulations were instituted in 2013, and transplant centers are expected to collect data for self-governing with outside CMS oversight. This layered approach encourages center compliance in order to avoid consequences. PMTI initiated PORTS and Morbidity and Mortality Sessions for all team members with cases, program issues, and trends discussed formally.

Decisions about practice

Description of the client

Mark is a 61-year-old, White man who presented at LTP after years of alcohol abuse. He suffered from alcoholic hepatitis and his liver failed to function properly. Alcohol abuse is the second cause of liver cirrhosis leading to liver transplant in the United States (Weinrieb, Van Horn, Lynch, & Lucey, 2011). Shortly before his hospitalization, Mark quit drinking. If he did not get the liver transplant, his life was in imminent jeopardy. Divorced, Mark has four children and was living alone prior to hospitalization. He completed some college and owned a small business but stopped working because his illness was severe enough for him to receive Social Security Disability Benefits, which provided a monthly allowance. Mark began drinking alcohol at a very young age and by his early 20s, was abusing it. He describes himself as a functional alcoholic with an addictive personality. At age 45, Mark attended a short rehab after family pressure to seek treatment, but he resumed abusing alcohol shortly after discharge.

Alcohol rehabilitation programs vary. One approach is intensive outpatient rehab (IOP), where individuals receive a combination of both individual and group counseling. I found local IOPs covered by Mark's insurance through the Substance Abuse and Mental Health Services Administration's website (SAMHSA.gov). Prior to his surgery, Mark said that he sought help in the recent past, controlling his environment by avoiding familiar friends, and re-establishing relationships with his supportive family. Mark denies any mental health diagnosis after being asked questions about anxiety, depression, coping strategies, former or current mental health issues, hospitalizations or emergency room visits related to emotional/behavioral health.

I met with Mark's sisters, Lori and Jessica, and his daughter-in-law, Britney, and they all expressed extreme concern about his poor health and recognized the seriousness of his medical condition. Mark and his family met with different members of the transplant team and were educated on all aspects of liver transplantation. They were made aware of a commitment to the medication regimen and lifelong care. Mark's sisters assured members of the team that they were dedicated to his recovery. They agreed to recruit family members for caretaking days and vowed to take Mark into their homes to help care for him, secure medications at the pharmacy, provide transportation, and ensure that he completed follow-up medical care and alcohol rehabilitation treatment after his transplant.

The evaluation process

Potential recipients arrive for an initial evaluation and are assessed by all the members of the liver transplant team, including the financial counselor, gastroenterologist, hepatologist, nurse coordinator, nutritionist, transplant surgeon, and social worker. Social workers recommend follow-up appointments for psychiatry, especially when addictions or active mental health issues are identified. Although it is important to have individuals be evaluated by an "addictive disorders specialist," the research in this field is growing, with the six-month abstinence rule being challenged. There is no evidence that a six-month abstinence period pre-transplant is needed in order to be successful post-transplant or that individuals have to be sober for six months prior to transplant (Rice & Lucey, 2013; Weinrieb, Van Horn, Lynch, & Lucey, 2011). Regardless, this is a huge cultural shift in the expectations for listing of a potential liver transplant recipient.

The social workers use the Stanford Integrated Psychosocial Assessment for Transplantation (SIPAT) as part of their evaluation process (Maldonado et al., 2012). The SIPAT, a new tool which was introduced at the Society for Transplant Social Work Conference in 2012, was embraced by the transplant community. The SIPAT places a number value on the social worker's psychosocial assessment of the adult recipient. It is considered a valid tool, with numbers indicating a low to high risk category; this number is then communicated to the team at the listing meeting and placed in the medical record. In the future, the Penn Medicine LTP social workers hope to collect data for an internal review of outcomes and compare them to the social worker's documentation of SIPAT scores. Mark's score of 20 placed him in the category of "good candidate" and indicated recommending proceeding toward listing, although monitoring of identified risk factors would be required, including a history of addiction and relapses.

Goals, objectives, and contracting

The role of the social worker in every transplant program is mandated by CMS. The liver transplant team consults with the social workers to mitigate psychosocial risk factors to promote better health and good outcomes, as is expected in all solid organ transplant programs (Thomas, 2014). Social work evaluates patients' transplant candidacy from a psychosocial standpoint. Thus, our goals are to understand Mark's mental health, alcohol abuse, and other addictions, and the social support network for his post-transplant recovery. If the evaluation is not urgent, or the potential recipient is stable, social work often has time to work with the patient and family to address these issues. We can facilitate referrals to intensive outpatient counseling, individual or family counseling, and continue education opportunities. We discuss the importance of strong social support and resources such as transportation and funds to support post-transplant recovery. The strong relationship that we develop with patients builds trust over time and allows for more readily established goals. During the initial meeting or evaluation, we identify support persons to aid recipients' physical recovery from surgery and provide them the emotional support needed to abstain from alcohol and complete treatment following transplant surgery. This relationship is essential because most contracts to abstain from alcohol or drugs, to complete an IOP, or to communicate difficulties or recidivism, are based on verbal commitments between the recipient and the social worker.

Because Mark was already very ill by the time he presented, I was unable to build such a strong relationship or to enroll him in the IOP that was recommended by the psychiatrist. There was no time to enroll Mark in the recovery maintenance treatment programs that help to facilitate a sober transplant journey and, hopefully, a sober life-long journey. I did not have time to assess his ability to adhere to any alcohol rehab treatment. Pre-operatively, with Mark's permission, I worked hard and fast with his family. We set two objectives: Mark's two sisters would remain readily available and active in his care and Mark would agree to enroll in an IOP post-operatively once the medical team cleared him to begin treatment. See Figure 15.1 for Mark's ecomap.

The liver transplant team has not utilized formalized written contracts; instead, we use extensive verbal agreements. Written contracts were discussed in the past, but the team has not embraced them because potential transplant recipients and families' strengths, weaknesses and tensions on how to proceed with goals and objectives sometimes affect their ability to negotiate terms. A verbal contract is the commencement of a trusting relationship that allows us to meet transplant candidates and families where they are, to avoid stagnation and build on resilience.

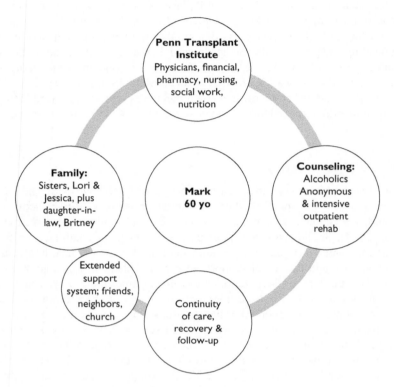

Figure 15.1 Ecomap for Mark

Meeting place and use of time

Mark was evaluated in his hospital room. He was too sick to attend the one-day outpatient liver transplant clinic where patients and families meet together. At this clinic, members of the team led by the transplant coordinator, a registered nurse, educate patients and their families about the evaluation, testing, listing, waiting, and transplant periods.

Some recipients require urgent intervention and are transplanted quickly. Expedited evaluations leave little time for social workers to address issues prior to listing and transplant. The goal is to support recipients and families in having a good transplant outcome. Some potential recipients arrive at the emergency room or are transferred from other hospitals to be evaluated immediately because of the threat of imminent death, whether related to a genetic disorder, contagious disease, or drug and/or alcohol addiction. Sometimes patients in this condition are newly diagnosed. Mark was evaluated on admission. In order for Mark to be urgently listed and prepared for transplant, the team had to be flexible in anticipating the last-minute changes in schedules, and types of procedures and staffing that would enable us to complete all necessary tests and assessments. Social work revisited the patient alone and with family multiple times for continuous re-evaluation, information gathering, education, expectation-setting, and verbal contracting.

Strategies and interventions

During the multiple times I met with Mark and his family to discuss post-transplant care and the expected recovery process, Mark's sisters spoke of their commitment to support him physically and emotionally so they could address his addiction as a family. Mark agreed and planned to enroll in a program to help him fight his alcohol addiction. I was able to advocate for Mark's transplant listing at the weekly multi-disciplinary listing meeting because the family was present, engaged, and offered a firm, verbal commitment toward caretaking and support. I felt confident in my assessment and advocated for Mark with the hope he would move forward with transplantation, noting his motivation to be transplanted and to live a sober life. Next, I began to investigate viable agencies to work with Mark and his family.

Case/care management

The pre-transplant and post-transplant care models require equal attention and provide similar team structure at our Institute. All transplant team members continue to care for and support Mark while he and his family go through the transplant evaluation, listing, waiting period, transplant, recovery, and post-transplant care. After the transplant, the focus changes to recovery support with the main objective to motivate and support patients to succeed and thrive. I support, counsel, and link patients with resources throughout the continuum (Figure 15.2).

Stance of the social worker

Mark was always surrounded by family members who vowed to support him through every step of the process, including inviting him to live with them while he recovered from his surgery. One of his sisters, Lori, even had a room at her house for him and volunteered to care for her brother full time for as long as he needed to recover and get back on his feet. Lori learned his medications and care requirements to support his full recovery. She took full responsibility for bringing him to his appointments and being the point person for his care. It was encouraging to know that his needs would be well met by Lori and other family members and to see that his family would be verbally and actively part of the journey.

After a lot of education from the medical team, Mark was discharged to Lori's house for recovery after the transplant. He was given medications, a visiting nurse, durable medical equipment such as a walker, and physical and occupational therapy. Once Mark got home, the visiting nurse taught Lori and other family members how to care for Mark. The family members rotated to provide supervision and to transport Mark to all his follow-up appointments. They made sure he took his medications as prescribed and accompanied him to all his follow-up appointments. As he became independent and healthy, they developed a plan to transition him from his sister's house back to his own apartment. They made sure that he was confident in his ability to care for himself. In addition, the family helped Mark stay connected to an alcohol abstinence treatment program. I modeled the trust relationship and knew it was essential as the basic tool for Mark to change and the family system to support Mark. I validated Mark's hard work and commitment and acknowledged his challenges. I was able to provide resources for drug and alcohol counseling as well as individual and group counseling.

Reassessment and evaluation

Mark recovered from his hospitalization and surgery, and after a few months of living with his sister, he returned to his apartment to live on his own. Since his transplant, he has enrolled

LIVER TRANSPLANT PROGRAM
Community of Support Worksheet

The Penn liver transplant team recommends patients identify two to three people for each area of support:

Θ **Primary Caregiver**
- Direct care
- Decision making
- Helps patient to identify Power of Attorney (may be the primary caregiver)

Θ **Advocate for Potential Donors**
- Identify living donor

Θ **Medical Care**
- Medications
- Blood sugar
- Blood pressure

Θ **Personal Support**
- Emotional
- Spiritual

Θ **Daily Activities**
- Cooking
- Cleaning
- Laundry
- Child care

Θ **Transportation**
- Follow-up appointments

Θ **Errands**
- Groceries
- Medications

Θ **Finances**
- Bills
- Banking

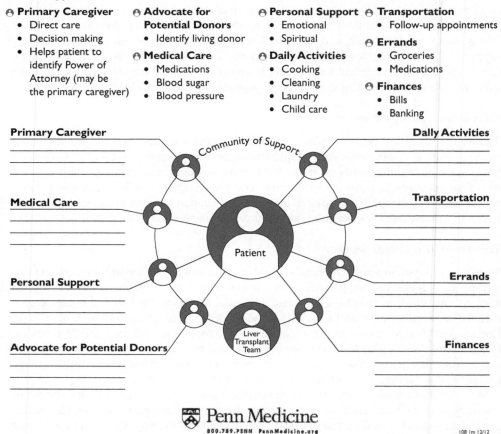

Penn Medicine
800.789.PENN PennMedicine.org

108 1m 12/12

Figure 15.2 Community of support worksheet

in counseling and works hard every day to maintain his sobriety. On occasion, I continue to reach out to support, provide resources, and listen to Mark. Many resources are available from charitable organizations that assist with prescription co-payments to foundations that work with patients and families raising funds for medical expenses.

Termination occurs in transplant with a transfer to another center or bereavement referrals due to death. The transplant relationships within the liver populations tend to be life-long. Transplant recipients can transfer their care to another center for many reasons, one of which is relocation to another part of the country.

Case conclusion

I am less involved now that Mark is at home and engaged with a treatment program. Mark also has a very supportive and engaged family. Mark will continue to see his hepatologist and transplant team members every six months and, eventually, annually. This provides additional opportunities to assess, teach, provide concrete resources, and/or emotional support.

Differential discussion and discussion questions

Ethical issues persist in relation to liver transplantation and Mark's case was complex. His recidivism and recent alcohol use became a sticking point for some of the team members. Mark's case was unique because he was evaluated, listed, and transplanted within weeks after presenting to the LTP. In hindsight, was it ethical to proceed with listing without mandating a successful IOP placement first? Should we have developed a written contract prior to listing a patient? Does the family support transplant in an active user? How do we explain the team's decision to move forward? Should we always consider the entire waitlist when looking at an individual candidate, such as Mark? If so, would Mark have ever been transplanted?

Some overarching program-specific questions deal with re-transplantation candidacy with more scrutiny, such as a recipient showing signs of non-adherence. How is non-adherence measured? How many times, and how many organs are reasonable to transplant? How much co-morbidity can be tolerated at the time of listing? What should the age limit be? Should we transplant candidates with active alcohol or drug addiction? If research demonstrates the benefit of transplanting those with acute alcoholic hepatitis, how will the transplant community defend its position to transplant if it is met with a public backlash? Should mental health issues be documented as treated and stable over a period of time prior to listing, even if death could occur while waiting? How much weight should psychosocial issues play in a decision to move forward, if any? How do we continue to be supportive of our teams, if we meet resistance against empathy for a particular person? These questions are debated and discussed vigorously at many transplant centers on a regular basis.

The team actively listed Mark because his MELD score was above the threshold; thus, he met the medical criteria for transplant. The team continues to advocate for all patients meeting medical criteria, and provide a strong presence after transplant to support any transplanted patient who requires additional psychosocial supports or interventions.

References and resources

ACA (2010). Patient Protection and Affordable Care Act. P.L. 111–148, 124 Stat. 119 (2010).

Axelrod, D. A., Milliman, D., & Abecassis, M. M. (2010a). U. S. Health Care Reform and Transplantation. Part I: Overview and impact on access and reimbursement in the private sector. *American Journal of Transplantation*, *10*(10), 2197–2202. doi: 10.1111/j.1600-6143.2010.03246.x

Axelrod, D. A., Milliman, D., & Abecassis, M. M. (2010b). U. S. Health Care Reform and Transplantation. Part II: Impact on the public sector and novel health care delivery systems. *American Journal of Transplantation*, *10*(10), 2203–2207. doi: 10.1111/j.1600-6143.2010.03247.x

CMS (Centers for Medicare & Medicaid) (2015). Certification and compliance: Transplant. Retrieved from www.cms.gov/Medicare/Provider-Enrollment-and-Certification/CertificationandComplianc/Transplant.html

Gedaly, R., McHugh, P., Johnston, T., Jeon, H., Koch, A., Clifford, T. & Ranjan, D. (2008). Predictors of relapse to alcohol and illicit drugs after liver transplantation for alcoholic liver disease. *Transplantation*, *86*, 1090–1095. doi: 10.1097/TP.0b013e3181872710

Gift of Life Donor Program: The Region's Organ & Tissue Donor Program. Retrieved from www. donors1.org/learn2/organs/liver

Government Accountability Office (2008). GAO-08-412, a report to the Ranking Member, Committee on Finance, US Senate: Accountability, Integrity, Reliability (2008, April). Organ Transplant Programs. Federal agencies have acted to improve oversight, but implementation issues remain. United States Government Accountability Office. Retrieved from www.gao.gov/assets/280/274897.html

Hays, R. E., LaPointe Rudow, D., Dew, M. A., Taler, S. J., Spicer, H., & Mandelbrot, D. A. (2015). The Independent Living Donor Advocate: A guidance document from the American Society of Transplantation's Living Donor Community of Practice. *American Journal of Transplantation, 15*, 518–525. doi: 10.111/ajt.13001

Lucidi, V., Thierry, G., Moreno, C., & Donckier, V. (2015). Liver transplantation in the context of organ shortage: Toward extension and restriction of indications considering recent clinical data and ethical framework. *Critical Care, 21*. doi: 10.1097/MCC.0000000000000186

Maldonado, J. R., Dubois, H., David, E. E., Sher, Y., Sermsak, L., Jameson, D., & Witten, D. (2012). The Stanford Integrated Psychosocial Assessment for Transplantation (SIPAT): A new tool for the psychosocial evaluation of pre-transplant candidates. *Psychometrics, 53*, 123–132. doi: 10.1016/j. psym.2011.12.012

Milliman Research Report (2014 December). 2014 U.S. organ and tissue transplant cost estimates and discussion. Retrieved from www.milliman.com/uploadedFiles/insight/Research/health-rr/1938HDP_20141230.pdf

National Committee to Protect Social Security and Medicare (2015). Retrieved from www. ncpssm.org/Medicare/QAMedicarePartD/ExtraHelpforLowIncomeSeniors/Answer/ ArticleID/936/22-What-is-the-low-income-subsidy-LIS-also-known-as-Extra-Help

Neuberger, J., Ferguson, J. & Newsome, P. (Eds.) (2013). *Liver transplantation: Clinical assessment and management*. New York: John Wiley & Son. doi: 10.1002/9781118675915

NOTA (National Organ Transplant Act 1984). Section 301 (c)(2) of NOTA, 42 U.S.C. §274e(c)(2).

O'Mahony, C. A. & Gross, J. (2012). The future of liver transplantation. *Texas Heart Institute Journal, 39*, 874–875.

OPTN (Organ Procurement Transplant Network) (2015). Data reports. Retrieved from http://optn. transplant.hrsa.gov/converge/latestData/rptData.asp

OPTN/UNOS Liver and Intestinal Organ Transplantation Committee (2014). Redesigning liver distribution to reduce variation in access to liver transplantation. Retrieved from http://optn.transplant. hrsa.gov/ContentDocuments/Liver_Concepts_2014.pdf

Rice, J. & Lucey, M. (2013). Should length of sobriety be a major determinant in liver transplant selection? (Current Opinion). *Organ Transplant, 18*, 259–264. doi: 10.1097/MOT.0b013e32835fb94b

Rodriguez, J., Nelson, D., Hanto, D., Reed, A., & Curry, M. (2013). Patient-reported immunosuppression nonadherence 6 to 24 months after liver transplant: association with pretransplant psychosocial factors and perceptions of health status change. *Progress in Transplantation, 23*(4), 319–328. doi: 10.7182/pit2013501

Rustad, J., Stern, T., Prabhakar, M., & Musselman, D. (2015). Risk factors for alcohol relapse following orthotopic liver transplantation: A systematic review. *Psychosomatics, 56*(1), 21–35. doi: 10.1016/j.psym.2014.09.006

Thomas, C. (2014). Role of the social worker and the transplant center QAPI committee. *Nephrology News & Issues, 28*(6), 40–41.

UNOS. Donation and Transplantation: Transplant Trends (2015). Retrieved from www.unos.org/ donation/index.php

Weinrieb, R. M., Van Horn, D. H. A., Lynch, K. G., & Lucey, M. R. (2011). A randomized control study of treatment for alcohol dependence in patients awaiting liver transplantation. *Liver Transplantation, 17*, 539–547. doi: 10.1002/lt.222.59

Wong, R., Gish, R., & Ahmed, A. (2014). Hepatic encephalopathy is associated with significantly increased mortality among patients awaiting liver transplantation. *Liver Transplantation, 20*, 1454–1461. doi: 10.1002/lt.23981

Returning veterans, constrictive bronchiolitis, and Veterans Administration services

A war-related illness and injury study center

Kathleen Ray and Rachel E. Condon[1]

Context

The war-related illness and injury study centers (WRIISCs) serve veterans with deployment-related health concerns and medically unexplained symptoms (Lincoln et al., 2006). Established in response to a 1999 National Academy of Sciences recommendation to create study centers focused on post-deployment health regardless of conflict, the WRIISC opened its first two locations in 2001 in Washington, DC, and East Orange, New Jersey. In 2008, the Palo Alto, California center was opened to provide additional access to veterans in the western United States. The New Jersey WRIISC is located on the East Orange campus of the Veterans Administration (VA) New Jersey Health Care System. It is a specialty outpatient program that utilizes a multi-disciplinary team of physicians, nurses, psychologists, neuropsychologists, and social workers. The New Jersey WRIISC coordinates with local hospitals as well as the veteran's local hospitals. The mission of the WRIISC is to "develop and provide expertise for veterans and their health care providers through clinical evaluation, research, education, and risk communication" (Lange et al., 2013, p. 705). This mission is achieved by a multi-disciplinary team who:

- provide clinical services to veterans with deployment-related health concerns and illnesses to improve their health-related quality of life;
- advance knowledge of ways to care for veterans with medically unexplained symptoms to improve their health-related quality of life;
- advance knowledge of and improve communication among veterans, the health care community and researchers regarding deployment-related health concerns and illnesses; and
- advance knowledge of medically unexplained symptoms in veterans and other populations.

It is projected that there are almost 22 million veterans currently in the United States. Since the start of conflicts in Iraq and Afghanistan, 2.7 million troops have been deployed in Operation Enduring Freedom (OEF), Operation Iraqi Freedom (OIF), and Operation New Dawn (OND) (Dougherty et al., 2015). In fiscal year 2013, 8.92 million veterans were enrolled in the Department of Veterans Affairs Health Care System, with almost 4 million receiving VA disability compensation (VA Benefits & Health, 2014). The U.S. Department of Veterans Affairs utilizes specialty clinics to provide veterans with access to "expert knowledge that optimizes treatment in unique or complicated courses of care" (Health Benefits, 2015). Specialty clinical services ensure the veteran's comprehension of the illness and coordinate the overall care they receive. The comprehensive exam at WRIISC is given by clinicians who are solely focused on that particular veteran for that time. Veterans seen at the WRIISC come from all conflicts and have multiple concerns including post-traumatic stress disorder (PTSD), mild traumatic brain injury (mTBI), gastrointestinal problems, and respiratory symptoms.

OEF/OIF/OND veterans as a group are experiencing an increase in both cardiovascular and pulmonary disease. Morris, Lucero, Zanders, and Zacher (2013) report that 69.1% of OIF/OEF/OND veterans stated they had respiratory illnesses after deployment, with number of deployments being associated with an increase in respiratory symptoms. Many veterans' diagnoses include asthma and chronic obstructive pulmonary disease (COPD) despite their daily exercise and overall high levels of physical fitness. OEF/OIF/OND veterans may have been exposed to geological dusts, sand storms, burn pits, exhaust emissions from vehicles and machinery, as well as industrial air pollution, and these conditions may have contributed to the rise in respiratory disorders (Morris et al., 2013).

At the WRIISC, veterans with respiratory and pulmonary symptoms can receive a 3 or 4 day individualized and comprehensive medical assessment of their health concerns with a focus on deployment-related exposures. In order to be eligible for the program, veterans must have unexplained symptoms after adequate primary and secondary work-ups have been completed at their local facility without a clear diagnosis. Veterans are referred to the WRIISC by their primary care provider (PCP) when the PCP believes a further assessment is warranted. The WRIISC is often able to pay for the hotel and transportation costs depending of the level of veteran's service connected disability. Service connected disability refers to disabilities incurred or aggravated during active military service. The evaluation consists of a review of the medical record, an extensive history and physical examination, a psychological interview, neuropsychological screening, exposure assessment, fitness testing, a social work assessment, and health education. If available, a spouse or parent may accompany the veteran for the evaluation (Findley, 2010).

Policy

The commitment to supporting disabled soldiers in the United States dates back to 1636, when the Pilgrims of Plymouth Colony passed a law that the colony itself would support disabled soldiers. Throughout history, assistance programs, medical and hospital treatments, specialized housing, and insurance were created for soldiers. The Veterans Bureau was created in 1921 as an effort to combine programs that were available for all World War I veterans (U.S. Department of Veterans Affairs, n.d.). President Herbert Hoover, signed Executive Order 5398 in 1930, which created the Veterans Administration, combining the Veterans' Bureau, the Bureau of Pension, and the National Homes for the Disabled Volunteer Soldiers into one federal agency, working to provide care to all veterans. In 1988, President Ronald Reagan raised the Veterans Administration to a cabinet-level executive department. One year later, President George H. W. Bush renamed the Veterans Administration the Department of Veterans Affairs (U.S. Department of Veterans Affairs, n.d.).

In the beginning of the OEF/OEF conflict, returning veterans were allowed 2 years of health care services with the VA system upon discharge and enrollment into the VA. President George W. Bush signed the National Defense Authorization Act (NDAA) of Fiscal Year 2008 to extend health care to 5 years after military discharge. This was noted as an important change in policy for veterans who did not immediately enroll with the VA and did not experience deployment-related issues until after the 2-year coverage was expired (Findley, 2010).

The WRIISCs follow VA policies and general treatment authority, including requirements that the veteran have an assigned VA primary care physician and is enrolled in the VA health care system. To be seen at the WRIISC, the veteran must also be medically and psychiatrically stable and believed to be able to benefit from a WRIISC evaluation.

Technology

Computerized patient record system

The VA uses a computerized patient record system (CPRS) that allows VA health care professionals to view a veteran's medical record, including the prescription history and laboratory results from any VA health care location. Clinical reminders for follow-ups or screenings are also made available through this system (Findley, 2010). CPRS allows for continuity in care for the veteran throughout all VA locations.

MyHealtheVet

Since its creation in 2005, veterans have been able to manage their health care through a patient portal known as MyHealtheVet, an e-health web-based portal (www.myhealth. va.gov/). Most widely used for its prescription refill abilities, MyHealtheVet can track blood pressure, sleep schedule, and dietary habits. These data can be put into a graph for the veteran to see progress and encourage a healthy lifestyle. Veterans are able to see the majority of the health care notes entered into CPRS.

MyHealtheVet includes a tool called "Secure Messaging" that allows for patient–provider contact through electronic messages. Secure messaging allows the veteran and provider to have contact and address non-urgent needs via a home computer, enhancing continuous patient-centered care. This system also promotes veteran engagement in health care services and health. Veterans report that secure messaging creates better communication with the primary care team by addressing health-related questions, test requests and results, medical refills and questions, and appointment management (Haun et al., 2014).

Telehealth

The Veterans Health Administration (VHA) is considered a leader in Telehealth-based treatment. Provided to the veteran either in their home via personal computer or at their local VA health care center through teleconference, Telehealth can either occur synchronously in a real-time video-conference or asynchronously in stored messages such as voice recordings or medical images which can be accessed at another time (U.S. Department of Veterans Affairs, 2015). In fiscal year 2008, approximately 230,000 veterans received care via Telehealth and another 40,000 enrolled in the home Telehealth program. This program is particularly beneficial to those with mobility difficulties or for those who reside far away from a VA site (Tuerk et al., 2010). By increasing access to care and continuing to focus on patient-centered health care, the VA is utilizing Telehealth to help achieve the goal of continuous access (Hogan, Wakefield, Nazi, Houston, & Weaver, 2011).

CRIS-CAT

The social work staff at the New Jersey WRIISC utilize the Community Reintegration of Injured Service Members (CRIS-CAT) scale to collect measures of reintegration. The CRIS-CAT is a computer-generated evaluation tool that assesses three areas of community reintegration: extent of communication reintegration, perceived limitations in community reintegration, and satisfaction in community reintegration (Resnik, Plow, & Jette, 2009).

Organization

As of July 2013, the National Center for Veterans Analysis and Statistics (NCVAS) reported 151 VA medical centers, 819 community-based outpatient clinics, and 300 vet centers in the United States. There are 23 Veterans Integrated Service Networks (VISNs), or regions, in which the VA funds services including nursing homes, residential treatment programs, and comprehensive homecare programs for more than 8.9 million veterans (VA Benefits & Health, 2014). In 2014, the VA requested a budget of US$152.7 billion overall, with US$86.1 billion in mandatory funds and US$66.5 billion allocated to discretionary funds. Programs such as women-specific medical care, mental health, and OEF/OIF/OND health care and non-VA fee care were allocated almost 17.5 billion. The financial budget also includes expanding access to care and benefits, allocating US$460 million to Telehealth. OEF/OIF/OND veterans received an increase of funding of 13.8%, which was the largest increase in the VA budget (FY 2014 President's Report, 2013).

The VA employs the most master's level social workers in the United States (Strong et al., 2014). In 1926, the Veterans Bureau, now known as the Department of Veterans Affairs, created a social work department with just 14 employees, dedicated to keeping social services within the VA. Today, there are over 11,000 social workers in the VA to provide assistance to veterans, their family members, and caregivers. These social workers can assist veterans with application for concrete resources within and outside the VA and are often employed as clinical providers (U.S. Department of Veterans Affairs, 2012). Social workers at the WRIISC work with the multi-disciplinary team to evaluate and assess veterans. Members of the team have the power to affect the outcome for the veteran through their evaluations and recommendations.

Description of the typical client: Framework

The framework used by social work staff at the WRIISC is based on the construct of reintegration based on the World Health Organization International Classification of Functioning, Disability and Health (Resnik & Allen, 2007) (Figure 16.1). The staff see reintegration as both an event (when the veteran returns from deployment) and as a process (how the veteran reintegrates back into the community over time). Generally, veterans are not evaluated at the WRIISC until time has passed from deployment. Many health symptoms associated with deployment can take time to develop and cause interruption in the veteran's life. The WRIISC completes a full assessment that evaluates each domain of this model: body function, body structure, activity, environmental factors, and personal factors. Medical staff evaluate function, structure, and activity. Psychology and neuropsychology evaluate activity, personal factors, and some environmental factors. Social work performs its assessment of the environmental and personal factors domains; even more importantly, we look at the overall model to evaluate the connection among all the different domains and help develop

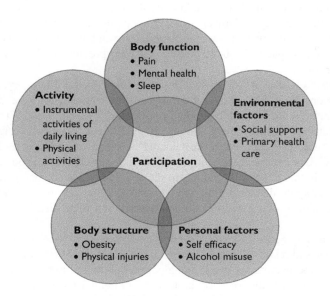

Figure 16.1 World Health Organization Framework of Reintegration. Developed by D. Helmer
using information from Ustün, Chatterji, Bickenbach, Kostanjsek, & Schneider (2003)

an appropriate treatment plan to improve the overall quality of the veteran's life. This often
includes medical, psychological, lifestyle, and resource recommendations.

Decisions about practice

Definition of the client

RF is an OEF/OIF Army Reserve Veteran. She is a White, single female who is 40 years
old, never married, and has no children. RF was referred by her PCP to the WRIISC after
experiencing both abdominal and respiratory symptoms that she believes are related to her
two deployments to southwest Asia in 2004 and 2011 as a heavy equipment construction
specialist. During both deployments, RF suffered from multiple upper and lower respiratory
infections with the recurrent use of antibiotics and was released from her deployment tour
in 2011 when she developed a chronic cough and dyspnea (shortness of breath), as well as
abdominal pain. RF presents as an intelligent, well-groomed woman. She decided to participate in the evaluation by herself. She took notes during the evaluation and asked relevant
questions. She was nervous and eager for answers about her symptoms.

RF's top concerns for her visit to the WRIISC were: chronic rhino sinusitis, cough and
dyspnea, hoarseness, throat closing, and dysphagia. Her goal for her WRIISC evaluation was
to receive a diagnosis and treatment recommendations regarding her pulmonary concerns. Up
until her evaluation, RF believed that she had not received a conclusive diagnosis; her PCP
had referred her to mental health services believing there was a psychological component to
her physical symptoms.

Health and fitness played a large role in RF's lifestyle prior to her symptoms. She enjoyed
participating in recreational and social activities such as hiking, weight lifting, dancing,

running, skiing, and speed skating. During her deployments, RF typically ran 5–10 miles each day while carrying 80–100 pound gear. However, her dyspnea decreased her physical activity. She tried to adapt to her health problems in her personal life and at work; however, she believes that her daily activity capacity is 50–80% lower than her previous abilities due to shortness of breath on exertion.

During her evaluation at the WRIISC, RF disclosed that she experienced military sexual trauma (MST) from her superior officer. She states that during her time with that unit, she felt uncomfortable and anxious, but did not report the incident out of fear of repercussions. The officer ceased the assaults after she confronted him, although he is believed to have molested other women in the unit. RF was also exposed to mortar attacks which caused injuries to two of her fellow soldiers. RF has experienced multiple flashbacks of that event, reported difficulty sleeping, and hypervigilance. Prior to coming to the WRIISC, RF was diagnosed with PTSD. RF was concerned about disclosing her MST as she felt she was immediately judged as having a mental health problem and her medical symptoms were dismissed as psychosomatic.

RF is employed full-time as a general foreman in a contracting company. She has been in a relationship for over a year and reports that her boyfriend and friends have provided her with support. RF is currently experiencing some additional stress due to her mother's deteriorating health. Her mother is 67 years old, recently underwent a kidney transplant, is permanently disabled, and is currently in remission from leukemia. RF has been responsible for all of her mother's medical care. She remains active in community activities and continues to serve in the National Guard. She is a recruiter for the National Guard and often goes to local colleges to speak to the students. During those talks, she is required to carry different types of materials that often weigh a lot. RF denies substance abuse or alcohol abuse as a coping mechanism. It is clear that RF is experiencing multiple life stressors. She is concerned about her current health situation, coping with her diagnosis of PTSD, and her mother's declining health. She has a support system that consists of her boyfriend, along with military and civilian friends.

Goals, objectives, and contracting

During RF's comprehensive evaluation, the medical staff recommended that she follow up with pulmonary function tests with and without bronchodilator and diffusing capacity for carbon monoxide (DLCO). They referred her to an ear, nose, and throat specialist (ENT) to check for vocal cord dysfunction or upper airway dysfunction. She was given a diagnosis of probable constrictive bronchiolitis, scarring of the small airways resulting in airway narrowing. The diagnosis was confirmed later by lung biopsy. The biopsy demonstrated features associated with deployment to southwest Asia (King et al., 2011).

RF had a full psychological exam with neuropsychological testing. She was functioning very well and the psychologist felt she was managing her PTSD very well through ongoing therapy at her local VA. The psychologist believed her anxiety and depressive symptoms were due to her declining physical health and that the focus of the recommendations should be about the veteran's medical conditions and not focused on her previous diagnosis of PTSD. The psychologist acknowledged that the veteran was a victim of MST.

From the social work perspective, I observed that the veteran was struggling to maintain a lifestyle that her medical condition could no longer sustain. RF had a self-concept that revolved around her independence and her ability to take care of others. She was on construction sites where she inhaled construction dust that exacerbated her pulmonary problems. Most of her social activities revolved around physical exercise and high-intensity sports. She was the primary caregiver for her mother who needed a great deal of care. To be able to optimize her well-being, lifestyle changes and developing a new sense of self-concept would be necessary.

RF had very specific goals in coming to the WRIISC. She wanted to get a clear diagnosis of medical problems, an understanding of the current treatment, and her prognosis. She wanted validation that her symptoms were "not in her head" as she had previously been led to believe. In this case, it was helpful that the veteran's goals and the staff's abilities and understanding of the case were the same. RF was distressed that her symptoms were viewed as psychosomatic by previous health care providers. Although she struggled with PTSD and had a history of MST, she had made excellent progress with her therapy and did not believe her symptoms were caused by these issues. The staff at the WRIISC agreed. The staff had seen many OEF/OIF veterans with similar pulmonary concerns.

Veterans' treatment plans are developed in two steps: first, the multi-disciplinary team meets to discuss individual provider recommendations and then a "roadmap" is created to discuss diagnoses, prognoses, and prioritized steps to maximize the veteran's well-being. As the WRIISC social worker, I often act as the advocate for the veteran in this meeting, especially addressing the feasibility of the "roadmap." Extenuating circumstances can make the information difficult to hear or the steps difficult to implement. The second step is another multi-disciplinary meeting that includes the veteran to discuss our findings and to get input from the veteran about their understanding of our recommendations and how she feels about implementing the recommended steps. The WRIISC staff believe that if the veteran is not aware and in agreement with the treatment plan, then most likely the veteran will not follow through with the recommendations. The objectives and goals are presented verbally at the final meeting, which has a casual tone, and provides the veteran with the opportunity to ask questions and make comments.

For this case, it was decided a second meeting with the social work staff was necessary. During that meeting, RF voiced both her relief and concern that she had a chronic illness with no known treatment. We believed it was important for her to start making lifestyle adjustments to sustain her current level of functioning. This was a very difficult recommendation for her to accept. She was hoping to get a clear diagnosis and treatment recommendation; she did not expect to be told she had a chronic condition that would necessitate lifestyle changes.

Use of contract

The contract formed with WRIISC patients consists of a "roadmap" or set of recommendations in the summary evaluation. The veteran receives a mailed copy and a copy is entered into CPRS. The team recommended follow-up medical appointments and a host of lifestyle changes. At the time of final meeting, the veteran was not in a frame of mind to take in all the lifestyle changes that were recommended. At the second social work meeting, the team agreed that I would work with RF via Telehealth to implement lifestyle changes. RF had a mental health provider at her local VA to continue PTSD treatment. It was decided that the evidence-based treatment of problem-solving therapy (PST) would be utilized over a 12 week period of time to help the veteran make the necessary changes to her lifestyle. This treatment decision was made in conjunction with RF and her mental health provider.

Meeting place

During a WRIISC evaluation, I meet with the veteran in a private office or in a small conference room, allowing full privacy in a quiet setting. All meetings with the evaluation team are held in a conference room, equipped with a whiteboard and computer. Follow-up phone calls and Telehealth appointments are made from my office.

Use of time

The WRIISC evaluation lasts between 3 and 4 days. Each discipline has a block of time with the veteran that follows a schedule. The schedule is flexible, based on the needs of the veteran. Social work typically sees a veteran for an hour and half in person. Follow-up phone calls can last anywhere from 10 minutes to 1 hour depending on the needs of the veteran.

Strategies and interventions

This veteran was offered PST via Telehealth specifically for anxiety and difficulties implementing lifestyle changes. PST is an evidence-based psychosocial intervention, usually considered under a cognitive behavioral umbrella, used to improve one's ability to cope with both minor (e.g., chronic daily problems) and major (e.g., traumatic events) stressors. The major treatment goals include the adaptation of a positive orientation towards problem-solving and the effective implementation of problem-solving behaviors (Nezu, Nezu, & D'Zurilla, 2013). This therapy is currently offered at the VA in person and via Telehealth for 1 hour per week for 12 sessions. Because RF lived in another part of the country, Telehealth delivery was used. RF was comfortable with this recommendation and she appreciated the focus on problem-solving in contrast to working on emotional difficulties.

The PST was very successful once RF was able to accept that changes were necessary. The 12-week model was extended because RF needed two sessions to discuss her anger and frustration about acknowledging her chronic illness. Once she was able to accept her chronic conditions, she was able to use the PST model to make changes in her life. The first change the veteran put into place was to get care for her mother. She contacted the local senior citizens program for meals on wheels, visiting nurses for medical concerns, and she met with a financial advisor to make long-term plans for her mother. Once she felt her mother was cared for, she was able to focus on her own needs.

RF's National Guard and work duties both involved physical work. She was able to contact both organizations and arrange less physical duties. It is likely she will need to separate from the National Guard as she will continue to struggle to meet the physical requirements. She is working on an exit strategy with her commanding officer. RF is confident she will be able to meet her new civilian work requirements. In planning for the future, I suggested that she apply for service connection disability that will provide her with the necessary VA medical care to treat her chronic pulmonary condition but also to provide financial resources in the future if she discovers her condition prevents her from continuing her civilian work.

The hardest recommendations for her were the limitations and changes to her exercise and social activities. Previously, she was extremely active and spent most of her free time participating in extreme sports. She was able to enroll in a VA-sponsored yoga class for OEF/OIF/OND veterans that enabled her to try a new exercise routine and to be with other veterans who were trying new VA programs. This class and her new connections led RF to try other types of complementary and alternative modalities, such as meditation and guided imagery. After the sessions of PST were complete, RF felt able to problem-solve effectively without the guidance of a therapist.

Case/care management

After the evaluation, a comprehensive report is sent to the veteran within two weeks. The report is written in an easy-to-follow layout and lay language. I contact the veteran for a follow-up phone call 1 month, 2 months, 6 months, and 12 months after their initial evaluation. At that time, progress made towards recommendations and barriers to achieving goals are discussed. The veteran has the opportunity to discuss any problems, concerns, or questions, and if needed, those can be redirected to another team member. A CRIS-CAT is completed at 2, 6, and 12 months to measure the veteran's perception of reintegration. The follow-up phone calls are documented in CPRS so that the entire team at the WRIISC, as well as the veteran's medical team at their local VA, can be aware of the progress. RF slowly implemented the recommendations and her CRIS-CAT score improved. At 12 months, she felt more satisfied with her participation in her community: work, military, family, and leisure activities.

Stance of the social worker

The social worker often fills dual roles. I am an employee of the VA system and a part of the multi-disciplinary team at WRIISC, but we also function as an advocate for the veteran. I am the liaison between the veteran and her home VA, WRIISC evaluation, and outside services. RF was having a difficult time accepting her diagnosis of constrictive bronchiolitis. I pointed this out so time in our team meeting could be devoted to helping her accept the diagnosis and answer relevant questions instead of focusing exclusively on the "roadmap." This was helpful to RF and ultimately to the team as we knew that with a comprehensive understanding of her illness, the veteran could become her own best advocate.

I also had to advocate for RF with her home VA. Up until that point, RF's illness was not clearly understood and the veteran was not receiving care specifically for her pulmonary problems. Prior to the veteran's evaluation at the WRIISC, there was a treatment emphasis on her psychological conditions and not her pulmonary symptoms. The comprehensive evaluation assisted the local VA in tailoring the veteran's treatment. With the change in focus of treatment and a new diagnosis, RF will be able to apply for service connected disability. RF also reports that she feels listened to and that the VA finally understands and is able to serve her needs.

Use of outside resources

Because the veterans seen at the WRIISC have ongoing long-term medical problems, outside resources are often used in conjunction with VA services. In this case, RF wanted more information regarding constrictive bronchiolitis. She was referred to National Jewish Health (www.nationaljewish.org) due to their work in lung disease and to the Burn Pit Registry (Airborne Hazards, 2015), a national VA service. She was also referred to her local order of the Military Order of the Purple Heart (www.purpleheart.org/), a non-VA organization created by Marines that can be very helpful with services for veterans, including help with applying for service-connected disability. RF was referred to local visiting nurse services to get care for her mother. She was also offered local recreational activities that are either free or low cost for veterans, including yoga, acupuncture, and massage.

Reassessment, transfer, termination, and case conclusion

RF and I started termination work at the beginning of the 12-week PST intervention. The evidence-based treatment was time-limited and time was spent each week discussing end of treatment. The veteran continued her supportive counseling at her home VA to supplement any psychological needs that arose during the PST treatment. I remained in touch with the local VA social worker to discuss gains and setbacks. The combination of treatment modalities was very successful. At the end of the 12-week program, RF stated she felt very capable of managing her life changes. I continued with previously scheduled follow-up phone calls per the WRIISC schedule and RF continued to progress well.

Differential discussion

This case brings to light the importance of medical concerns and lifestyle changes and reminds us not be solely focused on PTSD and MST. It is misleading to think that mental health dysfunction explains physical symptoms without a full assessment. Providers can spend most of their time addressing these very important issues but can miss the work necessary to improve overall quality of life. RF was so relieved to receive a medical diagnosis for her worsening pulmonary functioning. Her evaluation and the "roadmap" allowed RF to make significant lifestyle changes and to enjoy her life. She has become an advocate for other veterans who have pulmonary symptoms and who have not yet been diagnosed properly. RF believes that her evaluation at the WRIISC started the process necessary for her to get the help and care she needed to live a productive life.

Discussion questions

1   What are your beliefs about why veterans receive more comprehensive health care than average citizens and how do you view this through a social justice lens?
2   Discuss the hazards of focusing on mental health diagnoses over physical health diagnosis. How can you advocate assuring both get competent treatment?
3   What interventions might you use to work with people receiving a life-changing diagnosis? How would you modify your typical stance?

Note

1   This chapter reflects the knowledge and opinions of the authors, not the Department of Veterans' Affairs of the United States.

References

Airborne Hazards and Open Burn Pit Registry (2015). Retrieved from https://veteran.mobilehealth. va.gov/AHBurnPitRegistry/#page/home

Dougherty, D. D., Lee, S., Fonseca, V. P., Wolters, C. L., Schneiderman, A. I., Peterson, M. R., & Ishii, E. K. (2015). Health care use among Iraq and Afghanistan Veterans with infectious diseases. *Federal Practice, 32*, 36–41.

Findley, P. A. (2010). Returning veterans, traumatic brain injury, and Veterans' Administration Services. In T. Schwaber Kerson & J. L. M. McCoyd (Eds.), *Social work in health settings* (3rd edn.), (pp. 179–189). New York: Routledge.

FY 2014 President's Report (2013, April). In *FY 2014 president's report* (Vol. 1, pp. 1–23). Retrieved from http://comptroller.defense.gov/Portals/45/Documents/defbudget/fy2014/FY2014_Budget_Request_Overview_Book.pdf

Haun J. N., Lind, J. D., Shimada, S. L., Martin, T. L., Gosline, R. M., Antinori, N., et al. (2014). Evaluating user experiences of the Secure Messaging Tool on the Veterans Affairs' Patient Portal System. *Journal of Medical Internet Research, 16*(3), e75. doi: 10.2196/jmir.2976

Health Benefits (2015, March 17). Retrieved from www.va.gov/healthbenefits/access/medical_benefits_package.asp

Hogan, T. P., Wakefield, B., Nazi, K. M., Houston, T. K., & Weaver, F. M. (2011). Promoting access through complementary eHealth technologies: Recommendations for VA's home telehealth and personal health record programs. *Journal of General Internal Medicine, 26*, 628–635. doi: 10.1007/s11606-011-1765-y

King, M. S., Eisenberg, R., Johnson, J. E., Newman, J. H., Tolle, J. J., Sheller, J. R., et al. (2011). Constrictive bronchiolitis in soldiers returning from Iraq and Afghanistan. *New England Journal of Medicine, 365*(3), 222–230. doi: 10.1056/NEJMoa1101388

Lange, G., McAndrew, L., Ashford, W., Reinhard, M., Peterson, M., & Helmer, D. A. (2013). War related illness and injury study center (WRIISC): A multidisciplinary translational approach to the care of veterans with chronic multisymptom illness. *Military Medicine, 178*, 705–707.

Lincoln, A. E., Helmer, D. A., Schneiderman, A. I., Li, M., Copeland, H. L., Prisco, M. K., et al. (2006). The war-related illness and injury study centers: A resource for deployment-related health concerns. *Military Medicine, 171*(7), 577–585.

Morris, M. J., Lucero, P. F., Zanders, T. B., & Zacher, L. L. (2013). Diagnosis and management of chronic lung disease in deployed military personnel. *Therapeutic Advances in Respiratory Disease, 7*(4), 235–245. doi: 10.1177/1753465813481022

Nezu, A.M., Nezu, C. M., & D'Zurilla, T. J. (2013). *Problem-solving therapy: A treatment manual.* New York: Springer.

Resnik, L. J. & Allen, S. M. (2007). Using International Classification of Functioning, Disability and Health to understand challenges in community reintegration of injured veterans. *Journal of Rehabilitation Research and Development, 44*, 991–1006. doi: 10.1682/jrrd.2007.05.0071

Resnik, L., Plow, M., & Jette, A. (2009). Development of CRIS: Measure of community reintegration of injured service members. *Journal of Rehabilitation Research and Development, 46*(4), 469–480. doi: 10.1682/JRRD.2008.07.0082

Strong, J., Ray, K., Findley, P. A., Torres, R., Pickett, L., & Byrne, R. J. (2014). Psychosocial concerns of veterans of Operation Enduring Freedom/Operation Iraqi Freedom. *Health and Social Work, 39*(1), 17–24. doi: 10.1093/hsw/hlu002

Tuerk, P. W., Fortney, J., Bosworth, H. B., Wakefield, B., Ruggiero, K. J., Acierno, R., & Frueh, B. C. (2010). Toward the development of national telehealth services: The role of veterans' health administration and future directions for research. *Telemedicine Journal and E-health: the Official Journal of the American Telemedicine Association, 16*(1), 115–117. doi: 10.1089=tmj.2009.0144

U.S. Department of Veterans Affairs (n.d.). History – VA History. Retrieved from www.va.gov/about_va/vahistory.asp

U.S. Department of Veterans Affairs (2012). History VA Social Work. Retrieved from www.social work.va.gov/about.asp

U.S. Department of Veterans Affairs (2015). VA Telehealth Services. Retrieved from www.tele health.va.gov/

Ustün, T. B., Chatterji, S., Bickenbach, J., Kostanjsek, N., & Schneider, M. (2003). The International Classification of Functioning, Disability and Health: A new tool for understanding disability and health. *Disability Rehabilitation, 25*(11–12), 565–571.

VA Benefits & Health Care Utilization [Fact sheet]. (2014, December 23). Retrieved from www.va.gov/vetdata/docs/pocketcards/fy2015q1.pdf

Chapter 17

Work with undocumented immigrants

When serious illness intersects with no insurance

Patricia A. Findley

Context

Description of the setting

The Rutgers FOCUS Wellness Center (FOCUS) is a primary care clinic located in Newark, New Jersey. Funded in January 2012, and opened officially that March, this nurse-led program is a grant-funded interprofessional collaboration of the schools of nursing, social work, and pharmacy. Each discipline uses the site for student instruction, with an emphasis on collaborative care. In New Jersey, nurse practitioners are authorized to write prescriptions and they run FOCUS. Physicians are not on site, but as with any of the other consultants, they are available by phone.

Because the clinic is grant funded, it is able to provide some charity care, and it is also licensed to receive private insurance payments as well as Medicare and Medicaid. FOCUS also accepts sliding fee private payments. Clients can schedule visits for their primary health care needs (e.g., wounds, blood pressure monitoring, illnesses, and immunizations), mental health counseling services, prescriptions for medication, and case management. However, many clients come for visits on a walk-in basis. Clients may just make 1–2 visits, but many come regularly, particularly for counseling by the social worker or for medication follow-up with the medical team members.

Mental health visits are most often with the social worker for case management and counseling. A psychiatric nurse practitioner (PNP) is also part of the team and provides psychiatric assessments, therapy, and medication management for psychiatric diagnoses. The FOCUS PNP also has trained expertise in alternative medicine practices, allowing her to offer Reiki, a Japanese technique for stress reduction and relaxation that also promotes healing. She also practices pranic healing, where the prana or energy is used to heal ailments in the body by manipulation of the person's energy field. Given the PNP's mind–body focus, she works very closely with the social worker.

FOCUS is located near a very busy train station on the edge of a university campus, in an economically challenged neighborhood. The primary clientele are Spanish-speaking immigrants with very low incomes. The neighborhood is crime-ridden and violence is a constant threat. FOCUS has security cameras throughout the clinic space connected to the city police; the university police make random security checks.

Policy

Immigration status, especially of undocumented individuals, is a constant theme at FOCUS as they are at increased risk for poor physical, psychological, and social health outcomes and inadequate health care (Derose, Escarce, & Lurie, 2007). There are longstanding structural barriers and policies that restrict access to health care for these immigrants, the most notable is the Personal Responsibility and Work Opportunity Reconciliation Act of 1996 (PRWORA, 1996). Under this policy, documented immigrants may not use federal programs such as Medicaid and Children's Health Insurance Program (CHIP) until they have been in the United States for 5 years. Undocumented immigrants are not entitled to any health care coverage. Only emergency care (i.e., use of the emergency room at a hospital or disaster relief), immunizations, and general programs that protect life or safety such as soup kitchens or emergency shelter are available, with some charitable exceptions. Furthermore, the policy requires that the income of the immigrant's sponsor as well as the income of the immigrant be considered in the Medicaid or CHIP application (Riedel, 1998).

This leaves most recent immigrants and their children unable to access health care. In a study that examined the National Survey of America's Families in 1997, using data collected after the implementation of the PROWRA, immigrants and their children were found to be less likely to have a usual source of health care (Ku & Matani, 2001). They also found that being a noncitizen was associated with a 2.5% reduction in Medicaid coverage, an 8.9% decrease in job-based insurance coverage, and an 8.5% increase in the probability of being uninsured, compared with individuals born in the United States.

It has also been hypothesized that immigrants are less likely to access mental health care in the United States. Chen and Vargas-Bustamante (2011), using data from 2002–2006, estimated the impact of immigration status on mental health care utilization among patients with depression or anxiety disorders. They found that immigrants were significantly less likely to take any prescription drugs, but not significantly less likely to have any physician visits compared to citizens born in the United States.

Another important policy that impacts health care access for immigrants is the Illegal Immigration Reform and Immigrant Responsibility Act of 1996 (IIRIRA, 1996). This policy requires legal immigrants to demonstrate that they are not at risk of being financially dependent of public benefits. The determination of risk for becoming a public charge considers the person's age, health, resources, family status, financial status, education, skills, and receipt of any past benefits (Riedel, 1998). This last component, the receipt of any past benefits, was not clearly defined in the policy. This caused significant consternation among immigrants, leading many immigrants to avoid application for health care benefits for which they would have been eligible. Finally in 1999, new guidelines were issued by Immigration and Naturalization Services to clarify that benefits that are exempted from consideration of the public charge determination include Medicaid, CHIP, and services from nutrition services (e.g., Women, Infants, and Children, WIC, school lunch programs) and other services and programs allowable under PROWRA such as emergency room services, disaster relief, and educational assistance.

The restrictions and lack of clarity around the public policies have caused fear and mistrust regarding the receipt of health care services in the United States by immigrants, both documented and undocumented. Some estimate the 11–12 million undocumented immigrants live without health care coverage and not only suffer ill-health themselves, but risk passing infectious diseases along to others (www.undocumentedpatients.org/).

The Patient Protection and Affordable Care Act (ACA, 2010) does make provision for qualified (documented) immigrants to purchase health care coverage in the Healthcare.gov Marketplace Exchange (www.healthcare.gov/immigrants/), but few have the wherewithal to afford the coverage. Immigrants are much less likely than U.S.-born citizens to receive employer-based insurance, and efforts are being made to increase education around access to employer-based insurance, and the value of insurance itself (Derose, Escarce, & Lurie, 2007). Education about access to the state-funded programs such as Medicaid and CHIP under the ACA is also growing (Buettgens & Holahan, 2010). However, under the ACA, undocumented immigrants are barred from the exchanges and are also prohibited by law from all of the benefits of health reform and are not allowed to purchase coverage, even with their own money (Buettgens & Holahan, 2010).

Technology

FOCUS uses an electronic medical record (EMR). The building is wireless to allow staff to document or review records/test results from any location in the building. The record combines the notes into an interdisciplinary note that is ultimately signed off by each clinician and finally by the supervising nurse practitioner. The clinicians are careful to avoid using the technology in a room with a patient if it makes him or her uncomfortable. Providers talk with the patients, not around the technology to the patients. Some patients appreciate seeing the graphic depiction of their lab results to visualize their progress over time.

Organization

FOCUS can operate somewhat outside of the health care system due to its grant funding. We can treat individuals without insurance and those who are undocumented immigrants. FOCUS fills an important gap in the overall health care system. Without FOCUS, many of the clients who are seen would never have accessed health care in Newark. This ability gives FOCUS credibility with clients. FOCUS is typically the last resort, so many clients are desperate for care by the time they arrive at our door.

The interprofessional providers discuss these issues in team meetings. The providers maintain a stance that each will treat the clients/patients with dignity and respect. This is not out of the norm for this group. Many clients tell us that this first place where they have providers look them in the eye, smile, and show genuine interest in their situations. The FOCUS team realized their efforts were meaningful. The bulletin board in the staff area is filled with notes of gratitude from patients as well as students for their time at FOCUS; this is the testament that keeps the team focused on providing this challenging care that is filling an important gap.

Description of the typical client

The average client at FOCUS is a 42-year-old female who has experienced violence in the home or in the community, and has a chronic health condition such as diabetes, heart disease, asthma, or depression. Nearly all have at least one psychosocial need such as food insecurity, issues with housing or rent, lack of health insurance, and poverty. Some have severe mental health issues or experience substance abuse. The majority are Hispanic immigrants. The majority of the clients are referred through word of mouth from a friend or neighbor. However, other referrals have been growing through informal partnerships with several social services agencies. Such agencies include one that works with women who are victims of domestic violence, a Hispanic day center that has a soup kitchen and teaches English as a second language courses, and even the university hospital that can only provide emergency care.

Clients are typically first seen by a nurse to assess medical needs; however, the team at FOCUS have been working to quickly identify which issues may be best treated by one of the other disciplines (e.g., pharmacy or social work). Most importantly, the team members strive to collaborate with one another and with the client, sometimes even sitting in the same room together when discussing the client's need. For example, the nurse may recommend a medication for the client, and then will consult with the pharmacist with the client present to discuss issues such as medication compliance and allergies. Occasionally, the social worker will join the nurse, the pharmacist, and the client to discuss payment for the medication, concerns over taking medication, or to aid the adjustment by the client to the illness or condition for which the medication is prescribed. This interprofessional work group can include family members or friends as allowed by the client. Fortunately, many of the team members are bilingual and bicultural, so they can assist with language translation.

Decisions about practice

Definition of the client

Vilma Delgado is a 29-year-old Latina woman from Ecuador living in the United States since 2000. She lives with her husband, Ramon, and two children ages 6 years (son, Adolfo) and 3 years (daughter, Sofia). Alberto, the father of the 3-year-old lives in Ecuador; Ramon is the father of the 6-year-old. Vilma does not speak English, is undocumented, does not have any other family in the area, and does not have medical insurance. Ramon is working and is the only source of income for the family. He works in construction and he is seldom able to accompany Vilma to appointments at FOCUS.

Medical

Vilma was referred to FOCUS by a staff member of a Hispanic social service agency that has been involved with the family providing assistance with transportation, food, and medicine. They sometimes translate for Vilma when she has appointments. Upon arriving at FOCUS, Vilma had an open wound on her leg and difficulty walking due to leg and lower back pain. She was concerned about her health and her ability to care for her very active children.

With Vilma's consent, medical records were requested from the university hospital where she was last treated. From the records, the providers at FOCUS discovered that Vilma had been diagnosed with cancer, a synovial sarcoma, 3 years earlier. She reported having three surgeries to treat the sarcoma and two plastic surgeries to aid in wound healing. She had recent chemotherapy and her last chemotherapy session was just two weeks prior to her FOCUS visit. She had just been told (the prior week) that the chemotherapy was not working anymore. A PET scan revealed lung masses growing in number and size despite the chemotherapy. She handed a business card to the FOCUS social worker that indicated she was to return to see a surgeon regarding an amputation of her affected leg in June, three months from our meeting. Vilma was unclear about her prognosis and confused about what health care plan she was to follow.

Psychosocial

Vilma's mother and seven siblings live in Ecuador. Vilma came to the United States 4 years ago. She is married to Ramon, also from Ecuador, and is undocumented. Both are Roman

Catholic and have less than a high school level education. They live in a small, neat apartment close to FOCUS.

It was clear the stresses of Vilma's and Ramon's marriage and financial situation began years ago. Because of the financial stress, Vilma and Ramon had decided to separate, hoping that if Vilma were "single" she may have access to more public services. Nevertheless, they agreed to continue living under the same roof. While still living in the same household with Ramon, Vilma met someone (Alberto) who was very supportive and helped her a lot both financially and emotionally. Vilma became pregnant by Alberto, but she was still married to Ramon and wanted to remain with him. Alberto decided to return to Ecuador, leaving before Sofia was born. Ramon was present at the time of the birth and they decide to "try again" to make a family with both children. Ramon cares for both Adolfo and Sofia as his own children.

Vilma mentioned that her father had died at age 46 from "lung problems" when she was seven months pregnant with Sofia. She had been very close to him and had not seen him since she came to the United States. She reported feeling depressed after her father died; she also reported that the depressive symptoms worsened after she had Sofia. She gained a lot of weight and was more isolated and disengaged from Ramon. He started to drink more and became verbally and emotionally abusive. Their financial situation was getting worse; Vilma was unable to work due to her health and childcare responsibilities. Ramon was working as a construction worker, but the season had been rainy so he was frequently removed from the schedule and, thus, unpaid. Both were angry and frustrated at each other for their current plight.

Ramon's family was not as open to Sofia as Ramon was towards her. Ramon's family rejected Vilma and her newborn child because she cheated on Ramon, a sin in the eyes of the Catholic Church. Two years later when Vilma was diagnosed with cancer, his family told her "It was punishment from God for what she did to him." This devastated Vilma, yet Ramon stands beside her. In the face of her cancer diagnosis and ongoing grief over the loss of her father, her mental health is deteriorating.

Despite her contact with the health care system, Vilma was never offered mental health counseling due to her lack of insurance. Vilma was depressed, angry, frustrated, and overwhelmed with her situation. At FOCUS, the social worker set up a meeting with a nurse practitioner, Vilma, and Ramon. At the meeting, the nurse practitioner explained Vilma's medical condition and the social worker assisted with translation. In that team/family meeting, Ramon and Vilma began to "hear" how critical Vilma's condition was and understood the devastating prognosis that Vilma only had six months to live. They were never given the opportunity to sit together with health care providers to discuss Vilma's situation. They were beside themselves with grief. They had no plans for the children and were painfully aware of the difficult situation they were going to face. They knew that they needed to start planning and making arrangements.

Goals

The immediate goal for the social worker was to provide supportive counseling to Vilma and Ramon. The entire health care team held a "huddle" to discuss the care of Vilma and her family. The social worker had to emphasize culturally sensitive care when a nurse made a comment wondering just "what was Vilma thinking" when she had the second child out of wedlock, making the child a "burden on the system" in the United States. One goal was to maintain compassionate and culturally sensitive care for Vilma and her family.

Contracting and developing objectives

The interprofessional team developed a team evaluation and care plan that was then discussed with Vilma by the social worker. She was able to translate for her and incorporate Vilma's wishes into the plan. Vilma expressed concern about her children. We set up a team meeting with Vilma and Ramon to discuss the overall plan of care and future planning for the entire family. Ramon had to cancel a team meeting twice due to sunny weather; he struggled to balance Vilma's needs and earning money to deal with their financial situation.

Vilma divulged that she had not spoken to her family in Ecuador about her illness. That geographically distant family had been a source of support for her until the illness. The inability to talk about her situation with her family added to her stress. Although Vilma expressed gratitude to the social worker for support, she was becoming concerned that her increased frequency with the health care system could lead to deportation, a common fear among immigrants without documentation (Arbona et al., 2010). Like many immigrants, she had delayed contacts with the health care system due to that fear (Arbona et al., 2010). Her fear of deportation and her inability to share her situation with her family forced Vilma to isolate and to attempt to manage her stress and health situation on her own. This tendency towards isolation is another common issue for immigrants; social workers should explore isolation and connections (Furman et al., 2009) to enable mobilization of support where possible.

The evaluation's medical goals focused on pain management and medication management. Nursing and pharmacy worked together to identify the best medications for her. Together, they helped to coordinate an administration schedule, educate Vilma on the medications, and establish a culturally consistent nutrition plan. The social worker's main focus became the financial situation of the family and the future planning for the children. Weekly therapy focused on issues identified by Vilma, namely, issues of grief, anger, resentment, and guilt, especially in regards to God. Education about developing a Power of Attorney and a Living Will was planned and marital counseling was also offered.

Use of contract

The contract is formed with the clients at FOCUS through discussion with the social worker, either alone, or in collaboration with one or both of the other disciplines. Frequently, the social worker will lead the team, particularly if there are multiple components to the contract. Often, it is the social work role to follow up with the client to ensure steps are taken. The work is verbal and implied, but the client is reassessed at every appointment to establish progress, to determine if there is a need to change plans, and to discuss barriers to implementation of the care plan. Vilma came for regular appointments and included Ramon when the weather allowed his presence. Frequently, the children would accompany the couple to their visits. Sometimes the children were included in the sessions, and many times, a friend or a FOCUS staff member would sit with the children in the waiting room to play with them during the visits.

Meeting place

The meeting space was usually in the social worker's private office at FOCUS. Occasionally, the team would meet with Vilma and Ramon at the same table used for team meetings in our clinical space. Vilma preferred the privacy of the office space because, even though soundproof, the team meeting space was in a room with a bank of windows along one side that faced the waiting room.

Use of time

Appointments at FOCUS are scheduled through an electronic scheduling system within the medical record. Typically, each clinician is given time for an initial assessment. All social work visits are allotted an hour. Patients are seen as needed, sometimes once a week, sometimes once a month, and sometimes not for several months. FOCUS is able to schedule patients with multiple clinicians simultaneously. However, many of the interdisciplinary encounters with Vilma were more spontaneous in nature. For example, one day the nurse was examining Vilma's leg wound and Vilma began to cry. The nurse was able to walk through the small clinic to the social worker's office to invite her to come into the examination room to meet with Vilma while the nurse changed the dressings. Several times, on rainy days, Vilma would show up with Ramon to be seen. With awareness of Vilma's prognosis, schedules were flexed to accommodate Vilma and her family.

Strategies and interventions

The FOCUS social worker takes a generalist case management approach in working with the interprofessional team. Figure 17.1 depicts Vilma's ecosystem as we worked with her. The ecosystem perspective is similar to a person-in-environment perspective with the focus on the client in his or her environment. It then extends the approach by giving attention at levels of systems such as the macro, mesosystem, exosystem, and microsystem levels of interventions (Langer & Lietz, 2015; Sincero, 2015). We intervened at four different levels of relationship: *microsystem*, interventions were directly with the individuals, Vilma and Ramon; *mesosystem*, intervention directed towards the client's microsystem (work with the family, churches, health care providers); *exosystem*, the structures surrounding the client (the culture, health care organizations, state laws); and the *macrosystem*, the greater societal context, including federal laws and social norms about immigration. At the center is Vilma herself where she brings all of her own individual characteristics such as age, language, immigration status, and gender which, in turn, can influence or be influenced by the other systems. As the case is discussed, the roles of the interrelated systems will become clearer.

As a case manager, the social worker follows up and integrates the recommendations from the team huddle for the client. Patient education is a significant component of the social worker role, particularly if the individual is identified as a social work client. The team expects the social worker to follow up, facilitate service brokering, and coordinate services. Phone contact is sometimes impossible as many clients at FOCUS cannot afford a home or mobile phone.

Stance of the social worker

Working with an immigrant population requires a culturally sensitive approach as an overlay to all of the generalist practice principles social workers are trained to employ. Nearly 13% of the entire population in 2010 were non-U.S.-born in 2009–2013 (U.S. Census, 2013). As of July 1, 2013, there are 54 million people of Hispanic origin in the United States, making these individuals the nation's largest ethnic or racial minority. They comprise 17% of the U.S. population (U.S. Census, 2013). Also according to the 2010 Census,

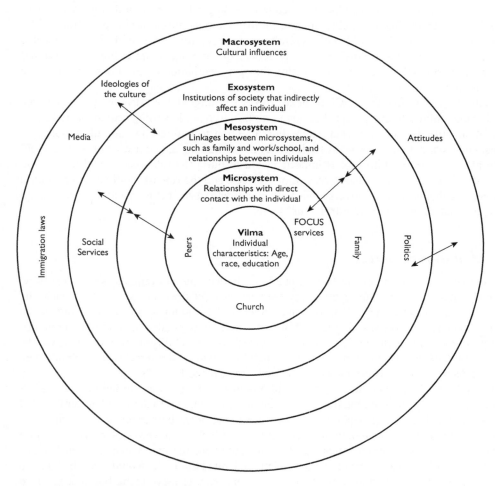

Figure 17.1 Ecosystem map for Vilma

New Jersey is home to more than 1.5 million Hispanics, with 18% of Newark's population claiming Hispanic origin.

Such growth in our immigrant population requires social workers to be culturally competent. Culturally competent practice means that one is aware of characteristics such as race, ethnicity, and culture, and understands specific cultural, language, social, and economic nuances and respects them (NASW, n.d.). Developing cultural competence as a social worker means using self, but understanding one's own attitudes and beliefs as well as how those attitudes can impact the worker's ecosystem, and attitudes about the diverse group as whole. Johnson and Yanca (2010) suggest that it is also important to understand the history of the diverse group within the context of the United States, including stereotypes, discrimination, and oppression the group may have experienced. We need to understand how our formal systems (the health care system for instance) may reinforce the discrimination and oppression some groups experience in contrast to the privileges and advantages the dominant group receives. Johnson and Yanca (2010) also suggest that understanding the immigrant group, including the culture, beliefs, and customs of the group is critical. Using social work values, we social workers need to develop knowledge regarding relationship building, assessment, planning, action, evaluation, and termination skills that meet the cultural expectations of the client (Potocky-Tripodi, 2002). For example, in some cultures, it would be inappropriate for a male worker to be assigned to a single, female client. Some cultures are more reserved with their emotional expression, so pressing for open ventilation of emotions would not be appropriately culturally sensitive.

In the case of Vilma, the FOCUS social worker is bilingual, born originally in Colombia and is quite culturally competent. Furman et al. (2009) have identified Latinos as requiring special attention by social workers, including attention to immigration and migration concerns, understanding how to assess for levels of acculturation, and educating ourselves about cultural values. Being bilingual is important, but to build the relationship and understand the cultural context of the illness, receipt of services, and the role of family require cultural competence that is built in conversations with clients and in an openness and non-judgmental approach that allows us to learn from our clients.

Use of outside resources

The use of outside resources to help Vilma was challenging and required some creativity. Given her immigration status, many of the agencies we typically used as referrals, such as the visiting nurse association (VNA), were not allowed. The lead nurse practitioner contacted a former student who was working for a different VNA: although also bound by the immigration policies outlined earlier, her non-profit agency had the ability to provide charity care, even to undocumented immigrants. We planned to activate the referral when Vilma's care became such that she was no longer able to make the trips to FOCUS.

We helped Vilma share her diagnosis and prognosis with her Ecuadorian family in a telephone call and Vilma soon felt the desire to go home to Ecuador to die with her family. That trip would be challenging because finances were a significant barrier and she was afraid to go back to her country without taking her children. Both children were U.S. citizens because they were born in the United States, but Ramon would need to travel with her to take care of the children. Vilma feared that once Ramon left the United States, he would never be allowed to return. His family lived in Newark and he did not want to leave them, but he also loved Vilma. They both struggled with this decision.

FOCUS made an arrangement with a storyteller for Vilma to complete a legacy project (Allen, 2009). Rachel was an award-winning storyteller, teacher, writer, and humanitarian based in New York City and her role within FOCUS was to help Vilma tell her life story. The goal was to create a document of Vilma's stories, thoughts, and wishes to give to Vilma's children. Rachel was not bilingual and worked with Vilma and the FOCUS social worker to create the book while the social worker monitored Vilma's emotional response to the storytelling experience. Vilma was pleased, yet sad, at the product of the experience. She knew her children would value it much later in their lives. It also allowed Vilma a beginning sense of closure on a journey that was emotionally and physically painful.

Finally, we connected with the School of Law at the nearby university. A professor and his student came to FOCUS, where Vilma and Ramon were comfortable, to discuss planning for the future of the children. This was extremely emotionally challenging for the couple. During the meeting, we could see the children playing in the waiting room with a nursing student. The bleak situation was difficult for all, including for the health care provider team.

Termination/conclusion

Vilma became quite ill; her functional status declined considerably over two weeks. She now knew she wanted to go home to Ecuador to die with her mother and siblings. We contacted Vilma's church to discuss the difficult dilemma and enlisted several church members to help pay for a plane ticket for Vilma and a companion from the church. This meant Ramon would not have to leave the United States. We called ahead to the airport to arrange for a wheelchair to get Vilma to the gate in the most comfortable fashion. We were only able to do our termination work with Vilma over the telephone as she needed to leave so abruptly. Vilma expressed her gratitude for all the team had done to help her. Vilma was scheduled to leave the next day on the plane home to Ecuador. The team wished her well.

No word came the following week, yet the team was unsure if they would hear any news at all. Late Friday, that same week, the Hispanic social service agency that introduced Vilma to us relayed to FOCUS that Vilma had traveled to the airport for her flight, but in the taxi she complained of extreme pain. The accompanying church member took her to the hospital emergency room. Vilma died in the hospital 2 days later.

Differential discussion

We learned a lot from this case. Following the news of Vilma's death, the team realized how emotionally involved we all had become with Vilma and her family. The team shared Vilma's hopes for reunification with her family of origin to bring peace and closure. We were saddened and a bit demoralized by Vilma's death in the United States. We now attend to self-care techniques as part of the general in-service schedule for the FOCUS team.

The team was able to discuss, albeit informally, the care decisions for and with Vilma. The team felt grateful that Vilma came to FOCUS; we knew the broader health care system would not have treated her with the dignity and respect that we were able to provide her given our ability to provide charity care. We were glad for the work we got to do with her despite her status as an undocumented immigrant. Ideally, laws that penalize immigrants will change. Maybe stories such as this will help others change the policies that hurt immigrants, documented or undocumented. We were able to be creative to work with this family to provide supportive care, despite the challenges of federal policies that created barriers to providing the best care we could offer.

Discussion questions

1   If you were the president, how might you direct the Immigration and Naturalization Service to develop policies that might affect patients who experienced health conditions like Vilma's?
2   What are your thoughts about how scarce low-cost health services might be equitably distributed to undocumented people in the face of groups such as workers making minimum wage who struggle to afford medical insurance? What do you believe your social justice ethic requires you to do in such situations?
3   If you had a patient who died under frustrating circumstances, how might you and your team members work to process the loss as a group?

References

ACA (2010). Patient Protection and Affordable Care Act. 42 U.S.C. § 18001 et seq. (2010).

Allen, R. S. (2009). The legacy project intervention to enhance meaningful family interactions: Case examples. *Clinical Gerontology, 32*(2),164–176. doi: 10.1080/07317110802677005

Arbona, C., Olvera, N., Rodriguez, N., Hagan, J., Linares, A., & Wiesner, M. (2010). Acculturative stress among documented and undocumented Latino immigrants in the United States. *Hispanic Journal of Behavioral Sciences, 32*(3), 362–384. doi: 10.1177/0739986310373210

Buettgens, M. & Holahan, J. (2010). *America under the Affordable Care Act.* New Jersey: Robert Wood Foundation.

Chen, J. & Vargas-Bustamante, A. (2011). Estimating the effects of immigration status on mental health care utilizations in the United States. *Journal of Immigrant and Minority Health, 13*(4), 671–680.

Derose, K. P., Escarce, J. J., & Lurie, N. (2007). Immigrants and health care: Sources of vulnerability. *Health Affairs, 26*(5), 1258–1268. doi: 10.1377/ hlthaff.26.5

Furman, R., Negi, N. J., Iwamoto, D. K., Rowan, D., Shukraft, A., & Gragg, J. (2009). Social work practice with Latinos: Key issues for social workers. *Social Work, 54*(2), 167–174.

IIRIRA (1996). Illegal Immigration Reform and Immigrant Responsibility Act of 1996, Division C of P.L. 104–208 (1996).

Johnson, L. C. & Yanca, S. J. (2010). *Social work practice: A generalist approach.* Boston: Allyn and Bacon.

Ku, L. & Matani, S. (2001). Left out: Immigrants' access to health care and insurance. *Health Affairs, 20*(1), 247–256. doi: 10.1377/hlthaff.20.1.247

Langer, C. L. & Lietz, C. A. (2015). *Applying theory to generalist social work practice: A case study approach.* Hoboken, NJ: John Wiley & Sons.

NASW (National Association of Social Workers) (n.d.) Diversity and cultural competence. Retrieved from https://www.socialworkers.org/pressroom/features/issue/diversity.asp

Potocky-Tripodi, M. (2002). *Best practices for social work with refugees and immigrants.* New York: Columbia University Press.

PRWORA (1996). Personal Responsibility and Work Opportunity Reconciliation Act of 1996, P.L. No. 104–193, 912, 110 Stat. 2353–2354 (1997).

Riedel, R. L. (1998). Access to health care. In S. Lolue (Ed.), *Handbook of immigrant health* (pp. 101–124). New York: Plenum Press.

Sincero, S. M. (2015). Ecological systems theory. Retrieved from http://explorable.com/ecological-systems-theory

U.S. Census Bureau (2013). Retrieved from www.census.gov/newsroom/facts-for-features/2014/cb14-ff22.html

An integrated health care approach to promote smoking cessation for persons with serious mental illness

Judith A. DeBonis, Lisa de Saxe Zerden, and Anne C. Jones

Context

According to the Centers for Disease Control and Prevention (CDC, 2015), cigarette smoking is currently the single greatest cause of preventable illness and death in the United States. Several decades of public health efforts have provided strong evidence showing that smoking harms nearly every organ in the body and is the most important modifiable risk factor for coronary heart disease, stroke, several types of cancer, and pulmonary disease. As a result, the rate of cigarette smoking has steadily declined for almost 50 years (CDC, 2013a). However, persons with serious mental illness (SMI) continue to smoke at rates nearly double those of the general public (CDC, 2013b) because they typically receive little encouragement to stop smoking, have poor access to smoking cessation programs, and receive mixed messages about smoking from the agencies and institutions providing mental health services. Therefore, many persons with SMI continue to have high rates of tobacco use, especially cigarette smoking, and suffer the related consequences, including a life expectancy that is shortened by 25 years (Scott & Happell, 2011). Most people who smoke want to quit (CDC, 2015), and individuals are more likely to be successful at quitting smoking when they have both support for their efforts and access to effective smoking cessation treatments (Williams et al., 2011).

Description of the setting

Located in southern California, Didi Hirsch Mental Health Services is one of the largest community-based mental health agencies in Los Angeles, providing exceptional mental health and substance-abuse treatment services to more than 90,000 children and adults each year. The agency offers an array of services, including crisis intervention/stabilization, counseling, residential treatment, case management, delinquency prevention programs, and the nation's first free, accredited, 24/7 suicide prevention crisis line (www.didihirsch.org).

The newest of the agency's services is the Healthy Inglewood Project (HIP), which is designed to increase access and expand physical health services for clients with SMI. Housed in the Didi Hirsch Wellness Center, HIP provides clients with access to a health care team that integrates and coordinates primary health care and behavioral health care services, creating a true medical home for HIP clients. HIP provides clients with access to primary care, specialty referrals, care coordination, support groups, therapy, psychiatry, wellness groups, and cognitive enhancement therapy.

Policy

The passage of the Patient Protection and Affordable Care Act (ACA) in 2010 set the stage for changes in the health care system by providing incentives to encourage the development of integrated systems of care to improve access to services, enhance quality of care, and lower costs. The integrated model of care is defined as "a coordinated system of care that provides both medical and mental/behavioral health services to address the whole person" (Hogg Foundation for Mental Health, 2008). The ACA also placed a renewed emphasis on prevention of disease and illness, allocating US$15 billion in funding for prevention programs, ranging from smoking cessation to combating obesity (ACA, 2010). Although policies have been effective in decreasing smoking rates in the public by implementing smoking bans in public buildings and facilities, increasing taxes on cigarettes, and limiting exposure to secondhand smoke (Fiore et al., 2004), the rates of cigarette smoking among persons with SMI have continued to exceed the national average, indicating that this population will benefit from preventive health services such as smoking cessation (Williams et al., 2011).

Historically, smoking cessation services have included brief interventions typically offered through primary care providers or public health agencies (rather than behavioral or mental health agencies), and targeted to smokers who are highly motivated to quit smoking. However, for smoking cessation programs to be effective among persons with mental illness, the programs require adaptations to meet the unique needs of these individuals (Williams et al., 2011).

Technology

Most definitions of integrated health care include the electronic medical record (EMR) as an essential component of good care. EMRs provide efficient, timely sharing of medical records and service information between systems that collaborate as part of the health care team (World Health Organization, 2014). The inclusion of smoking assessments in the EMR along with monitoring of other vital signs of health (e.g., blood pressure, weight) can help to ensure that tobacco use is routinely addressed as a crucial component of a person's overall health (McCullough, Fisher, Goldstein, Kramer, & Ripley-Moffitt, 2009). Collecting "dosage" data in the EMR, such as the number of cigarettes smoked per day, enables providers to track smoking patterns and to use these data to motivate smokers to consider change (Holroyd-Leduc, Lorenzetti, Straus, Sykes, & Quan, 2011).

Mobile phone technologies offer new avenues for supporting clients making behavioral changes, such as quitting smoking and include an ever-expanding range of functions that can be used to provide individual support (Free et al., 2013). Given the increasing access to mobile devices, persons wanting to quit smoking can receive reminders to change a nicotine patch or take a medication, be prompted to practice a relaxation technique to lower stress, or track the amount of money saved over time with each reduction in the number of cigarettes smoked.

Another effective technology that the health team can use to motivate clients' smoking cessation is the breath carbon monoxide (CO) monitor (CoVita, 2015). CO is one of approximately 4,000 chemicals delivered to the lungs every time a smoker inhales from a cigarette. CO binds easily with the red blood cells, occupying the spaces that are meant to be filled by oxygen molecules, which has multiple negative effects, including a faster heartbeat. CO levels reveal real-time feedback about the impact of smoking, and offer opportunities for a discussion about smoking behavior that may help motivate a client's commitment to behavior change (CoVita, 2015).

Organization

The mission of Didi Hirsch Mental Health Services is to "transform lives by providing quality mental health and substance abuse services in communities where stigma or poverty limits access." The agency undertook a 4-year grant-funded research pilot to design and test the HIP program's effectiveness in increasing access to culturally respectful and responsive care among clients with SMI. HIP uses an integrated model, providing a client-centered medical home that offers systematic coordination of primary and behavioral health care. Clients eligible to designate HIP as their medical home need to have a mental health diagnosis; the focus of care is on treatment and prevention of chronic medical conditions. Many HIP clients have more than two diagnoses, including a substance use/misuse disorder. Although most HIP clients initially come to the agency for mental health services, HIP encourages wider participation in the Wellness Center services, activities, fitness classes, and didactic health groups on nutrition and physical activity (www.integration.samhsa.gov/resource/pbhci-program).

Description of typical clients and situations

As HIP clients completed physical health screenings during the first year of the project, staff discovered that 68% of clients were identified as "at risk" for high blood pressure (hypertension). As a result, HIP then took several actions: (a) increased focus on physical health for *all* agency clients (b) initiated an agency-wide tobacco-free policy, and (c) added smoking cessation groups to HIP services. According to the HIP Integrated Health Coordinator (Ariel Peterson, personal communication, February, 2015), the initial smoking cessation groups were a "dismal failure," in part because the label of a Stop Smoking Group was unappealing to those not ready to quit. Although clients responded more positively to the new name of "Trash the Ash," HIP recognized that helping clients to quit smoking required individualized attention to the demographic makeup, cultural backgrounds, and specific smoking behaviors of specific consumers. For example, 64% of HIP clients identified as African American; 86% reported using tobacco in the past 30 days, 38% reported daily use, and 53% were designated as "heavy smokers" by CO monitor test results. Therefore, although the majority of African American clients could benefit from smoking cessation, those who were "heavy smokers" may need specific support to address nicotine withdrawal symptoms. Each person's readiness to quit, motivations and barriers must be assessed.

Many agencies and institutions serving clients with SMI have had a permissive culture toward smoking and have used cigarettes as client rewards. Thus, the organizational culture reinforces staff beliefs that allowing clients to smoke helps them focus on other, more important therapeutic goals. Staff may view denying smoking privileges as unreasonably harsh because, in their view, smoking is a client's one source of pleasure and relaxation (Williams et al., 2010).

Decisions about practice

Definition of the client

Lewis is a 58-year-old African American male with a history of homelessness and incarceration. He is muscular, tall, of normal weight, and speaks quietly, initially avoiding eye contact. His thoughts and speech are clear without signs of disordered thinking. During young adulthood, Lewis was diagnosed with paranoid schizophrenia and schizoaffective disorder. Lewis began smoking at age 12 and has been a heavy smoker for most of his life. When asked how many cigarettes he smokes each day, he replied: "The maximum I can."

Lewis was frustrated and upset because he was recently diagnosed with pre-diabetes and hypertension. The HIP physician assistant recommended that he make several lifestyle changes that would help lower his blood pressure and reduce his risk of developing diabetes (decrease salt intake, consider smoking cessation); the provider also advised eating well and exercising regularly. Lewis's ability to follow this advice was hindered by his living situation: his boarding home had a starchy menu and at one point he attempted to manage his pre-diabetes by eating only oatmeal and lost eight pounds in one week.

The Wellness Center staff took note of his weight loss and referred Lewis back to the HIP program where staff helped him to plan simple, balanced meals that he could prepare and afford on his budget. Soon after, Lewis became engaged in other Wellness Center activities, including a weekly health group where clients share their health goals with each other. Lewis later moved to a studio apartment so that he could exercise more control over his diet. Although concerned about his health, Lewis prefers not to take medications for his conditions. He does not trust doctors, and believes that hospitals experiment on persons of color. Members of his family have been diagnosed with cardiovascular disease and diabetes, and his mother died of complications stemming from her diabetes. Relatives also smoked cigarettes, but Lewis believes his family's history of chronic health conditions and premature death is due to unhealthy eating and a lack of physical activity – not smoking.

Lewis used physical activity while he was in prison and while he was homeless as a way to pass the time and feel good. He understands how exercise can boost his mood and confidence. Still, he needs more information about maintaining a healthful diet, learning to plan meals and cook, and trying new foods. Lewis is pessimistic about successfully quitting smoking. Although Lewis was forced to decrease his smoking while incarcerated, after each release from prison, he quickly resumed his previous level of smoking. Fortunately, his success in increasing his daily physical activity can serve as a foundation for future healthy behavior changes.

The application of several integrated health care principles supports smoking cessation efforts as part of the overall care plan for Lewis. First, the integrated health model stresses a comprehensive bio-psycho-sociocultural-spiritual assessment. For Lewis, this whole-person approach uncovered potential health risks and offered him the opportunity to learn about lifestyle changes he could make to lower his health risks. Lewis' providers asked about his lifestyle choices and other health behaviors (smoking, diet, exercise, weight management). The positive impact of such inquiries on smoking cessation has been demonstrated in studies using the Surgeon General's "Five As Model" (i.e., Ask about smoking, Advise stopping, Assess willingness to stop, Assist those willing to stop, and Arrange follow-up). The study results are promising because some smokers may stop smoking simply because their doctor asked them about their smoking behavior (AHRQ, 2012).

Second, integrated models of care emphasize prevention and the importance of behavior and lifestyle changes related to diet, weight management, smoking cessation, and physical activity in order to improve health outcomes and lower risks that can prevent disease. According to Prochaska's Stages of Change theory (Pro-Change, 2014), change is a process that includes five stages: precontemplation (I won't), contemplation (I might), preparation (I will), action (I can), and maintenance (I have). Lewis, like many clients, is in a different stage of the change process for different behaviors. He adheres to a regular program of physical activity (maintenance stage), is ready to prepare to take action toward making changes in his dietary habits (preparation stage), but he is less ready to consider changing his smoking habits (precontemplation), despite awareness that smoking is not healthy. Lewis is clear that his reasons for smoking (pros) far outweigh the risks of smoking (cons). More important, because he is pessimistic about his ability to quit – in fact, he believes it is impossible to quit – he has not tried. For Lewis, the move from Prochaska's precontemplation to the contemplation stage could be a relatively small step that is easily facilitated by his care providers. The HIP staff could facilitate his progression to contemplation by providing information that reinforces the health consequences of smoking, and by giving Lewis consistent encouragement to talk with his care providers about options for quitting without pushing him to take action. Once Lewis has progressed to the contemplation stage, his care providers might initiate an examination of the pros and cons of smoking cessation as a way of addressing his ambivalence. By using motivational interviewing and solution-focused techniques, the care team can keep the conversation about smoking open, and help Lewis to recognize the connections between his current health conditions and smoking.

Third, integrated health care promotes the use of standardized instruments to screen and identify common conditions and risk factors in the population. Standardized instruments, such as the Fagerstrom Test for Nicotine Dependence on Cigarettes (Nova, 2014), can provide important information about the client's level of dependence on nicotine. This helps identify individuals who might benefit from nicotine replacement treatment; in addition, similar to the solution-focused approach, the test responses can offer suggestions for individualized strategies for small or easy changes in smoking behavior that can lead to bigger changes (DeJong & Berg, 2002).

Goals

Lewis' goal is to "stay healthy" and his behavior indicates concern about his health and willingness to make significant lifestyle changes to reach his goals. His commitment to his health goals motivated him to join HIP, come to the Wellness Center, to attend the weekly health group, and to meet with his team of providers. Like other HIP clients, new health goals for Lewis might emerge from recommendations made by any of his providers addressing the medical, behavioral, and emotional aspects of self-management (Lorig et al., 2012). For example, a social worker might offer education about relaxation techniques while the licensed vocational nurse (LVN) and registered dietician (RD) assists with healthy eating. The entire team works collaboratively to encourage progression toward goals.

Developing objectives and contracting

Ideally, integrated health settings promote a shared decision-making process related to goal-setting (Adams & Grieder, 2005). No decisions about the client's care are made without the participation of the client and the client participates fully in setting personal health goals. Lorig et al. (2012, p. 11) emphasized goals should focus on "what the person wants to accomplish" rather than goals identified by others. Just as health care providers are considered the experts on health conditions and treatments, clients are experts on their lives and what they are willing to do. Working as partners, care providers can help clients to identify small steps toward a goal that they are 70% confident can be accomplished successfully within one week. Lacking that level of confidence, the provider and client should modify the goal to make success more likely (Lorig et al., 2012).

Meeting place

The Inglewood Center, where the HIP program is housed, offered a variety of spaces for interacting with Lewis, including small, private offices and an informal recreation area. HIP services and the Wellness Center are open weekdays (8.30 a.m. to 5.00 p.m.), allowing scheduled or drop-in appointments. The Center also sponsors activities (e.g., grocery shopping, walks, field trips) and weekly therapeutic groups. Lunch is made by the wellness clients and served daily, offering additional opportunities for clients and staff to interact. Appointments with the physician assistant are scheduled for Tuesdays, when the other care team members (nurse, social worker, and program coordinator) also have office hours; each provider has a separate office in a private hallway with a small waiting room. This common day and central location of all care team members facilitates access to all providers who work as part of the clients' health care team (Figure 18.1).

Use of time

Given the structure of the HIP program, integrated care providers typically use brief interventions because the format fits well with the timing and flow of the clinical encounters (Pomerantz, Corson, & Detzer, 2009). A typical HIP appointment involves brief meetings with a variety of providers; the final stop is a review meeting with the social worker, intended to ensure that the client has accomplished his or her goals for the visit. The social worker may suggest using the Million Hearts Initiative program (http://millionhearts.hhs.gov/index.html)

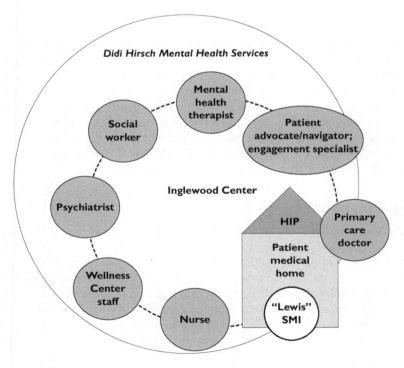

Figure 18.1 Healthy Inglewood Project's (HIP) integrated services for persons with serious mental illness: a "medical home"

aimed to reduce cardiac disease by allowing individuals to discuss the possible impact of a hypothetical lifestyle change on heart health.

Brief interventions in integrated settings use evidence-based practices designed to motivate at-risk individuals to change their behaviors and reduce their risk for behavioral health problems. In primary care settings, brief interventions typically last from 5 minutes (i.e., brief advice or a "warm hand-off" to another provider) to 30 minutes of brief counseling (SAMHSA, 2013) that might be scheduled as a series of 5–12 counseling sessions. Some of the most commonly used brief intervention therapies incorporate components of either cognitive behavioral therapy or motivational interviewing, or both (SAMHSA, 2013). Brief interventions in integrated primary care settings have been shown to be effective in increasing clients' self-management skills (Battersby et al., 2010) and reducing substance use (Henry-Edwards, Humeniuk, Ali, Monteiro, & Poznyak, 2003). The effectiveness of brief interventions for smoking cessation was clearly demonstrated in a critical review of 24 studies that included persons with mental illness or addictive disorders, and found post-treatment quit rates for smoking ranged from 35% to 56% (El-Guebaly, Cathcart, Currie, Brown, & Gloster, 2002).

Strategies and interventions

Brief interventions with demonstrated effectiveness in integrated care settings include the following key features: use of a solution-focused approach; set clearly defined goals related to specific behavioral change; incorporate client values and beliefs; include measurable outcomes; enhance self-efficacy; and use an active and empathetic therapeutic style. Smoking and smoking cessation have more than one workable solution and the collaboration of clients and providers is a key element in identifying the combination of treatments most likely to be successful. Our recommendations for assisting Lewis with smoking cessation draw from these key features and utilize motivational interviewing, consideration of readiness to change, and solution-focused techniques. These approaches support the combination of evidence-supported psychotherapy and pharmacotherapy interventions shown to increase success rates for smoking cessation (Williams et al., 2011). By empowering clients to recognize exceptions to their smoking problem (e.g., times when they are able to not smoke, times when they cut down the number of cigarettes smoked per day), they can discover their inner strengths and become hopeful that smoking cessation is possible (Table 18.1).

Stance of the social worker

Social workers in an integrated health care setting have the opportunity to use strengths-based, person-centered, person-in-situation approaches. If clients are not yet considering change, they might agree to talk with a provider about their smoking habits on the condition that the provider does not ask them to quit smoking. Respecting client self-determination helps to maximize clients' autonomy, competence, and reinforces a positive partnership. In addition, taking the following and guiding stance recommended by motivational interviewing increases trust between the practitioner and client and supports open dialogue (Butler et al., 1999).

Prochaska's Stages of Change model (Prochaska, Norcross, & DiClemente, 1994) offers specific interventions that correspond to the person's intent and readiness to take action and willingness to accept information and assistance. Smoking cessation programs are typically

Table 18.1 Supporting client's progression through the early stages of change

Stages of change	Precontemplation "I won't"	Contemplation "I might"	Preparation "I will"
Smoking behavior	Lewis' starting point: "Just don't ask me to quit....it seems impossible to quit....I've been smoking since I was 12!"	"Everyone knows smoking is bad for your health but I also know how I'll feel if I stop"	"I noticed that I can swap out a quick 10 minute walk for one cigarette"
What is needed to move to the next stage?	Break through denial Increase acceptance of relevance Build hope that change is possible	Address ambivalence Become armed with personal benefits and reasons for quitting	Recognize opportunities when changing the problem behavior seem more possible Choose a plan
Helpful strategies	Offer information Support, reinforcing changes already achieved on other behaviors Monitor CO levels to highlight the difference in CO ratings after a period of reducing even one or two cigarettes	Decisional balance (help client focus on pros of change rather than the cons) Build on motivation related to successful changes in diet/exercise	Experiment with options for cutting back on cigarettes Make a plan with a trusted provider
Effective practitioner stance	Nurturing parent using support and motivational interviewing techniques to encourage open dialogue about smoking	Socratic teacher encouraging the client to consider the advantages of smoking cessation and change as a possibility	Experienced coach who is there to give guidance, teach skills, and cheer you on when discouraged

Source: Adapted from Prochaska, J. O., Norcross, J. C., & DiClemente, C. C. (1994). Changing for good: A revolutionary six-stage program for overcoming bad habits and moving your life positively forward. New York: Avon Books.

aimed at taking action and making change (usually only 10–20% of the population are in the action stage), and often out of sync with the larger percentages of people in the precontemplation or contemplation stage. Providers who match interventions to the client's needs and stage can support a client in any stage to progress through the stages, and eventually take action to change unhealthy behaviors. Social workers who are familiar with a variety of intervention approaches and methods to quit smoking can more effectively tailor interventions to individual clients using a combination of approaches – some targeted to motivate, some targeted to cessation efforts, and some targeted to relapse prevention.

Providers who take a nurturing stance with clients in the precontemplation stage are more likely to encourage movement to contemplation (where Socratic questions can be effective in helping the client to explore the benefits and obstacles to quitting smoking). Changes in attitudes, feelings, and intentions during the early stages can lead to larger, lasting changes in behavior. By applying Prochaska's model, all clients can be included for participation in smoking cessation programs regardless of their motivation level or intent to change. Because essential learning and critical experience is gained from going through each stage, skipping stages is discouraged.

Use of resources outside of the helping relationship

The literature notes that collaboration among providers is essential for clients who are attempting to quit smoking and is especially important for clients with co-occurring mental health and physical health diagnoses. Without needed support, clients with SMI may not be successful with smoking cessation for several reasons: (1) because the change in smoking behavior may be complicated due to biological predispositions that can increase the use of nicotine; (2) a provider feeling that smoking cessation is beyond the scope of the client's mental health treatment; and (3) a myriad of other factors related to cognition, mood, and psychotic features (Morris, Waxmonsky, May, Giese, & Martin, 2009).

To support a client's movement to preparation and action, a medical home provides integrated supports that increase the likelihood of success. Ideally, a psychiatrist ensures that pharmacotherapy used for smoking cessation does not have unwanted side effects; the physician continues monitoring health parameters; and wellness group support provides ongoing monitoring and social support. The social worker can utilize the Million Hearts (http://million-hearts.hhs.gov/) program to help Lewis envision how smoking changes could lower his blood pressure and reduce his risk of diabetes. Using language to shift the discussion into the future – that is, referring to *when* change has been made, rather than *if* change will be – may help Lewis to focus on solutions (DeJong & Berg, 2002). Shifting to a future orientation enables him to move into the preparation stage and experiment with actions such as reducing the number of cigarettes he smokes each day. During preparation, Lewis might talk with the psychiatrist about the new medications for smoking cessation, or he may talk with his physician assistant about nicotine-replacement products, or actually try one, to help him manage his cravings.

Reassessment and evaluation

Current knowledge about smoking and the nature of behavior change suggests that any attempts at smoking cessation – whether the behavior change is sustained or not – should be viewed as an opportunity for gaining experience that can ultimately can lead to success. Although the overall goal is complete abstinence from smoking, providers should not overlook the importance of intermediate achievements that are signs of progress (reducing the number of cigarettes consumed per day, taking steps that support movement through a stage of change, or becoming "more ready" to take action). The social worker should ensure that there is ongoing reassessment of the client's status and evaluation of outcomes to inform and define future strategies. Recognizing the client's movement from one stage of change to the next is essential for building motivation, confidence, and sense of empowerment (Prochaska, Norcross & DiClemente, 1994).

Transfer and termination

Although HIP clients might move from daily involvement with the Wellness Center to community-based activities or employment, they are allowed to keep HIP as their medical home and use Didi Hirsch Mental Health Services as long as they are being treated for their mental health diagnosis. Once discharged from Didi Hirsch Mental Health services, clients are transferred to the provider's home location for primary care services. The HIP medical home model provides access to a continuum of care, including primary care, psychiatry, mental health therapy, and nursing support for management of chronic conditions and represents the ultimate goal of the ACA – access to a trusted source of health care and trusted providers for everyone.

Case conclusion

Changing smoking behavior is difficult and involves tremendous motivation and effort on the part of the person who smokes. For social workers and other health care providers to support this change requires that they create a working partnership with the client and offer ongoing encouragement, acceptance, and normalization of "failed" attempts." As for Lewis, his experience with the HIP care team was the first time a health care provider had asked about his smoking behavior and suggested that quitting was possible. Lewis' lack of hope that he could be successful was challenged by the stories he heard from other HIP participants who had quit smoking. The evidence he collected from his CO monitor readings increased his awareness that cutting back on a few cigarettes was positive for his overall health. With staff available for ongoing dialogue but not pushing him into "action" before he was ready, Lewis was able to accept that he was not doomed to failure; gradually he started swapping a few cigarettes a day for a quick walk. Recently he stated: "Six months ago, I'd have never believed that I wouldn't be constantly thinking about my next drag. Now I'm proud that I'm smoking less than half of the cigarettes a day that I used to!" While he reported it was not easy "giving up an old friend," he more recently has been considering trying a nicotine patch to see if he can "quit for good."

Differential discussion

Integrated care aligns well with the social work profession's values and mission – to enhance human well-being at the micro, mezzo, and macro levels (Rishel, 2015). Even so, important considerations must be taken into account before this model of care can be fully endorsed to improve the health of one of society's most vulnerable and neglected groups (Jones, 2000). For Lewis, the HIP integrated model offered a familiar setting (mental health provider) where he could access care for all of his health concerns. Building upon the limited trust established with his mental health providers, Lewis was able to gradually create a trusting partnership with a wider circle of health care providers, allowing him to take more control over his health. A primary consideration is the historic exploitation of minority groups, particularly African Americans, through clinical and research abuses (of which the Tuskegee syphilis experiment is the most commonly referenced), which has fostered an enduring mistrust of medical systems (Eiser & Ellis, 2007). This fact must be recognized by health care providers and dealt with sensitively in an open, non-defensive manner. Second, the integrated behavioral health medical home is not a stand-alone concept and can only work, as it did for Lewis, if it is strongly linked to other important community supports such as housing and food resources. Lastly, the concept of integrated health care and the medical home is still in its infancy and for many people with SMI, this type of positive, holistic service may not yet exist. Developing this kind of medical care system will take time and require social workers and other health care professionals to be flexible and accept some blurring of traditional professional boundaries. It also necessitates a paradigm shift that acknowledges the client as a fully-fledged member of the health care team. At Didi Hirsch, the HIP and Wellness Center continue to emphasize the importance of a comprehensive, whole-person approach to care, partnering with clients and supporting them to achieve all of their health care goals.

Discussion questions

1   Smoking cessation clearly helps improve the health of individuals with serious mental illness (as well as all individuals). What other interventions might yield similar positive health benefits for a large group of people in the organization where you work?
2   How might you integrate smoking cessation support into a mental health setting? What changes would be needed at the micro, mezzo, and macro levels?
3   How would you engage medical and/or mental health colleagues to consider helping clients with smoking cessation as within their "scope of practice," especially when most clients who smoke will be in the precontemplation stage and lack motivation?

References

ACA (2010). Patient Protection and Affordable Care Act, 42 U. S. C. § 18001 et seq. (2010).

Adams, N. & Grieder, D. (2005). *Treatment planning for person-centered care.* Amsterdam, the Netherlands: Elsevier.

ARHQ (Agency for Healthcare Research and Quality) (2012). *Five major steps to intervention (The "5 A's").* Retrieved from www.ahrq.gov/professionals/clinicians-providers/guidelines-recommendations/tobacco/5steps.html

Battersby, M., Von Korff, M., Schaefer, J., Davis, C., Ludman, E., Greene, S. M., & Wagner, E. H. (2010). Twelve evidenced-based principles for implementing self-management support in primary care. *Joint Commission Journal on Quality and Patient Safety, 36,* 561–570.

Butler, C. C., Rollnick, S., Cohen, D., Bachmann, M., Russell, I., & Stott, N. (1999). Motivational consulting versus brief advice for smokers in general practice: A randomized trial. *British Journal of General Practice, 49,* 611–616.

CDC (Centers for Disease Control and Prevention) (2013a). Trends in current cigarette smoking among high school students and adults, United States, 1965–2011. Retrieved from www.cdc.gov/tobacco/data_statistics/tables/trends/cig_smoking/

CDC (2013b). *Adult smoking.* Vital signs series. Retrieved from www.cdc.gov/vitalsigns/smokingandmentalillness/index.html

CDC (2015). Smoking and tobacco use: Fast facts. Retrieved from www.cdc.gov/tobacco/data_statistics/fact_sheets/fast_facts/

CoVita (2015). *Smokerlyzer breath carbon monoxide (CO) monitors.* Retrieved from http://covita.net/pdfs/Datasheets/micro+datasheet.pdf

DeJong, P. & Berg, I. K. (2002). *Interviewing for solutions* (2nd edn.). Belmont, CA: Wadsworth/Cengage.

Eiser, A. R. & Ellis, G. (2007). Viewpoint: Cultural competence and the African American experience with health care: The case for specific content in cross-cultural education. *Academic Medicine, 82*(2), 176–183. doi: 10.1097/ACM.0b013e31802d92ea

El-Guebaly, N., Cathcart, J., Currie, S., Brown, D., & Gloster, S. (2002). Smoking cessation approaches for persons with mental illness or addictive disorders. *Psychiatric Services, 53,* 1166–1170. doi: 10.1176/appi.ps.53.9.1166

Fiore, M. C., Croyle, R. T., Curry, S. J., Cutler, C. M., Davis, R. M., Gordon, C., et al. (2004). Preventing 3 million premature deaths and helping 5 million smokers quit: A national action plan for tobacco cessation. *American Journal of Public Health, 94,* 205–210. doi: 10.2105/AJPH.94.2.205

Free, C., Phillips, G., Galli, L., Watson, L., Felix, L., Edwards, P., et al. (2013). The effectiveness of mobile-health technology-based health behaviour change or disease management interventions for health care consumers: A systematic review. *PLoS Medicine, 10*(1), e1001362. doi: 10.1371/journal.pmed.1001362

Henry-Edwards, S., Humeniuk, R., Ali, R., Monteiro, M., & Poznyak, V. (2003). *Brief intervention for substance use: A manual for use in primary care.* (Draft Version 1.1 for Field Testing). Geneva: World Health Organization. Retrieved from www.who.int/substance_abuse/activities/en/Draft_Brief_Intervention_for_Substance_Use.pdf

Hogg Foundation for Mental Health (2008). *Connecting body & mind: A resource guide to integrated health care in Texas and the U.S.* Retrieved from www.hogg.utexas.edu/uploads/documents/IHC_Resource_Guide1.pdf

Holroyd-Leduc, J. M., Lorenzetti, D., Straus, S. E., Sykes, L., & Quan, H. (2011). The impact of the electronic medical record on structure, process, and outcomes within primary care: A systematic review of the evidence. *Journal of the American Medical Informatics Association, 18,* 732–737. doi: 10.1136/amiajnl-2010-000019

Jones, C. P. (2000). Levels of racism: A theoretic framework and a gardener's tale. *American Journal of Public Health, 90,* 1212–1215. doi: 10.2105/AJPH.90.8.1212

Lorig, K., Holman, H., Sobel, D., Laurent, D., Gonzalez, V., & Minor, M. (2012). *Living a healthy life with chronic conditions. Self-management of heart disease, arthritis, diabetes, asthma, bronchitis, emphysema and other physical and mental health conditions.* Boulder, CO: Bull.

McCullough, A., Fisher, M., Goldstein, A. O., Kramer, K. D., & Ripley-Moffitt, C. (2009). Smoking as a vital sign: Prompts to ask and assess increase cessation counseling. *Journal of the American Board of Family Medicine, 22,* 625–632.

Morris, C., Waxmonsky, J., May, M., Giese, A., & Martin, L (2009). *Smoking cessation for persons with mental illnesses: A toolkit for Mental Health Providers.* Retrieved from www.integration.samhsa.gov/Smoking_Cessation_for_Persons_with_MI.pdf

Nova Southeastern University (2014). *Fagerstrom test for nicotine dependence on cigarettes.* Retrieved from www.nova.edu/gsc/nicotine_risk.html

Pomerantz, A. S., Corson, J. A. & Detzer, M. J. (2009). The challenge of integrated care for mental health: Leaving the 50 minute hour behind and other sacred things. *Journal of Clinical Psychology in Medical Settings, 16,* 40–46.

Pro-Change Behavior Systems, Inc. (2014). The Transtheoretical Model. Retrieved from www.prochange.com/transtheoretical-model-of-behavior-change

Prochaska, J. O., Norcross, J. C., & DiClemente, C. C. (1994). *Changing for good: A revolutionary six-stage program for overcoming bad habits and moving your life positively forward.* New York: Avon Books.

Rishel, C. (2015). Establishing a prevention-focused integrative approach to social work practice. *Families in Society: The Journal of Contemporary Social Services, 96*(2), 125–132. doi: 10.1606/1044–3894.2015.96.15

SAMHSA (Substance Abuse and Mental Health Services Administration)–HRSA Center for Integrated Health Solutions (2013). *Integrated care models.* Retrieved from www.integration.samhsa.gov/integrated-care-models

Scott, D. & Happell, B. (2011). The high prevalence of poor physical health and unhealthy lifestyle behaviours in individuals with severe mental illness. *Issues in Mental Health Nursing, 32,* 589–597. doi: 10.3109/01612840.2011.569846

Williams, J. M., Zimmerman, M. H., Steinberg, M. L., Gandi, K. K., Delnevo, C., Steinberg, M. B., & Foulds, J. (2011). A comprehensive model for mental health tobacco recovery in New Jersey. *Administration and Policy in Mental Health, 38,* 368–383.

World Health Organization and Calouste Gulbenkian Foundation (2014). *Integrating the response to mental disorders and other chronic diseases in health care systems.* Geneva, Switzerland: WHO Press. Retrieved from www.who.int/mental_health/publications/gulbenkian_paper_integrating_mental_disorders/en/

Aging

Chapter 19

In-home support for Junior

A study of collaboration, boundaries, and use of self

Reneé C. Cunningham

Context

Policy

Junior was a consumer in the In-Home Support Program (IHSP) at Center in the Park (CIP). The IHSP is a program of the Philadelphia Corporation for Aging (PCA), a private, non-profit organization that serves as Philadelphia County's Area Agency on Aging. PCA was created as a result of the Older Americans Act, the major federal vehicle for the organization and delivery of social and nutrition services to older adults and their caregivers in the United States (Older Americans Act, 2015). PCA contracts with five senior community centers, including CIP, to administer the IHSP. PCA wrote and continues to revise the manual for this program, and it audits all sites regularly to ensure contract compliance, including intake procedures, documentation, appropriateness of services, timeliness and accuracy of paperwork, proper fiscal management of the Discretionary Fund budget, and the contract budget. Two factors affect the delivery of IHSP services, the manner in which the governing policies and procedures are interpreted, the manner in which they are delivered, and the degree to which they are followed: (1) CIP's philosophy, mission, and long-standing history of serving older adults and meeting the needs of the whole person, and (2) the personal and professional values and ethics of each care manager charged with administering the program.

Other policies affecting Junior's life and care are the U.S. Department of Housing and Urban Development (HUD) rules and regulations that govern the eligibility and occupancy requirements of Section 202 buildings as Junior was a resident of such a building, hospital regulations that affected the length of time, terms, and conditions under which Junior could stay in the hospital, and ultimately the Medicaid stipulations that govern a nursing home's ability to admit and retain low-income residents, as a nursing home was Junior's final residence. Each policy and regulation and the agents charged with administering and enforcing them, worked together, and, in some cases, in direct conflict with each other; thus, each significantly affected the coordination of services and programs that were to benefit Junior.

Technology

Many dimensions of technology are vital to our consumers, including the medications, medical and home-care devices that keep them going. However, this section will focus on the PCA database that contains relevant information about each person who has been a program consumer. Before PCA used a computerized database, contact logs, assessments, and care plans were handwritten and maintained in a case file. Now, computerized information includes contacts, demographics, care plans, program involvement, the care manager's name and home visit dates. Care managers are responsible for data entry and, within 24 hours of contact, must enter contact notes in the database. All contact logs and tracking dates are monitored by the IHSP Supervisor at CIP as well as the Director of IHSP and the IHSP Specialist at PCA.

Organization

A nationally accredited, non-profit senior community center, CIP has provided comprehensive programs and services to people age 55+ since 1968. We help older adults experience the positive rewards, opportunities, challenges, and losses of aging through realization of our mission: "Center in the Park promotes positive aging and fosters community connections for older adults whose voices are critical instruments in shaping its activities and direction" (Center in the Park, 2015). We offer a variety of programs such as: the IHSP, a Housing Counseling Program (information, assistance, referral and advocacy regarding housing-related issues for people of all ages), an Ombudsman Program (advocate and give voice to older consumers of long-term care services), a Neighborhood Energy Center (assist people of all ages with applying for energy-related benefits and entitlements, facilitate individual heating and energy grants, provide conservation workshops), and a Center Counseling program (assist CIP members 55+ with benefits, entitlements, personal concerns, information, and referral).

CIP has over 6,000 members ranging in age from 55 to 102, including 1,000 who are homebound. Primarily, we serve consumers from a large geographic area including counties outside of the city and in a neighboring state, but the majority of our membership comes from immediately surrounding zip codes. In this area, approximately 40% of older adults live alone compared to about 30% of all Philadelphia elders, and approximately 25% live in poverty – double the statewide average. The demographics of the IHSP consumers closely mirror those of the Center participants, with CIP delivering supportive services to low-income, homebound older adults. The over-arching goal of the IHSP is to help older adults "get back on their feet." In order to qualify for IHSP services, older adults must be over 60 years of age, homebound, and able to independently perform their own activities of daily living (ADLs) (i.e., bathing, dressing, grooming, etc.). For qualifying older adults, we are able to provide a wide range of services to meet one-time or ongoing needs with the goals of assisting them in maintaining independence in their homes and preventing further deterioration.

The program uses a "Discretionary Fund", provided by PCA and managed by each site, to deliver those services which the consumer and his or her care manager agree are needed, and which are then approved by the supervisor. In some cases the supervisor must first seek the approval of the IHSP Specialist at PCA before giving final approval for an expenditure. Consumers are reassessed for continued appropriateness on a yearly basis and events-based reassessments are carried out as needed.

For the duration of this case, I worked closely with the Visiting Nurse Association of Greater Philadelphia (VNA), an independent non-profit home-care agency which serves Philadelphia and its surrounding areas. The position of Community Liaison was created at the VNA to help identify isolated individuals in need of home-care services with the goal of helping them remain in their place of residence as long as physically and safely possible. The Community Liaison provides services with the client's consent and with authorization from their physician and their medical insurance. Professionals from the VNA and CIP do not always agree about every decision in the course of care.

Description of typical clients

Typical IHSP clients are between the ages of 72 and 77, can bathe and dress independently, and are independent in their ability to perform most instrumental activities of daily living (IADLs), such as managing finances, using the telephone, and managing medications, but need some assistance (due to functional limitations) with transportation and meal preparation. Referrals come from a variety of sources but, most often, the elder or a family member calls CIP. The intake worker determines with a phone interview whether potential clients seem appropriate for IHSP. If they seem to meet the eligibility criteria, the intake is assigned to a care manager (CM) who visits the home for the initial assessment. During that assessment the CM determines if clients are eligible for benefits and entitlements, and with clients' permission the CM assists the client with the necessary applications. The client and the CM discuss the client's goals, the scope of the IHSP and what it is possible to provide, such as bathroom grab bars, a home repair, a new refrigerator if needed, and an application for the area's door-to-door community paratransit for which IHSP can pay, and/or a senior companion if clients are isolated due to homebound status. For example, if clients need assistance with meal preparation because they can no longer stand at the stove for long periods of time due to arthritis, home-delivered meals would be ordered (seven frozen meals delivered once per week). IHSP care managers collaborate with PCA (to arrange for meals), the client's family and informal supports, and any formal supports (such as doctors, visiting nurses, other social workers).

Decisions about practice

Description of the client situation

Junior was a client in the IHSP receiving home-delivered meals with occasional housekeeping services and financial assistance with past due bills for 3 years. I met Junior prior to becoming his care manager and I supervised his previous care manager. I was familiar with his situation, having reviewed his case file several times. At the time I became his care manager I was the senior supervisor of CIP's Social Services Department, supervising the six IHSP social workers, a supervisor for another program, and the Social Services Department secretary. I reported directly to the associate director of Social Services and Housing, who focused primarily on macro-level social service and housing issues and Center operations and allowed me to oversee most of the general day-to-day department affairs. In addition, I carried a small caseload of consumers who had complicated issues who needed specialized attention, intensive care management and multi-system coordination.

Definition of the client

Junior was a 72-year-old homebound African American man who suffered from non-insulin-dependent diabetes, hypertension, mild short-term memory loss, arthritis, allergies, and lower extremity edema, which was a direct result of congestive heart failure (CHF). An alcoholic who had been in recovery for many years, Junior continued to smoke cigarettes. During the time we worked together he admitted that he was also addicted to crack, and until recently, had smoked it for years. Junior received a modest amount of Social Security income and lived by himself in a senior housing complex. He was a retired sanitation worker and was forced to leave his job due to a leg injury he sustained while working. The apartment that Junior lived in was a HUD 202 building and, therefore, his rent was subsidized. As a result, his rent never exceeded 30% of his income and most of his utilities were included.

Family was vitally important to Junior and he maintained contact with several family members. His older brother Thomas was in his eighties, wheelchair bound, and lived in a nursing home. Junior and Thomas spoke on the telephone every morning and, until Thomas had several toes amputated due to complications from diabetes, he would come and stay with Junior on the weekends. Junior was also close to an older sister, Thelma, to whom he spoke regularly, and was also in regular contact with some of her children, namely her son, John. Junior had been divorced for many years. His ex-wife passed away some time after their divorce. He had five children, but was only in contact with one of them. He had two children with his wife and three others from an extramarital affair. He had been close to his only son who had died of a drug overdose 2 years before. One of the daughters from his marriage, Sandra, was the only one of his children with whom he kept in touch. He spoke to her regularly but had only been doing so for the past 2 or 3 years. She lived out of state, visited him monthly, and had often asked Junior to move in with her and her family so that she could better assist with activities that were difficult for him. Junior continually declined her offer as he wished to be independent. Sandra and John seemed to provide the most support to Junior, trying to make sure he went to medical appointments and providing some emotional support and socialization. That being said, Junior's basic needs not being met necessitated his referral to our program.

During my work with Junior, I spoke to Sandra several times on the telephone and worked closely with his nephew, John. They were satisfied with the services Junior received from the IHSP and were grateful for any assistance provided. Both Sandra and John regularly confided in me about their frustrations with Junior, as he was a proud man who relished his independence and was reluctant to accept help from anyone. Junior and I developed a strong bond and had an excellent rapport. His faith in me and trust in our relationship made it possible for me to have a significant impact on Junior's life; I was able to convince him to make positive changes where his family and doctors had been previously unsuccessful.

The hallmarks of an effective working relationship are trust, mutual respect, support, understanding, and empathy. Clients should know that their social worker is invested in them and will work with them to establish and meet their identified goals. Still, certain sociocultural barriers to the client–social worker relationship have to be overcome to establish good rapport. For Junior and me, there were major barriers of race, age, and socioeconomic status. For example, Junior was an older African American man and I was a White woman, young enough to be his grandchild. To work effectively with Junior, I had to understand the effects of oppression, discrimination, the impact of the Civil Rights Movement and what preceded it; the role of family, family dynamics, and the importance of kinship; an affiliation with a particular house of worship and congregation if one exists, and the pastoral relationship; and the health disparities that exist for African American older adults. It is important to understand how all of these circumstances affect clients' lives and decision-making. Another key to establishing a positive relationship with a client is authenticity; with a sincere desire to help a client, a social worker can overcome almost any barrier. Junior trusted me because he knew that I was invested in his well-being, I believed he could overcome the challenges he faced, and I would do whatever I could to help him. We worked well together. Our partnership was equal and friendly. We discussed mutual interests such as sports and music, and my use of self-disclosure helped him to feel less like a client and more like a partner (Barth, 2014).

My advocating for Junior was central to our work and strengthened his trust in me. I advocated with doctors, family members, institutions and even within the IHSP. Although Junior often made poor decisions and neglected his health and environment, he was competent to make those choices. Although I did not agree with some decisions, I respected his right to make them and to defend that right when it was threatened. I agreed with his family and doctors that Junior would be better off and perhaps even thrive in a more structured environment where someone could prompt him to take his medicine or eat properly, but a client's making a bad decision does not mean he lacks the capacity to make a "good" one. Despite the fact that the decisions he made often had deleterious effects on other aspects of his life and situation and were, at times, in direct conflict with his overall objectives and goals, Junior had the right to choose how he wanted to live. I believed it to be my role to advocate for his right to do that, but I continued to point out to Junior the times when his decisions conflicted with his objectives and how they jeopardized his ability to live independently. I also used his trust in me and respect for my position to try to convince him to make better choices.

Goals

Junior lived alone in a senior housing complex, with his most important goal being to maintain his independence. The objectives that were set forth by his family, physicians and me had to further this goal. As his social worker, however, I knew that our goal was conditional in that I could only help Junior to maintain his independence in the community as long as he was safe. When clients' safety and well-being are in direct conflict with their stated goals, I help them to alter their goals to match current circumstances. As Junior's health and circumstances deteriorated, it was necessary that he amend the goal.

Junior's other stated goals were to stay in the IHSP and retain me as his care manager. Clients whose cases are open for a long period of time inevitably work with several care managers as there is often turnover in entry level positions. Junior had worked with three different IHSP care managers prior to our work together. I was careful to make sure he understood the parameters of the IHSP and that he could continue in the program only as long as he met the eligibility standards. I assured him that if his circumstances necessitated his transfer to another program, I would maintain our relationship and would always do whatever I could to advocate for him. My response to the latter goal showed not only a disregard for, but a lack of understanding of, the importance of proper disengagement at the end of the client relationship. At the time, I felt justified doing so with two reasons: first, I was not only Junior's care manager; I was also the supervisor for the program and, as such, frankly speaking, I had more latitude. The other reason showed both my humanity and need for continued training; I felt genuine feelings of friendship toward Junior and wanted to do whatever I could for him, whether inside or outside the confines of the program.

Developing objectives and contracting

Various objectives were established and addressed in the years Junior had an active IHSP case at CIP. The main objectives were to: keep his apartment clean, better maintain his health, ensure he received proper nutrition, and make sure his bills were paid in a timely fashion. All of these objectives, if met, would ensure the achievement of his goal to maintain his independence. Many significant crises and challenges presented themselves as serious barriers to Junior's goal. Each time, he and I would verbally contract and assign specific tasks to get back on track. For example, I would agree to negotiate a payment arrangement for a past due bill, and he would agree to make a doctor's appointment. This was done on an "as needed" basis. In the time his case was active, Junior was able to have many objectives met that in turn helped him to meet this goal. When we first opened his case we ordered home-delivered meals because he was unable to cook for himself. We purchased furniture for his apartment because he was sleeping on a mattress on the floor and had only milk crates to sit on, and one time, when he had been mugged while walking to purchase money orders, we paid his rent and utilities.

Junior's health and functional ability began to deteriorate and his ability to remain safely in the community was called into question. Junior often visited me in the office, which would have jeopardized his eligibility for the IHSP had his case been reviewed by PCA. On one particular day, Junior arrived nearly breathless; his vision was blurred and his legs were swollen such that he could not get his socks on and had to leave his shoes untied. He told me that he had two doctor's appointments on this day (cardiologist and optometrist) and he walked several blocks after taking the bus to ask my opinion on which appointment he should keep. Junior was reluctant to go to the cardiologist because he was afraid he would be admitted to the hospital. He was adamant that he did not want to be admitted and had signed himself out against medical advice (AMA) on previous occasions. Furthermore, Junior was afraid that, if he was admitted, he would be forced to go into a nursing home. Junior had been told by doctors during previous hospital stays that they were concerned about his capacity to make decisions and that they felt he was unable to continue living on his own. His nephew John also threatened to "put him away" in a nursing home. I was able to convince Junior to go to the cardiologist, but had to promise that I would advocate for him, should anyone call his competency into question. Afraid that he would not make it to the appointment in his current state, I drove him to the cardiologist and informed them of his current state, noting that I was afraid he had CHF. While the doctor determined that Junior was in severe CHF, he was not admitted to the hospital and was instead sent home with a very complicated regimen of medications, mostly diuretics. Given his state when he arrived at the cardiologist's office, his complex medical conditions, and new diagnosis, I was incredulous that he was not admitted. When he arrived home, he called and said that he could not read the medication bottles he was given because his vision was still very blurry, likely a sign that his blood sugar was unstable. I contacted a colleague, Carol, who was the Community Liaison from the VNA, for consultation, support, to try to get an emergency home-care visit to assist him in setting up his meds. Carol agreed with me that Junior should have been admitted and contacted the cardiologist to get an order for home care so that she could go to Junior's home, check his vitals, and set up his medications for him. The cardiologist refused to approve the order, stating that she "went against her better judgment by allowing him to leave and not admitting him," said that he needed to be in the hospital, and advised that he go to the emergency room (ER). In over 15 years as a home visiting nurse Carol reported that this was the first time she had ever experienced a doctor refusing to approve home care.

I attempted to convince Junior to go the ER and, given the urgency, advised that he take an ambulance. He refused, wanting to protect his privacy and not wanting the people who lived in the building to think he was frail. Carol and I both tried unsuccessfully to reach Junior's primary care physician to approve the home care. Junior was not speaking to his nephew John and would not give me permission to call him, vaguely mentioning that they were having "problems." His daughter was also unavailable. I called Junior's neighbor, Ernestine, and asked her to read me the medication bottles and I instructed her as to which pills to give him immediately and which pills to set out on the counter for the evening. Junior said he felt okay and promised he would call 911 if needed. Ernestine promised me she would look in on him.

When I called him the next day there was a woman yelling in the background. I asked him who that was and he indicated that it was "the woman who cleans the apartment" and that she wanted money and drugs. I told Junior to tell her to leave, he did, and I could hear her refuse. I told him I was on my way to the apartment. I do not know what I thought I was going to do when I got there, but she left before I had to find out. When I arrived, Junior and I talked about his deteriorating health and need for immediate medical treatment. I spoke candidly to him and told him that if he did not do so he was going to die. He agreed to go, but only if I took him. It was on our ride to the ER that he confessed to me that he smoked crack and that his nephew, John, was the person who gave it to him. John allegedly gave crack to both Junior and "the woman who cleaned the apartment" so that she would "look after" him. We spent the entire day in the ER and he was admitted.

After his stay in the hospital, Junior required oxygen and a higher level of care than could be provided by the IHSP. I facilitated his transfer to a long-term care program through PCA and continued to work with Junior and his new social worker informally. Shortly after his transfer, it became clear that Junior could not live safely on his own. I discussed nursing home placement with him, and he agreed to enter a facility, provided he could be with his brother, Thomas.

Meeting place

Because IHSP clients are homebound, we are required to do home visits. Homebound does not mean that clients are completely unable to leave the home, but rather, that it is difficult for them and they require assistance to do so. Because Junior often took the bus to CIP and walked from the bus stop to my office he would, in the pure definition, not be appropriate for the IHSP. If at the time of my work with him the contact logs were entered in the computerized database, they would have been closely monitored by PCA, and it is most likely that I would have been forced to close his case. The lack of technology at the time worked in my favor, and I made the decision to keep Junior's case open, knowing that I would have a lot of explaining to do if that case was ever audited. It was a risk I was willing to take.

If I had given in to the urge to do Junior's reassessment in my office during one of his "drop in" visits, I would not have gotten a clear picture of his true situation. Without observing their environment, it is nearly impossible to envision clients' living circumstances. In Junior's case, my initial visit to his apartment shocked me. His apartment smelled strongly of urine; there were blood stains on his sheets; he had no food in his cabinets; and the only things in his refrigerator were a plate of rotten food and a few frozen meals from the IHSP. These are things he would have been too proud to admit if we had only met in my office; I might never have known the depth of his problems had I not seen his home.

Use of time

The IHSP is strengths-based, solution-focused, and primarily short-term. My approach has always been to be a boundary-spanner, that is, to push rules to their limits and a bit beyond in order to maximally advocate for my clients (Kerson, 2002). Junior's case had been open for approximately 4 years, and I worked with him for about 1 year. Though the IHSP requires phone contact every three months and two home visits per year, clients' circumstances often demand more frequent contact. I spoke to Junior weekly, sometimes daily, and, when in crisis, several times in a day. In the year we worked together he probably visited my office four times, and I visited him at home three times, and at the hospital, twice. Our visits lasted about an hour, but some were shorter, and some, several hours.

Strategies, interventions and case/care management

A strengths-based approach is a natural fit for work with older adults because they have many years of experiences, perspective, challenges, and resiliency to draw from when problems arise. Grounded in the belief that change happens only when one collaborates with an individual's aspirations, perceptions, and strengths, this approach provides techniques and tools to help social workers focus on a client's abilities instead of their pathology, illnesses, or problems (Ponnuswami, Francis, & Udhayakumar, 2012). In the IHSP we try to draw on clients' past experiences in overcoming difficult circumstances in order to help them make positive changes that will maximize their independence. Thus, Junior and I discussed previous situations where he was able to overcome an obstacle. Unfortunately, Junior's old ways of coping were often maladaptive. For example, he noted that when he faced difficult situations in the past he often drank or did drugs in an effort to avoid the conflict and its potentially painful resolution. However, we continued to discuss more positive solutions, and Junior was able to actively participate in the decision-making process, arrive at solutions that would improve his situation, and to the extent possible, remain in control of his circumstances.

Stance of the social worker

I took on many roles in my work with Junior: I was the conciliator when he was at odds with his family; I was the mediator when he was in danger of eviction; and I was his advocate when the hospital staff wrongfully deemed him incompetent. I was a sort of police officer when I sped to his apartment to remove a crack addict from his apartment. I was his medical professional when I explained his medical conditions and medications. I organized his bills, arranged to have his apartment cleaned, and delivered messages to his brother who worried when Junior did not answer the phone. In many regards what Junior and I developed was a friendship. Feelings of friendship are, in some cases, a natural byproduct of the helping relationship. There is a debate in the social work field about "dual relationships." There are some who believe dual relationships should be avoided at all costs. On the other side are those who say these relationships are situationally and contextually determined. They argue that being too dogmatic about avoiding dual relationships diminishes the essence and authenticity of social work (Dewane, 2010). A good rapport can have a very positive impact on the helping relationship and the client, but a social worker must always remember that the client relationship is imbalanced. At the time of my work with Junior I was still developing my professional identity. I found it difficult to remain professional at all times because I genuinely liked Junior and felt a personal stake in his well-being. Also, it was important to Junior that I was a "real person" and not just a service provider. While some social workers do not believe in the use of self-disclosure, it can be a key tool if it is used appropriately (Barnes, 2012; Barth, 2014).

Use of resources outside of the helping relationship

I spoke to and tried to work closely with every possible individual and agency to help Junior meet his goal and to provide for his growing needs. Junior's extended network of family and service providers was both helpful and problematic, in some cases helping and in others providing little or being in direct conflict with Junior's goal and objectives. In the ecomap in Figure 19.1, solid lines indicate an active helping relationship, dotted lines indicate individuals who provided purely emotional support and socialization, and dashed lines indicate a problematic relationship.

It may seem unusual to show the primary care physician (PCP) and cardiologist relationships as problematic, however, both physicians made it very difficult for Junior to maintain his well-being. The cardiologist chose not to admit Junior, showing poor judgment in my opinion and then, after allowing him to leave, and knowing he lived on his own, gave him a regimen of medications that Junior was clearly not capable of following. Realizing the mistake, she refused to authorize home care for Junior when that could have made a great difference in his ability to comply and remain independent. I also made many emergency calls to the PCP's office in an effort to relay Junior's rapid physical decline. The PCP showed no appreciation of the urgency and severity of Junior's health crisis, provided no advice or

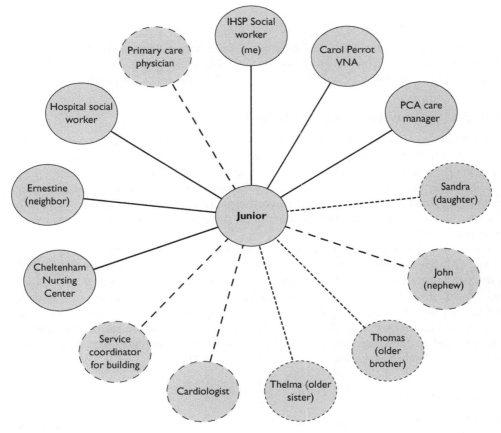

Figure 19.1 Ecomap for Junior

support to either Junior or I, and, by the time he authorized home care through VNA, Junior was already hospitalized.

I also worked very closely with Carol, the Community Liaison nurse from the VNA. In the situation that precipitated Junior's hospitalization, Carol affirmed what I already knew: that the health care system was failing Junior and that if I had not intervened and taken him to the ER, Junior would have died. Carol educated me about his medical conditions and how the lack of medical attention, improper nutrition, drug use, and poor self-care were affecting his overall health. She tried desperately to help me to navigate the health care system by speaking with his doctors and the hospital social workers. We had worked closely on several cases and her guidance was always invaluable. In my work with Junior she provided me the greatest support.

At times it is necessary to use everything you have at your disposal, both personal and professional. When it became clear that he should no longer live on his own, I knew a nursing home was the safest, most suitable place for Junior. Though I had already closed his case at this point I worked with his new social worker at PCA to give Junior all the information, pros and cons, in order for him to make that decision. Junior was willing to live in a nursing home if he could be in the same facility as his brother. My mother worked there, spoke to the admissions department, and helped facilitate Junior's admission. Junior was comforted to know he would be with his brother, and was pleased to know my mother would be there to look in on him.

Reassessment and evaluation

During my work with Junior, I conducted one official reassessment within the timeframe specified by the IHSP. In our time together, we were able to meet many objectives, and while Junior did eventually go into a nursing home, we met his goal for as long as we could.

Transfer, termination, and case conclusion

When Junior was released from the hospital, a higher level of care was warranted, and I referred him to PCA for a long-term care program. I knew that transitions of care are difficult for elders (Robison, Shugruo, Porter, Fortensky, & Curry, 2012). I was clear in our ongoing discussion that this may happen and, though he did not want to lose me as his social worker, he understood and agreed that he needed more assistance than the IHSP could provide. PCA assessed Junior and assigned him to an appropriate program, and after those services began, I closed his IHSP case.

Someone examining Junior's closed file will only get a taste of what he (and I) went through. My assessment does not include details about the client/care manager relationship. It will not say that I sat in the ER with him all day, or that this man, who was in severe CHF and in withdrawal from crack, offered to give me his seat. There is no place for me to write that Junior touched and broke my heart with his hardship and his ways. Closing his case was difficult for me. Junior remained in the community for a month before entering the nursing home. He did well in the nursing home and lived there with his brother Thomas for another 3 years before he died as a result of complications from CHF.

Differential discussion

If you had asked me when I closed Junior's case if I would have changed anything, in my hubris, I would have said there was nothing. But experience, training, and education have given me a new perspective. I should have looked into whether or not he was eligible for disability income as a result of his work-related injury. I should have conducted a home visit much sooner than I did; I would have had a better understanding of the severity of Junior's situation and could have begun adding services sooner. I never should have driven to his apartment to chase out the cantankerous crack addict; I should have had Junior call the police to have her removed. As a supervisor, I would never allow social workers to conduct them-selves in that way: it was a rash decision, showing poor judgment, a lack of professionalism, a lack of boundaries, and a lack of regard for my own safety. When I found out Junior's nephew John was supplying him with crack, I could have called the police and I could have called Older Adult Protective Services. I did not do these things because I allowed my rela-tionship with Junior to cloud my professional judgment. Junior asked me not to report John, and I was afraid of how it would affect him, was concerned for his safety when John found out, and I was afraid it would do irreparable damage to my relationship with Junior. He trusted me.

What I think about most in this case is my use of self and the setting of boundaries. I believe that my self-disclosure and the posture that I took with Junior, coupled with my genuine desire to help him, is what made our bond so strong and, furthermore, I credit this bond with the successful outcome of the case. I truly believe that Junior would have died if he had not come to see me the day I took him to the hospital (another breach, as we have a rule against transferring clients in our own vehicles). But in an effort to show Junior friendship, I compromised some of my authority and professionalism. I should have been more aware of myself and more in tune with how Junior made me feel and what impact our working rela-tionship had on me. Had I been more aware of these triggers, I would have likely conducted myself differently, and I would not have become so personally involved with him. As it is, Junior and I had a profound effect on each other, both personally and professionally, and I learned much from our work together.

Discussion questions

One can see ethical dilemmas and social justice issues throughout this work. Some of these issues have to do with autonomy vs. safety, but in the case of drug use, some have legal implications. Thinking through the many decisions that Junior and I made together:

1   What would you have done differently? Do you think professional boundaries were breached or stretched? Was there a dual relationship and if so, do you think it helped or hurt the client?
2   In relation to the organization, does one's role in an organization affect one's capacity to advocate for clients? Think here about the demands of being a practitioner, a supervisor or an administrator.

References and resources

Administration on Aging (AoA) (2015). Retrieved from www.aoa.gov

Barnes, M. (2012). Care, ethics, policy and politics. *Care in everyday life*: *An ethic of care in practice* (pp. 167–174). Bristol, U.K.: The Policy Press.

Barth, F. E. (2014). An integrative approach to therapeutic relationships. In *Integrative clinical social work practice*: *A contemporary perspective* (pp. 93–106). New York: Springer.

Center in the Park (2015). Retrieved from www.centerinthepark.org

Chapin, R. & Cox, E. O. (2002). Changing the paradigm: Strengths-based and empowerment-oriented social work with frail elders. *Journal of Gerontological Social Work, 36*, 165–179. doi: 10.1300/J083v36n03_13

Dewane, C. J. (2010) Respecting boundaries – the don'ts of dual relationships, *Social Work Today, 10*, 18. Retrieved from www.socialworktoday.com/archive/012610p18.shtml

Dybicz, P. (2012). The ethic of care: Recapturing social work's first voice, *Social Work, 57*(3), 271–280. doi: 10.1093/sw/sws007

Kane, R. L. (2010). Reimagining nursing homes. The art of the possible. *Journal of Aging & Social Policy, 22*, 321–333. doi: 10.1080/08959420.2010.507509

Kerson, T. S. (2002). *Boundary spanning: An ecological reinterpretation of social work practice in health and mental health systems.* New York: Columbia University Press.

Older Americans Act (2015). Retrieved from www.aoa.gov

Ponnuswami, I., Francis, A. P., & Udhayakumar, P. (2012). *Strengths-based approach to social work practice with older persons.* New Delhi: Allied Publishers. Retrieved from https://www.academia.edu/3470933/Strengths-Based_Approach_to_Social_Work_Practice_with_Older_Persons

Robison, J., Shugruo, N., Porter, B. A., Fortensky, R. H., & Curry, L. A. (2012). Transition from home care to nursing home: Unmet needs in a home-and community-based program for older adults. *Journal of Aging & Social Policy, 24*, 251–270. doi: 10.1080.08959420.2010.507509

Chapter 20

Geriatric social work in a community hospital

High-touch, low-tech work in a high-tech, low-touch environment

Sarah Maus and Toba Schwaber Kerson

Context

Description of the setting

Memorial is an independent 570-bed, acute care teaching hospital located in a suburb of a large city. The county where we are situated is wealthy; it has the third highest percentage of older adults in our state, one of the highest percentages of older adults in the nation. We serve parts of two adjoining counties, one of which includes a large, metropolitan area. While our patients are overwhelmingly White, we have significant Hispanic, African American, Portuguese, and Korean populations. Forty-seven % of our inpatient population is over 60 years of age. Our statistics reflect those of the nation in that the old old – those over 85 – are the fastest growing segment of this older population. A large home-care department provides services to our patients in the community, and we work closely with our Area Agency on Aging and a local network of over 60 extended care facilities.

Policy

Several policies influence our work. Perhaps the most significant is the Health Insurance Portability and Accountability Act of 1996 (HIPAA, 2009). Also referred to as the "Privacy Rule," HIPAA defines the kind of communication we are allowed to have with regard to our patients' health information. A second policy, Advance Health Care Directives, Act 169, signed into state law late in 2006, provides a comprehensive statutory framework governing advance health care directive and decision-making for incompetent patients (Johnson & Stadel, 2007). It makes available a set of standards for use in the health care setting to define legal incompetence and to seek determination from the courts for such (Doukas & Reichel, 2007). Included in this Act is a hierarchy created by the legislature that sets the order in which family and friends are to be used as health care representatives (American Bar Association, 2006). This is especially helpful to our medical staff who feel more comfortable with proper legal backing for decisions. In addition, our hospital has its own policy for Patient Rights and Responsibilities. Given to every patient upon admission, this brochure describes the rights of all hospital patients and the responsibilities of patients as partners in their care. It directs patients who have any questions or concerns to our Patient Relations Department.

Increasingly, we are seeing the effect of the changes brought about by the Affordable Care Act. The Centers for Medicare and Medicaid Services (CMS) is significantly altering the way in which hospitals and physicians are reimbursed. Emphasis is shifting from procedure-based to population health; admissions and readmissions to the hospital are closely reviewed. Patients who need inpatient care, but who do not meet certain requirements for admission, are placed in Observation Status until they are either discharged or their condition changes to allow for admission (Bagley & Levy, 2014; Moon, 2012). This affects out-of-pocket expense to the patient as well as reimbursement to the hospital.

Technology

The primary function of a social worker in an acute care hospital is discharge planning (Auslander, Soskoine, Stanger, Ben-Shahar, & Kaplan, 2008; Eaton, 2013; Rockwell, 2010). Tools to enhance communication are critical to the process (Backhaus, 2011). In addition to cell phones and e-mail, social workers use copiers, scanners, and fax machines to share pertinent information with institutions to which we are referring our patients and communicate within the system. Almost all documentation is electronic as we move towards the goal of total electronic medical records (EMR). Forms pertinent to our case study relate to professional consults, patient transfer, and discharge, and the formal application for a court competency hearing with essential medical interrogatories (Gibson, 2011; Moye, Butz, Marson, & Wood, 2007; Qualls & Smyer, 2007).

Communicating with geriatric patients involves several forms of technology. Because of the effects of aging on geriatric patients' sight, hearing, and comprehension, assessment of these faculties is critical (Brink & Stones, 2007). To whatever degree they choose or are able, it is also important to insure patients' involvement in their own medical care (Backhaus, 2011; Leung, 2011). We do this through engaging conversation, assuring that eye glasses and hearing aids are available and functioning, and providing patient rooms with orientation boards.

Organization

Approximately 10 years ago, Memorial combined its social work and case management departments and chose a registered nurse as the director. The administration believed that because both departments were responsible for discharge planning, it would be more efficient to have one director. Those who were left out of the transition were tapped to create a geriatric service line, and I am the Manager of Geriatrics. The mission of this entity is to improve and maintain the health status of our elderly community through both inpatient and outpatient geriatric and gero-psychiatric services. In our inpatient program, the Hospital Elder Life Program, we collaborate with the Department of Nursing to assure specialty geriatric inpatient care to "at risk" patients. The program has made health system staff more aware of the special needs of the frail elderly.

The nature of hospital social work has changed dramatically since the introduction of diagnosis-related groups (DRGs), and our hospital's Case Management Department reflects these changes. With length of stay a primary concern and with complicated and problematic discharges occurring more frequently within the elderly population, many of the less measurable social work functions fall to the geriatric service. The social workers who are affiliated with the geriatric service line have fewer time constraints and more flexible ways of measuring success than those within the Case Management Department because of the nature of our role within the hospital (Cantrell, 2007). For this reason, coordination of decision-making in relation to questions of patient competency is centered in our Senior Service Department rather than Case Management.

To ensure clear and timely communication, we work closely with attending and consulting physicians, floor nurses, and the physical therapists who help to determine what level of care our patients will need upon discharge. Also, we facilitate conversations when we learn of patients' and families' medical concerns. Open communication with the clinical staff guides our ability to inform patients and families, and to secure an appropriate and timely discharge.

Decisions about practice

Client description

Mrs. Esposito is a 79-year-old widowed woman who lives alone in her two-story row home in a city neighborhood. Her three grown children are married and live close by, and she has seven grandchildren. Always a homemaker during her working years, Mrs. Esposito depends on her deceased husband's Social Security check for financial support. Until Mrs. Esposito was diagnosed with lung cancer, she was independent in all activities of daily living, attended church every morning, kept a spotless house, and welcomed visits from family and friends. Recently, however, the family has noticed increased confusion, impaired short-term memory, and a change in her normally pleasant demeanor.

Brought to the emergency room by a daughter, Mrs. Esposito was experiencing a tingling in her arms and legs and had a brief loss of consciousness. Because of her cancer history, Mrs. Esposito was admitted to oncology for further tests and observation. Unfortunately, some time during her first night, she fell out of bed. While she did not experience any serious injury, she did have some pain and bruising. She was placed on a low bed with a bed alarm. Over the course of the next few days, Mrs. Esposito became more confused, was not oriented to time, and could neither identify that she was in a hospital, nor imagine why that would be so. An anti-anxiety medication that she had taken in the past was restarted, believing that some of her confusion might be due to withdrawal. Otherwise, her confusion was attributed to delirium, not unusual in hospitalized elderly persons, especially those who have already begun to experience some dementia (Scott & Barrett, 2007). As her anxiety and confusion worsened, she made attempts to leave the hospital, had frequent angry outbursts, and refused care. Mrs. Esposito was placed on 1:1 observation, where a staff member is assigned to sit with a patient at all times.

Once it became clear to Mrs. Esposito's physician that she would not be able to return to her previous living situation, social work was consulted. At first, Shelley, a case management oncology social worker, attempted to meet with Mrs. Esposito, but she became hostile and was not willing or able to participate in her discharge plans. Pam and Rita, the patient's daughters, were often in her room, so Shelley arranged to meet with them together. Both daughters explained that their absent brother was an active alcoholic and had not been interested in becoming involved in the past. He did not return phone calls so the meeting occurred without him.

As the discussion turned to changes that would need to be made in Mrs. Esposito's living situation, it became clear that both Pam and Rita were distraught (Raveis, 2007; Wolff et al., 2010). They believed that, aside from minor changes in memory and mood, their mother had been independent before coming to the hospital. They were not ready to accept that the changes they now saw were likely to be permanent. They were unwilling to participate in a discussion of discharge planning at that time, so the meeting adjourned with the idea that another one would take place later in the week.

Mrs. Esposito stabilized medically and, while still confused, she did go to physical therapy. Her confusion became intermittent and her doctors felt she could go to a skilled nursing facility. She had been in bed for many days; her legs were weak, her balance was bad, and her stamina non-existent. When Shelley next met with Pam and Rita, she gave them the names and phone numbers for several skilled nursing facilities with good rehabilitation programs, asking that they visit these facilities and choose one. She told them that she would take care of the discharge arrangements once they had decided on a destination.

When Pam and Rita returned with their decision, they met in Mrs. Esposito's room and told her of the visits that had been made on her behalf. Her daughters assured her that this was a temporary placement and that they had chosen a good facility. Mrs. Esposito became angry and hostile, insisting that she be allowed to go to her own home immediately upon discharge. She was adamant in refusing to go to a skilled nursing facility. When questioned about how she would be able to care for herself she simply stated that she would manage (Dwyer, 2005).

At this point, we decided that any further discussion with Mrs. Esposito would only cause undue distress. Reconvening in a conference room down the hall, Pam and Rita were in tears. They began to talk about their own health issues; Rita had been diagnosed with multiple sclerosis 5 years earlier, Pam had had lupus since early adulthood. Both of these chronic medical conditions had been under control until the stress of Mrs. Esposito's condition had caused an exacerbation of symptoms. Pam was in pain much of the time; Rita's mobility became more limited. They wanted to make their mother happy – she had done so much for them, often putting their wants and needs before her own while they were growing up. They knew that if Mrs. Esposito went home, she would need care that they could not provide. No one could financially provide for the 24-hour home care that Mrs. Esposito would need, although she would probably be eligible for some home services through the local office of aging. Mrs. Esposito was still intermittently confused; we hoped that in time she would see the wisdom of our plan.

Unfortunately, after several days, Mrs. Esposito was still confused and refused to consider placement. She no longer needed acute care, a fact that our case manager, who is responsible for utilization review, reminded us of daily. Shelley, the case management social worker, spoke with the attending physician and it was determined that Mrs. Esposito would need a guardian (Crampton, 2011). It was at this point that I was asked to become involved.

A geropsychiatrist was consulted who determined that Mrs. Esposito lacked the mental capacity to make informed decisions regarding her care. Pam and Rita held joint power of attorney, however this did not allow them to make decisions which she vehemently opposed. I coordinated the petition process with our legal department, making sure the interrogatories (specified written questions) by the psychiatrist and medical doctor were completed. The use of interrogatories allows the physician's opinion to be considered by the judge of the Orphans' court without the physician attending the proceedings. Pam would seek to be made guardian. Along with the hospital attorney, I would attend the hearing to represent the testimony.

It took a few days to gather the documentation necessary to petition the court. As we prepared our case, Mrs. Esposito grew sicker. Her cancer had spread and her prognosis was poor. Her attending physician did not believe she had long to live. We arranged for Pam and Rita to meet with our palliative care team. The palliative care team is consulted when curative medicine is no longer providing meaningful outcomes or when a patient would like to consider alternative care, mostly because the side effects of current care are significantly affecting quality of life. In the end, Mrs. Esposito went home with hospice care. This service was mostly covered by her insurance. Additionally, since her care would be time limited, her daughters believed that, amongst the extended family, her needs could be met. See Figure 20.1 for Ms. Esposito's ecomap.

Definition of the client

Social workers employed by the hospital serve several different clients. One thinks first of the patient. Usually, the patient comes with a family who can assist us in our work or sometimes make our work more difficult. Working within the hospital system, we are mindful of our relationships with all health professionals, staff, and administrators. Insurance carriers can also be seen as our clients, as they directly influence the hospital stay and discharge arrangements. In our case, Mrs. Esposito is at the center of the client system. We also worked with her children to help assure a safe discharge for their mother. We are responsible to the hospital administration to provide good-quality client satisfaction while efficiently managing our patient's case to avoid a discharge delay and thus assure reimbursement (Soskolne, Kaplan, Ben-Shahar, Stanger, & Auslander, 2010).

Mrs. Esposito was referred for social work intervention when the attending physician began to anticipate discharge. After our initial meeting, it was clear that she would need help in planning for her discharge. Because Pam and Rita were available and interested, they became an integral part of the client system. Their provision of background information and family history helped us to understand Mrs. Esposito and plan for her. Working with them gave us insight into the relative ability of the family to support our patient and helped to explain their emotional reactions throughout the discharge planning process.

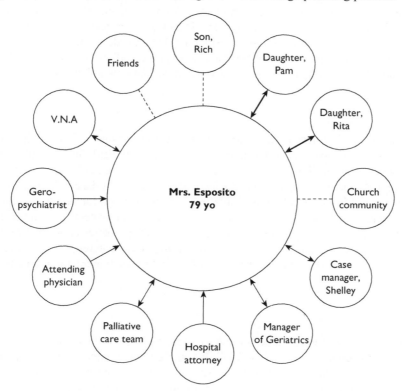

Figure 20.1 Ecomap for Mrs. Esposito

Goals

Our goal, as hospital social workers, is to coordinate a safe discharge for our patients. We provide them with the information and resources necessary to make choices. Patients are allowed to make unsafe choices; but because Mrs. Esposito was clearly unable to make a rational decision about her discharge, we involved her family. Our goal of a safe discharge remained the same, but the cast of characters with whom we had to coordinate this discharge grew.

Developing objectives and contracting

The only formal contract that exists is the one between the social worker and the hospital. Our job description determines the role we play with staff, patients, and families. Patients' satisfaction with our work has become a large part of our annual evaluation. Sometimes in opposition to this, but equally as important, is our ability to complete tasks in a timely manner. Hospital length of stay is monitored closely. Pressure is brought to bear on social workers who cannot effectuate a timely discharge when a patient is no longer in need of acute care.

Our unofficial contract is with our patients and their families. Representing ourselves as patient advocates within the hospital system, we promise them that their voices will be heard and that we will keep them informed of arrangements made on their behalf. We often feel as if we are walking a tightrope between the goals of the hospital and those of the patient and family.

In the case of Mrs. Esposito, we could not develop a contract with our patient. Her objective, to be discharged to her own home, could not be met because of the hospital's commitment to assure a safe discharge to those who lack capacity to make informed decisions. The contract we did develop was with her daughters. They were in agreement regarding our objective, which was to create a safe discharge destination, but, in order to make this a working relationship, we had to respect the time they needed to process all of the changes in their mother's condition while moving them forward towards a decision about her care.

Meeting place

Hospital social workers are often assigned to patients by floor or medical specialty. The initial meeting with Mrs. Esposito occurred in her room, which is typical. Subsequent meetings continued in her room until it became clear that this was causing her undue stress and anxiety. When we met separately with Pam and Rita, we were able to find a conference room on her floor that was not in use. Finding available space in the hospital for family meetings is often difficult. Once found, however, the ability to close the door protects us from interruption. Though medical staff, physicians in particular, are getting better about respecting the existence of a meeting in a patient's room into which they have entered, it is often only a seasoned social worker who has the temerity to insist on acknowledgment and etiquette in these situations.

Use of time

We saw Mrs. Esposito about every other day throughout her 12-day hospitalization. The length of the interaction depended upon her mood. When she seemed interested in engaging, we stayed for perhaps 20 minutes but when she was angry or agitated by the tenor of our conversation, we left rather quickly. Meetings with Pam and Rita lasted anywhere from

20 minutes to more than an hour, depending on the nature of the discussion and their ability to engage in the issues at hand. We met with them five times during their mother's stay.

Because of the confusing and conflictual nature of Mrs. Esposito's situation, I spent a lot of time coordinating the consultations needed to file for guardianship (Toaster, Schmidt, Lawrence, Mendiano, & Wood, 2010). Trying to catch up with busy physicians is difficult and a certain amount of telephone tag is to be expected. At one point, when Mrs. Esposito was less confused, the attending physician questioned the need for guardianship. After a particularly lucid conversation with her, the physician was convinced that it would be possible for her to return to her home with appropriate home care. The following day, I arranged a meeting in the patient's room with the physician and the case management social worker. We allowed the physician to lead the interview, but when we had information that would underscore Mrs. Esposito's irrationality, we gently exposed it. In this way we were able to show the wisdom of our plan without offending our patient. Had it been determined that Mrs. Esposito would go to a skilled nursing facility, Shelley would have spent time contacting the facility, faxing the chart copy, and arranging transportation.

Strategies and interventions

Working with older adults in an acute care hospital demands patience and constant "checking in." It was important at our first meeting that I take the time to get to know Mrs. Esposito – who she was before she became a patient, and what resources, including family, financial, and internal, were available to her. To do this, I make a pronounced effort to respect each patient's space. I introduce myself and explain my role in the hospital. I ask if it is all right if I sit near her bed as it is important that I am at face level. I make sure that she can see and hear me and I intersperse our conversation with questions to ascertain her level of comprehension.

Without this very intentional effort, it is easy to assume patients agree with everything we are saying. If that assumption proves false, our plans for the patient can unravel, often at the last minute. As Mrs. Esposito was only one of many patients to be seen, I had to make this interview as comprehensive as possible in a short span of time without making her feel rushed. An efficient, but personal and respectful assessment is key to a successful intervention. "Checking in" with older adults to be sure that they understand what is going on around them is very important. Mrs. Esposito neither saw nor heard well and often seemed to agree with medical staff either because she did not want to bother them or because she did not have the energy to care to understand. When she became angry and combative, it was important to recognize when our interaction was no longer helpful and to exit the room gracefully.

It was necessary to convene a meeting with the physician, his residents, Shelley, and me with Mrs. Esposito in her room to make sure that we were all in agreement with the plan. We were not interested in taking our patient's independence away from her, but after meeting with Pam and Rita, Shelley and I did not believe that Mrs. Esposito would be able to care for herself, and we knew the strain this would put on her daughters. With careful questioning, we were able to expose Mrs. Esposito's unrealistic expectations of both her and her daughter's abilities to manage in her home.

Stance of the social worker

As a patient advocate, I try to help the patient and family process the medical information they are being given in a way that allows them to make appropriate decisions about their future. It was important that Pam and Rita felt that they were being respected and treated like partners in the care of their mother. Although Shelley would have liked to have left the first meeting knowing that a choice would be made about a skilled nursing facility within the next few days, neither Pam nor Rita was ready. We always work to "meet clients where they are." To try to rush them into making a decision almost never works, and when it does it is often fraught with anxiety and doubt. Patients and caregivers are expected to process a lot of information in what seems to them a very short amount of time. Shelley and I have intimate knowledge of the discharge process and the choices that need to be made; however, this was all new to Pam and Rita. Additionally, we, as professionals, have no emotional connection to these decisions or their consequences – we go home to our own lives at the end of the day – so we must always be mindful of the process for others.

Resources outside of the social worker–client relationship

We have both internal and external consumers and resources available. Internally, the medical staff greatly influence our work in the timeliness and appropriateness of referrals, in their interactions with patients and families (which we might be called on to explain), and in their cooperation with paperwork and administrative functions necessary to accomplish the discharge. The social workers in our home-care department can be a great resource, both in their prior knowledge of the patient and for follow-up. We frequently request consultation with our palliative care and hospice teams as well as our pastoral care and physical therapy departments. Each of these entities help us to advocate for our patients and craft a comprehensive discharge plan. In guardianship cases, we work closely with our legal department. They submit the petition to the Orphans' court and schedule the hearing times. The legal team has many responsibilities, so there are times when we have to assert our agenda.

Our relationship with agencies outside the hospital, our external customers, is important to maintain as this maximizes good communication and ease of referral. Shelley works closely with the clinical admissions liaisons who represent the extended care facilities in our area. Her interaction with them determines her ability to place patients with challenging circumstances.

Because of their discretion and professionalism, our legal department maintains a good relationship with the Orphans' court, which makes it easier to obtain optimum hearing times. Meals on Wheels is another outside agency with which we interact regularly. Religious organizations, including the patient's individual place of worship, are a great resource. Had Mrs. Esposito been less delirious, we might have called on her parish priest to help in negotiating a safe aftercare plan for her. We have several faith-based thrift stores in our area and we rely on them for clothing, furniture, and food donations when necessary.

Reassessment and evaluation

With each new development in Mrs. Esposito's health status, we were required to reassess and revise our interventions. Initially, we thought we could work with our patient in selecting a rehabilitation facility for discharge. Next, we endeavored to work with Pam and Rita, but we realized that they would need to be given more time than we had anticipated to concur with our plan. Once they agreed with our plan, and it became evident that Mrs. Esposito never would, we needed to begin the guardianship process. When the physician questioned this plan, we had to reevaluate and test our assumptions. Finally, when Mrs. Esposito became gravely ill, we had to transfer her care to the case manager.

Transfer, termination, and case conclusion

Once it was decided that Mrs. Esposito would go home, the case manager became responsible for discharge arrangements, including hospice, home care, and transportation. We stayed in touch with her and her daughters until she left. We encourage patients to call us, even after discharge. Sometimes we hear from patients and/or relatives almost immediately after discharge, others, months or years later, and some, none at all. There does not seem to be any logic to this; the families I have worked the hardest for might never call, while those for whom I felt I was able to do very little make the grandest expressions of gratitude. Mrs. Esposito died in her home two weeks after discharge. Pam and Rita came to the hospital with chocolates for the nurses on her floor to thank the staff for their kindness towards their mother. They thanked Shelley and me and said that their mother had died peacefully with family around her.

Differential discussion

Often, it is only in retrospect that we know whether or not we have done a good job. I felt that the Esposito family had a good outcome, but this was not without anxiety and tension throughout. We wanted to fulfill Mrs. Esposito's wish to go home; neither her daughters nor Shelley or I wanted to send her to a skilled nursing facility against her will. However, we had to consider her safety and the fact that she was no longer thinking clearly. We also had to deal with the reality that her funds, as well as Pam's and Rita's ability to help, were limited. Ultimately, her advanced cancer allowed her to go home with hospice support. I believe her last days were more peaceful than months more in a facility would have been. I was happy to see Pam and Rita again and to hear, from them, of their mother's death. Even after the best of outcomes, families can feel that they were pressured to make choices they did not want to ever have to make and they can blame the social workers for that. Sometimes, as visible representatives of the hospital, we can become the targets of anger and blaming due to unresolved grief. We can also be the scapegoat of a health care system that is often neither fair nor equitable.

Though there is not a proven correlation – social work is, after all, a soft science – I believe that the way in which we relate to our patients and their families throughout the hospital stay has direct consequences for their ability to adapt to the overwhelming changes in their lives. The respect for their circumstances and empathy for their feelings, as well as an understanding that life is a process, allows them a safe space to absorb these changes and participate positively in their health care. In our case, Mrs. Esposito could not make good use of our interventions. Her dementia and subsequent delirium would not allow this. Though it meant additional stress on and patience from us, we were able to advocate for Pam and Rita and allow them the time they needed to make appropriate decisions. The fact that they came back and thanked us seemed to be evidence that they benefited from our intervention.

Furthermore, our ability to meet Mrs. Esposito's and her family's non-medical needs may further the hospital's financial objectives. In an increasingly competitive health care climate, patient satisfaction with regards to hospitalization is a critical area of concern. Indeed, as mandated by the Affordable Care Act, Medicare offers substantial financial rewards to hospitals that excel in ratings of patient satisfaction (Centers of Medicare and Medicaid Services, 2014). While determining the principal drivers of patient satisfaction is a complicated process, research suggests it has a key role for the way health care is delivered to patients in addition to what is delivered (Hamilton et al., 2013; Mira, Tomás, Virtudes-Pérez, Nebot, & Rodríguez-Marín, 2009). As illustrated here, social workers' skill set positions them to help hospitals increase patient satisfaction, and, in the process, contribute to the hospital's financial goals.

Discussion questions

1   What are some of the psychosocial aspects of pursuing guardianship for a patient? Why might the hospital, patient, and/or family want to avoid the guardianship process if possible?
2   Palliative care is a growing specialty in the hospital. Why do you think that is so?
3   How does even the highest level health care policy affect the work being done by social workers in the hospital? What stressors can be caused by policy created by persons not frequently involved in the practical application of a policy?

References

American Bar Association (2006). *Legal guide for Americans over 50* (2nd edn.). New York: Random House Reference.

Auslander, G. K., Soskoine, V. Stanger, V., Ben Shahar, I., & Kaplan, G. (2008). Discharge planning in acute care hospitals in Israel: services planned and levels of implementation and adequacy. *Health & Social Work, 33*, 178–188. doi: 10.1093/hsw/33.3.178

Backhaus, P. (2011). *Communication in elderly care: Cross cultural perspectives*. London: Continuum.

Bagley, N. & Levy, H. (2014). Essential health benefits and the Affordable Care Act: Law and Process. *Journal of Health Politics, Policy and the Law, 39*, 441–465. doi: 10.1215/03616878-2416325

Brink, P. & Stones, M. (2007). Examination of the relationship among hearing impairment, linguistic communication, mood, and social engagement of residents in complex continuing-care facilities. *The Gerontologist, 47*(5), 633–641.

Cantrell, R. L. (2007). Common care: Toward a more acceptable option of care of the frail elderly. *Social Work in Public Health, 23*(1), 61–73.

Centers of Medicare and Medicaid Services. (2014). *HCAHPS: Patient's Perspectives of Care Survey.* CMS.gov.

Crampton, A. (2011). Population aging and social work practice with older adults: Demographic and policy challenges. *International Social Work, 54*, 313–329. doi: 1177/0020872810396257

Doukas, D. J. & Reichel, W. (2007). *Planning for uncertainty: Living wills and other advance directives for you and your family*. Baltimore, MD: Johns Hopkins University Press.

Dwyer, S. (2005). Older people and permanent care: Whose decision? *The British Journal of Social Work, 35*(7), 1081–1092.

Eaton, C. K. (2013). Discharge planning with older adults in Minnesota Hospitals. *ProQuest.* Thesis University of Michigan, Ann Arbor, MI, AAI3522977.

Gibson, L. (2011). Giving courts the information necessary to implement limited guardianships: Are we there yet? *Journal of Gerontological Social Work, 54*, 803–813. doi: 10.1080/01634372.2011.604668

Hamilton, D. F., Lane, J. V, Gaston, P., Patton, J. T., Macdonald, D., Simpson, H. R. W., & Howie, C. R. (2013). What determines patient satisfaction with surgery? A prospective cohort study of 4709 patients following total joint replacement. *BMJ Open, 3*, 1–8. doi: 10.1136/bmjopen-2012-002525

HIPAA (2009). Health Insurance and Portability and Accountability Act of 1996 (HIPAA). Retrieved from www.hhs.gov/ocr/privacy

Johnson, Y. M. & Stadel, V. L. (2007). Completion of Advance Directives: Do social work pre-admission interviews make a difference? *Research on Social Work Practice, 17*, 686–696. doi: 1177/1049731506299011

Leung, T. T. F. (2011). Client participation in managing social work service – An unfinished request. *Social Work, 56*, 43–52. doi: 10.1093/sw/56.1.43

Mira, J. J., Tomás, O., Virtudes-Pérez, M., Nebot, C., & Rodríguez-Marín, J. (2009). Predictors of patient satisfaction in surgery. *Surgery, 145*, 536–541. doi:10.1016/j.surg.2009.01.012

Moon, M. (2012). Medicare and the Affordable Care Act. *Journal of Aging and Social Policy, 24*, 233–247. doi: 10.1080/08959420.2012.659111

Moye, J., Butz, S. W., Marson, D. C., & Wood, E. (2007). A conceptual model and assessment template for capacity evaluation in adult guardianship. *The Gerontologist, 47*(5), 591–603. doi: 10.1093/geront/47.5/591

Qualls, S. H. & Smyer, M. A. (2007). Changes in decision making capacity in older adults: Assessment and intervention. In J. Moye & M. Braun (Eds.), *Assessment of medical consent capacity and independent living* (pp. 205–236). Hoboken, NJ: John Wiley & Sons.

Raveis, V. H. (2007). The challenges and issues confronting family caregivers to elderly cancer patients. In S. Carmel, C. A. Morse, & F. M. Torres-Gil (Eds.), *Lessons on aging from three nations*, Volume II. *The art of caring for adults* (pp. 85–97). Amityville, NY: Baywood Publishing Company.

Rockwell, J. (2010). Deconstructing housework: Cuts to home support services and the implications for hospital discharge planning. *Journal of Women and Aging, 22*, 47–60. doi: 10.1080/08952840903489052

Scott, K. R. & Barrett, A. M. (2007). Dementia syndromes: Evaluation and treatment. *Expert Reviews of Neurotherapeutics, 7*(4), 407–422.

Soskolne, V., Kaplan, G., Ben-Shahar, I., Stanger, V., & Auslander, G. K. (2010). Social work discharge planning in acute care hospitals in Israel: Clients' evaluation of the discharge planning process and adequacy. *Research in Social Work Practice, 20*, 368–379. doi: 10:1177/1049731509338934

Toaster, P. B., Schmidt, W., Lawrence, S., Mendiano, M., & Wood, E. (2010). *Public guardianship: In the best interests of incapacitated people.* ABC-CLIO.

Wolff, J. L., Giovannetti, E. R., Boyd, C. M., Reider, L., Palmer, S., Scharfstein, D., et al. (2010). Effects of guided care on family caregivers. *The Gerontologist, 50*, 459–370. doi: 10.1093/geront/gnp124.m

Chapter 21

A framework for working with people with early-stage dementia

A relationship-focused approach to counseling

Phyllis Braudy Harris and Kathleen "Casey" Durkin

Context

Over the last 20 years, the approach of health care professionals working with people in early-stage dementia and their families has evolved from first working mainly with family members, to then focusing on the needs of the person, to now working with the whole family structure in a relationship-centered (versus a caregiver-centered) approach (Harris & Keady, 2006). This chapter discusses the clinical case of a man who referred himself to counseling for assistance in dealing with the impact of a diagnosis of Alzheimer's disease (AD) on himself and his family. Dementia is a clinical syndrome and an all-encompassing term used to connote a loss of memory or other thinking skills that affects a person's ability to perform everyday activities. It is caused by a variety of conditions, with AD being the most common cause of dementia. AD is a progressive, irreversible dementia estimated to affect 5.2 million people currently in the United States and 13.8 million by 2050, if prevention or effective treatment is not found. One in nine people age 65 and older (11%) has AD and about one-third of people 85 and older (32%) have AD. It is also the condition that older adults are most afraid of getting (Alzheimer's Association, 2014). Thus, AD is a significant and mounting concern for older adults, their families, the community, and the country. In April 2012, The World Health Organization published *Dementia: A Public Health Priority* (WHO, 2012). The purpose was to raise awareness world-wide and encourage action on national and international levels (Waite, 2012).

Policy

Working with people living with dementia and their families takes place within an ever-growing public concern and national awareness about AD. In 2011, following the lead of many European countries, the U.S. National Alzheimer's Project Act was signed into law, resulting in the creation of the National Plan to Address Alzheimer's Disease. The plan outlines a set of initiatives to provide improved tools for clinicians, assist care partners and individuals with dementia, raise public awareness about the disease, and advance research. It also sets a research goal to "Prevent and effectively treat Alzheimer's Disease by 2025" (Alzheimer's Association National Plan Milestone Work Group, 2014; U.S. Department of Health and Human Services, 2014). One of the major hurdles of this initiative is to find the resources to adequately fund it. In addition, in the summer of 2013, the Centers for Disease Control and Prevention (CDC) joined with the Alzheimer's Association to release *The Health Brain Initiative: The Public Road Map for State and National Partnerships, 2013–2018*. The report outlines how state and local public health agencies can promote cognitive functioning and address cognitive impairment (Alzheimer's Association and Centers for Disease Control and Prevention, 2013). Now, with the Affordable Care Act, people with a pre-existing diagnosis of dementia cannot be denied health care insurance coverage, and paid caregivers and nurses' aides (in nursing homes and skilled nursing facilities) are mandated to undergo dementia care training (Bryan, 2013). Thus, in the last 4 years there has been much movement in passing health care policy to support people living with dementia and their care partners.

Policies were initiated because of the enormous burden American families shoulder emotionally, physically, and economically in caring for a family member with dementia. Eighty-five percent of dementia care is provided by family members. In 2014 it was estimated that the out-of-pocket costs alone for caring for a family member with dementia reached US$36 billion. In addition, more than 15 million Americans provide 17.7 billion hours of unpaid care giving for people with Alzheimer's and other dementias, which averages out to 21.9 hours of care per care partner every week (Alzheimer's Association, 2014; Gitlin & Schulz, 2012).

Technology

The last 10 years have brought major biomedical technological advances in the diagnosis of AD. These have resulted in the pinpointing of biomarkers in the body that can indicate the presence or absence of the disease. These biomarkers are identified through brain imaging technology that includes: magnetic resonance imaging (MRI), computed tomography (CT), and positron emission tomography (PET scanners), and also the presence of certain proteins in the cerebrospinal fluid (CSF). This allows a person to be diagnosed much earlier in the disease trajectory (Alzheimer's Association, 2015a). Because of the availability of this technology and other advances in the field, in 2011 the National Institute on Aging (NIA) released the new NIA/Alzheimer's Association Diagnostic Guidelines for Alzheimer's Disease. The previous criteria for clinical diagnosis and research were developed in 1984.

New guidelines have expanded the stages of AD to include periods before the actual symptoms of the disease are behaviorally noticeable. It is now believed that the changes in the brain due to AD occur years before visible behavioral symptoms. Now, AD stages are defined as: (1) preclinical (presymptomatic) Alzheimer's, (2) mild cognitive impairment (MCI) due to Alzheimer's, and (3) dementia due to Alzheimer's (Jack et al., 2011). The first stage is when the biomarker changes in the brain are evident before symptoms affecting memory, thinking, or behavior can be detected by affected individuals or their physicians. The second stage is evident when there are mild changes in memory and thinking, which can be measured on mental status tests; however, the person's everyday activities are not disrupted. In the third stage, impairments in memory, thinking, and behavior affect a person's ability to function independently on a daily basis (Alzheimer's Association, 2015d). The development of these categories has not been without controversy; since there is no known cure for AD, early detection tests might do more harm than good (Lock, 2013; Pimplikar, 2010).

There are four accepted anti-dementia drugs: Aricept, Exelon, and Razadyne (donepezil, rivastigmine, and galantamine/galanthamine) for early-stage and Namenda (memantine) for middle- to late-stage dementia. For some people, for a limited time, one or a combination of these drugs may slow down the symptoms. However, given that the cause of AD is still unknown, no present-day treatment stops the deterioration of brain cells (Alzheimer's Association, 2015b; NIA, 2014a). Because people can have meaningful lives with dementia, especially in the early stages, those with dementia and their families are urged to use psychosocial interventions to maintain the quality of their lives. Such interventions include counseling, support groups, environmental modifications, adult daycare, and keeping physically, mentally, and socially active (Alzheimer's Association, 2015c; Woods & Clare, 2008). In addition, new advancements in technology have assisted in maintaining quality of life. Location-based mapping services allow family members to monitor a person's location, while the individual with dementia can remain independent (Alzheimer's Association, 2015e; Burrow & Brook, 2012). In addition, social media blogs and on-line support groups provide information, education, and emotional support to both the person living with dementia and their care partner (Alzheimer's Association, 2015f; Carey, 2014). Today, prevention and keeping the brain healthy are emphasized. Though there is no known effective way to prevent dementia, the NIA has developed recommendations and an on-line toolkit for older adults to assist in maintaining a healthy brain (NIA, 2014b). Recommendations include healthy eating, physical exercise, social engagement, and mental stimulation.

Organization

The case discussed below takes place within a loose organizational structure starting with the memory assessment unit of a well-known local hospital where Mr. Adams was diagnosed with early-stage AD. As stated earlier, Mr. Adams was the one who noticed the changes in himself and self-referred. Once he had received the diagnosis which confirmed his suspicions, he referred himself to the local chapter of the Alzheimer's Association to further his education about the disease, its trajectory, its treatment, and its impact. After meeting a few times with the staff at the Association he was referred for private counseling as the staff thought he would benefit from this type of intervention and the Association did not offer this service. Thus, except for the restraints of third party insurance providers, the social worker (CD, co-author of this chapter) did not have many organizational restraints on her provision of service to Mr. Adams. Because of the variability in the disease and how it expresses itself, there is no "typical" person with AD.

Decisions about practice

Description of the client

Mr. Adams is a college-educated African American gentleman and a long-time community activist and engineer. He describes himself as a leader, from beginning as a student body president in junior high school, to college fraternity president and becoming the director of a Civil Rights program. He holds the distinction of being the first African American to become a member of a distinguished group of corporate professionals. Mr. Adams is very proud of his children's accomplishments: all three children graduated from college, with his son holding a master's degree from a prestigious university and one daughter holding a master's degree from a local private university. The remaining daughter had proved herself to be an accomplished business person and mother. This background serves to describe the fabric of Mr. Adams' personality (as well as his family's): a self-starter and a highly motivated man who throughout life demonstrated proactive thinking and planning. About 4 years ago, he began to notice changes in his behavior, which precipitated his making an appointment with a memory and aging clinic. He had been separated from his wife for many years.

Meeting place and use of time

Before meeting with people who are experiencing memory loss, it is optimal to ensure that they have been evaluated neurologically. If this has not occurred, part of the counseling "contract" must be a referral for a neurological evaluation. There are times when individuals who are concerned about their memory will seek counseling. Through counseling, they will gain support to make the appointment knowing that they will not need to whether a possible diagnosis of dementia alone. Then, when agreeing to work with a person with dementia or any type of memory loss, it is critical for the social worker to identify a regular time and place (e.g., same time and day weekly). This provides the opportunity for the person to develop a set routine and ensures her or his ability to keep appointments. Also, meeting in the same location (office) can provide a sense of comfort and familiarity, which is especially important for a person with memory loss.

In this case example, I, CD, provided a welcoming environment: plants, objects for fidgeting, comfortable seating, and bottled water to increase a sense that Mr. Adams and his family were held in high regard. Also important here is clear signage within the therapist's office building and elevators (including exit, bathroom and parking area signs). Research suggests that providing counseling within the home may also be considered as the person with dementia or care partner may experience difficulties with transportation or other unforeseen complications (Hill & Brettle, 2006; Whitlatch, Judge, Zarit, & Femia, 2006).

Stance of the social worker

Dementia's course and the reactions of family members vary greatly. Bowers (1987) and Harris (2001) review different styles of care that daughters and sons (respectively) provide for parents with dementia. Bowers identified "preservative care," which supports this relationship-focused approach in psychotherapy, maintaining the person with dementia's family connections, dignity, hope, and sense of control. Although it was initially indicated for use later in the disease, preservative care fits our concept of working with people with dementia and their families in the early stages as well. This will be further illustrated through the discussion of goals and strategies below. In addition, Keady and Nolan (2003) identify stages perceived by the person with dementia. These include slipping, suspecting, covering up, revealing, confirming, surviving, disorganization, decline, and death. The first eight stages and the "preservative care" concept are pertinent to this relationship-focused approach.

CD's stance is warm, respectful, valuing, and accepting. She helps clients to comfortably express their thoughts, feelings, and fears and to join her and each other in planning. In this way, clients preserve one another's dignity and resiliency and allow for successful adaptation and integration. Partly because the presentation of the illness is so varied, social workers must remain flexible and responsive to the changing needs of this population (Hill & Brettle, 2006). In addition, therapists have to take the lead in the first meeting to discuss confidentiality alone with the person with dementia and then with the family group. Social workers must also help those with dementia and their care partners to understand that it is urgent to develop and maintain a proactive stance, and consistently support one another to practice, repetitively, new communication and coping skills.

At this time, the vast majority of people with dementia are from a generation that was taught not to voice its concerns, fears, or even desires. Their adult children, many of whom are baby boomers, have a different mindset and believe talking therapies are a helpful and a sometimes necessary tool. For these reason, the social worker respects the older adult's perspective but, through psychoeducational discussions, can help the older adult to understand that therapy will greatly add to the goal of preserving independence and control. The authors have found a relationship-focused approach with inclusion of care partners to be very effective (Hill & Brettle, 2006; Whitlatch et al., 2006).

Goals, developing objectives, and contracting

The goals when working with a person with memory loss are similar and yet differ from typical psychodynamic psychotherapy. The similarities lie within representative goals for this modality. These include, but are not limited to, enhancing self-esteem, developing good coping skills, developing a trusting relationship, and working through previous issues, including loss (Hausman, 1992). The differences are significant, with particular focus on the need to involve family members during the course of treatment. The rationale for involving family members needs to be clearly explained to the people with dementia as a method of validating their sense of their own perspectives. The social worker needs to engage the people with AD to understand that sometimes, due to this destructive disease, there may be times when they may miss some crucial facts. In order to be of greatest help, family members may share critical information that will help the people with AD to maintain better control of their lives as well as to identify the coping strategies that will preserve people with AD's sense of self.

As the social worker begins to work with the person with dementia and the family members, this team can serve to identify and reinforce any opportunities to foster resiliency (Harris & Durkin, 2002). Table 21.1 illustrates ways in which the social worker can efficiently help the person and engage family members to support the development of valuable coping strategies.

In goal-setting, maintaining a positive sense of personhood is paramount (Kitwood, 1997). People with dementia in the early stages often struggle with grief over their losses of independence and heightened fears of further incapacitations (Kasl-Godley & Gatz, 2000). Goals should include helping the person maintain as much self-control as possible. The initial goals for Mr. Adams and his family members were: (1) improved open and honest communication among them, and (2) the development of positive coping strategies for Mr. Adams to enhance his sense of self and accept a realistic level of independence. Together, if we could create a safe environment in which Mr. Adams did not cover up the difficulties that were causing him stress, he would more likely tell us when and where he needed assistance. This would improve his quality of life and allow his family to feel that their father was safe. Outcomes were measured qualitatively by tracking these goals in each session. Additionally, together, we tracked community resources used (see Figure 21.1). The combination of open/honest communication with increased coping strategies and use of community resources resulted in decreased isolation and a stronger support system overall. This allowed Mr. Adams to remain safely and independently in his apartment.

Mr. Adams came to his first session with his son and two daughters. In the waiting room I explained that I would first meet alone with Mr. Adams and I would then invite the adult children to join us. Seeing me alone first allowed Mr. Adams the opportunity to state his wishes and to "have an objective person to talk with." During that individual time, I explained that I would respect Mr. Adams' wishes and thoughts, and together we would decide how to weave his family members in and out of the therapy. I conveyed to Mr. Adams that I saw him as a person who had made and could continue to make many contributions to our society.

Table 21.1 Harris and Durkin's relationship-focused approach to develop positive coping strategies

Coping strategy	Social work action steps for working with a person with dementia	Social work action steps for working with family members to help a person with dementia
Acceptance of diagnosis	Allow the person with dementia to share what brought him or her to the session, symptoms and concerns, and actions taken to deal with them Allow time for questions and discussion of physician's diagnosis Provide opportunities in a safe environment for expression of feelings including frustration, anger, guilt, blame, hopelessness, and humiliation Help the person with dementia move toward acknowledgment of the dementia diagnosis Discuss how diagnosis has affected family and other relationships Make referrals to Alzheimer's Association local chapter or Online Support Community for: education, and early-stage support groups	Help family to hear the person with dementia's account and concerns Listen to major caregiving concerns Make referrals to another therapist to help individual family member(s) with issues related to changes in their relationship, role transition, anticipatory losses, and caregiver stress Encourage family to secure accurate information on etiology of the diagnosis Help family members to acknowledge that the person with dementia can be a partner in making decisions Encourage the person with dementia and family to discuss together possible actions steps to handle mutual concerns
Disclosure of diagnosis	Discuss privacy and how to choose who to tell Suggest keeping a journal Develop opportunities during sessions to practice new skills for talking about the diagnosis	Help family to develop understanding that a person with dementia in early stages needs to have control and they should decide together who, when, and how significant people need to be told Encourage family to anticipate out loud what any potential reactions may be and how to respond Suggest keeping a journal
Role transition acceptance	Address feelings related to loss of career/family and/or social roles and independence Evaluate and refer for treatment of depression and/or anxiety Reframe loss as a relief and an opportunity vs. failure (e.g., This is your time to be taken care of . . .) Refer for possible inclusion in clinical drug trials (allows for feelings of altruism) Help the person with dementia consider meaningful volunteer work or early-stage adult day care or clubs Discuss still possible meaningful roles In the family	Help family member(s) identify roles/tasks so that the person with dementia can continue meaningful participation in the family and elsewhere Identify roles of primary care partners and other supports Help family identify people in their lives who can take on caregiving tasks to lessen their stress (examples include who helps with medication, transportation, meals, cleaning, etc.) Prepare for breakdowns in plans and discuss the need to be understanding of one another

(continued)

Table 21.1 (continued)

Coping strategy	Social work action steps for working with a person with dementia	Social work action steps for working with family members to help a person with dementia
Strength identification	Help the person with dementia to identify lifelong strengths as well as new strengths – look for examples of resiliency and adaptation Explore, discuss and help the person with dementia identify previous positive coping strategies	Encourage family to focus on and reinforce the strengths of the person with dementia Help family to identify lifelong strengths and new strengths of the person with dementia – look for examples of resiliency and adaptation Work with the person with dementia and family member(s) to compose a list of their individual and family strengths and accomplishments and read these together regularly
Proactive approach: Taking control	Engage the person with dementia as a capable person and partner in the treatment planning process Encourage the person with dementia to take proactive stance Promote the person with dementia putting together a file of all medical, financial, and legal documents to share with family member(s) Consider various forms of technology that may allow new coping skills (emails; blogging; shared calendars, GPS, etc.)	Encourage family to include the person with dementia in all levels of planning; demonstrate this in sessions Discuss openly the desires of the person with dementia; encourage the person with dementia or family to arrange for durable power of attorney, advance directives or living will; organize all financial documents, medical information, and legal documents Encourage the family to utilize technology that will allow all family members access to an interactive calendar to always be up to date with any changes or additions in appointments, etc.

During this first session, Mr. Adams assumed control, explaining his current situation with his diagnosis of AD, involvement as a participant in an AD research center, and recent completion of an educational lecture series at the Alzheimer's Association. I told Mr. Adams that I could see that he prided himself on his ability to be realistic and proactive on his own behalf. After about 25 minutes, I suggested we invite his son and daughters to join us. Before I left the office I clearly stated what I planned to tell his children and asked him if this was acceptable, and if there was something he would prefer me to leave out or add. I purposefully wanted Mr. Adams to understand he and I needed to be partners in how and why we involved family members in this relationship-based modality.

As the three children settled in, I teased Mr. Adams that he was obviously a VIP, as an entourage had accompanied him. The entire group chuckled and this purposeful use of humor allowed an ease to exist within the group. I sat the son and both sisters facing their father so he could see them and me from his seat. I took the lead and gave a thumbnail sketch of my discussion with Mr. Adams. I asked the son and daughters if this was their "take" on Mr. Adams' situation or had we missed any important details. They agreed I had an accurate summary and commended their father for seeking professional help. The children explained to their father that they wished to be as supportive as possible and felt some added safety themselves in having a "professional" walk them through some difficult situations.

Mr. Adams had explained to me earlier that there had been a situation where he had mixed up his medications, and thus his family had safety concerns. Although Mr. Adams had a complete rationalization for how he mixed up his medications, he added he would feel more secure with a new and safer medication plan. Together with his son and daughters, we devised a new medication schedule that identified who would stop by Mr. Adams' apartment daily to monitor his medication. Two of the three children could add this into their own daily routines. All agreed that this would support Mr. Adams in his wish to remain living alone in his apartment and give the children "some peace of mind." I also mentioned that there probably were other areas of his life where working together like this with his family could assist him in remaining independent as long as possible, and we could discuss these at future meetings.

I contracted with Mr. Adams that we would meet for six sessions, which would also allow for family members to join us for parts of our sessions. I explained that at the end of these six sessions, together we would evaluate if Mr. Adams wished to continue or if together we thought we might take a break and he could use me on an as-needed basis. This would allow both Mr. Adams and his children some predictability and control. I explained that contracting in this way would help us to plan our time and work together.

Strategies and interventions

Table 21.1 shows interventions for social workers to assist the person with dementia to develop positive coping strategies for preserving a sense of self and to promote a realistic independence. It uses a strengths-based philosophy. Some of these strategies were used with Mr. Adams and his family; the authors have used others with other clients. This table illustrates how the social worker in a relationship-focused approach should remain inclusive of people with dementia and their care partner in the treatment approach. Previous research on ways health care professionals and family members can help persons with dementia develop positive coping strategies (Harris & Durkin, 2002) has prompted these same authors to develop this relationship-focused approach.

Mr. Adams' words exemplify the development of these positive coping strategies.

ACCEPTANCE OF DIAGNOSIS

As I thought about my situation, as I move through the twilight years, I do so with neither dread nor apprehension, I do so with the assurance that the quality of life is going to be good for me. Good for me because of my attitude as I grew up, good for me because I'm surrounded by a really loving and devoted family that I can depend on . . . it is these forces plus my attitudes that will get me through this . . . being angry and not accepting reality is not going to change the fact that you've got a problem.

ROLE TRANSITION ACCEPTANCE

One of the things I learned is it's [dementia] not gonna go away. Whatever the problem is, it's not going to get better by being left to its own devices. This is why I try to be honest with my kids. They can help me stay strong. I think the family needs to accept that this individual is not handicapped or has his mental capacity just diminished and be able to accept that, adjust to that instead of becoming upset about it, accommodate that difference. It certainly makes a lot of difference that I am blessed with my son and daughters . . . So, I'm blessed and even when I'm feeling a little sorry for myself, and worry, I remember that they are making lots of arrangements for me. . . . It ain't what happens to you that really matters, it's what you decide to do about it.

PROACTIVE APPROACH (TAKING CONTROL)

Seriously, I've decided I'm going to have a very highly regimented life. In other words, what to do, who to see, why, it's very simple. That's the way I'll organize. You know: 8:00 showers, shave, blahblahblah, breakfast, etc.

Words from Mr. Adams' family also illustrate themes in this relationship-focused approach:

STRENGTHS IDENTIFICATION

There's a lot, Dad, that I know you struggle with, like sometimes writing out your checks, but I still want to talk about my business proposals with you. You still offer words of wisdom and I appreciate your listening.

ROLE TRANSITION ACCEPTANCE

As Dad points out, we are stepping in and helping out in areas, and sometimes there's somewhat of a feeling of role reversal in a way that's kind of awkward. Sometimes we disagree but it doesn't seem like it's really a big deal.

Use of time

Mindful that the person with dementia may sometimes (but not always) lose track of time, the social worker should begin each session using routine with a verbal cueing of warm-up techniques. In this case, I would ask Mr. Adams to bring me up to speed with how his week had gone, specifically repeating the coping strategies he had planned to practice during the week. If there were a visible concern, I would respectfully register this. For example, once, for the second week in a row, I noticed Mr. Adams wearing clothes that appeared to have small food stains on them. His appearance was always important to him, which reinforced his positive sense of self. I shared with him my concern that maybe he just was not getting the chance to keep up with his laundry and perhaps we could involve his children in helping out.

The social worker needs to be mindful of how much time is being used in the counseling session and help the person with dementia have a sense of time remaining. Helping the family group develop a routine and a rhythm of the sessions should include the warm-up, getting concerns on the table, tracking goals, and then wrapping up the session with a clear plan of any necessary changes in caring and assisting the person with dementia. The therapist needs to prepare the family group for the end of the session vs. feeling "Where did the hour go?" The therapist can simply state: "We are about half way through our session," and then later, "We have about five minutes remaining, let's review our plan for this upcoming week."

Use of outside resources

As described earlier, Mr. Adams was a proactive, "take the bull by the horns" type of person, as he liked to describe himself. As an engineer, he had always prided himself on being able to fix almost anything in his home. He confided that following a "snafu" where he almost made a grave mistake in repairing his hot water heater, he immediately enlisted help from the local senior center. He began with home repair help and gradually enlisted other supports through this resource. After confiding in his long-term internist about his suspicions that he may have some cognitive decline, as evidenced by his home repair debacle, coupled with experiencing moments of complete confusion, he was referred to the memory assessment center of a local hospital, as discussed earlier in the chapter. His suspicions were confirmed and he accepted the referral to the local chapter of the Alzheimer's Association. Table 21.1 specifically addresses how the social worker in a relationship-focused approach can encourage the use of outside resources that promote role transition acceptance, strengths identification, and, most importantly, a proactive approach taking control. The ecomap in Figure 21.1 illustrates the strong network Mr. Adams has at his disposal.

Reassessment, evaluation, and termination

This area underscores the ethical responsibilities involved with this at-risk group. This specialized dementia population requires termination to begin, as with most clients, in the first meeting. Because of the unknown speed and trajectory of this disease, reiterating the contracted number of sessions each time is critical, as is the ability to re-contract for additional sessions. The ethical considerations of the capacity of the person with dementia cannot be overlooked. At the point when the social worker feels the person with dementia can no longer use the counseling session to reduce emotional stress and aid in developing positive coping strategies, the need for termination is fundamental.

In order to be cognizant of when termination is appropriate, reassessment and evaluation need to be a constant part of the weekly counseling sessions. This consists of comparing the agreed-upon goals and action steps to the person with dementia's weekly progress. Given the person with dementia's memory loss, this reassessment and evaluation needs to be an important part of every session. The person with dementia should be encouraged to record the counseling session and to listen to it during the week. Use of the recording provides a "supplemental memory aid," reminding the person with dementia of the goals that need to

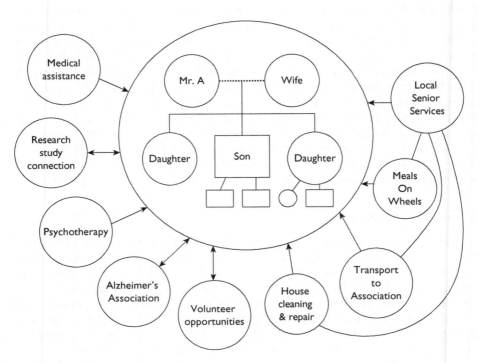

Figure 21.1 Ecomap for Mr. Adams

be accomplished. The family can assist by reminding the person with dementia about the recording.

As part of the reassessment, certain questions relevant for this specialized population need to be asked, such as:

- Given the person with dementia's strengths and his or her disease process, do the agreed-upon goals continue to be realistic?
- Have the goals been broken down in small enough steps and been explained in under-standable terms?
- Do family members' observations support the reported outcomes?
- What can family members do to support these outcomes?

When the decision to terminate has been reached, the stance of the social worker shifts to helping the person with dementia know that the social worker will always be there for him or her and their care partners, should future needs develop. The stance of the social worker also includes possibly acting as a bridge to a case management service, either privately or through a community agency. This involves discussing and defining case management and leading the family to learn all their options. As in most clinical cases utilizing sound clinical boundaries, the clinician is not necessarily going to be informed of the progression of the disease and effects on the person with dementia following termination.

Case conclusion

A diagnosis of dementia dramatically changes the lives of those diagnosed and their family members. It is a devastating disease with an irreversible negative trajectory. Yet people can still live lives of quality and of meaning. Social workers working with people in the early stages of the disease and their family members can make a difference in the lives of their clients through the use of counseling. The relationship-focused approach discussed above allowed the person with dementia and his carers to become partners in the future decision-making and planning of their lives. Together, they all felt as if they were sharing control, preserving Mr. Adams' dignity and sense of selfhood, and coming to an acceptance of necessary interdependence upon each other. All of this was being undertaken with the aim of maintaining a realistic independence for Mr. Adams as long as possible. Together they mapped out how they planned to cope through the next stages of this journey of dementia. Mr. Adams reflected: "I feel like I'm Chairman of the Board and I have the best board of directors one could wish for."

Discussion questions

1   Dementia tends to change family roles so that children must provide more care for their parents. How would you work with children who are less willing to accept this role than Mr. Adams' children were?
2   Private practice allows social workers the time and autonomy to provide individualized care and support. What ethical issues do you see for this model?
3   Once dementia progresses, need for family support remains. What sorts of social work care could you envision providing as Mr. Adams' AD continues to progress?

References

Alzheimer's Association (2014). Alzheimer's disease facts and figures. *Alzheimer's and Dementia, 10*(2), 1–75.
Alzheimer's Association (2015a). Steps to diagnosis. Retrieved from www.alz.org/alzheimers_dis ease_diagnosis.asp
Alzheimer's Association (2015b). Medications for memory loss. Retrieved from www.alz.org/alzhei mers_disease_standard_prescriptions.asp
Alzheimer's Association (2015c). Treatments for Alzheimer's disease. Retrieved from www.alz.org/ alzheimers_disease_treatments.asp
Alzheimer's Association (2015d). New diagnostic criteria and guidelines for Alzheimer's disease. Retrieved from www.alz.org/research/diagnostic_criteria/overview.asp
Alzheimer's Association (2015e). About comfort zone. Retrieved from www.alz.org/comfortzone/ about_comfort_zone.asp
Alzheimer's Association (2015f). Alzheimer's and dementia caregiver center. Retrieved from www. alz.org/care/overview.asp
Alzheimer's Association and Centers for Disease Control and Prevention (2013). *The healthy brain initiative: The public health road map for state and national partnerships, 2013–2018*. Chicago, IL: Alzheimer's Association.
Alzheimer's Association National Plan Milestone Work Group (2014). 2014 Report on the Milestones for the U. S. National Plan to Address Alzheimer's Disease. *Alzheimer's and Dementia, 10*(5), Supplement, S430–S452. doi:10.1016/j.alz.2014/08.103

Bowers, B. J. (1987). Inter-generational caregiving: Adult caregivers and their aging parents. *Advances in Nursing Science, 9*(2), 20–31.

Bryan, Derek (2013). How the Affordable Care Act will affect dementia patients. Retrieved from www.dementia.org/resources/affordable-care-act-and-dementia-patients

Burrow, S. & Brook, D. (2012). Atdementia: An information resource on assistive technologies that help support the independence of people with dementia. *Dementia: The International Journal of Social Research and Practice, 11*(4), 553–557. doi: 10.1177/1471301212437822

Carey, E (2014). The best Alzheimer's blogs of the year. Retrieved from www.healthline.com/health-slideshow/best-alzheimers-dementia-blogs

Gitlin, L. N. & Schulz, R. (2012). Family caregiving of older adults. In R. T. Prohaska, L. A. Anderson, & R. H. Binstock (Eds.), *Public health for an aging society* (pp. 181–204). Baltimore, MD: Johns Hopkins University Press.

Harris, P. B. (2001). The voices of husbands and sons caring for a family member with dementia. In B. J. Kramer & E. H. Thompson (Eds.), *Men as caregivers: Theory, research & service implications* (pp. 213–233). New York: Springer Publications.

Harris, P. B. & Durkin, C. (2002). Building resistance through coping and adapting. In P. B. Harris (Ed.), *The person with Alzheimer's disease* (pp. 165–186). Baltimore, MD: Johns Hopkins University Press.

Harris, P. B. & Keady, J. (2006). Editorial. *Dementia: The International Journal of Social Research and Practice, 5*(1), 5–11.

Hausman, C. (1992). Dynamic psychotherapy. Retrieved from www.alzforum.org/dis/tre/drt/dynamic.asp

Hill, A. & Brettle, A. (2006). Counseling older people: What can we learn from research evidence? *Journal of Social Work Practice, 20*(3), 281–297.

Jack, C. R, Albert, M. S., Knopman, D. S., McKhann, G. M., Sperling, R. A., Carillo, M. S., Thies, B., & Phelps, C. H. (2011). Introduction to the recommendations from the National Institute on Aging and the Alzheimer's Association workgroup on diagnostic guidelines for Alzheimer' disease. *Alzheimer's & Dementia, 7*(3), 257–262. doi: 10.1016/j/jalz.2011.03.004

Kasl-Godley, J. & Gatz, M. (2000). Psychosocial interventions for individuals with dementia: An integration of theory, therapy, and a clinical understanding of dementia. *Clinical Psychology Review, 20*(6), 755–782.

Keady, J. & Nolan, M. (2003). The dynamics of dementia: Working together, working separately, or working alone. In M. Nolan, U. Lundh, G. Grant, & J. Keady (Eds.), *Partnerships in family care: Understanding the caregiving career* (pp. 15–32). Maidenhead: Open University Press.

Kitwood, T. (1997). *Dementia reconsidered.* Buckingham: Open University Press.

Lock, M. (2013). *The Alzheimer's conundrum.* Princeton, NJ: Princeton University Press.

NIA (National Institute on Aging) (2014a). Alzheimer's medication fact sheet. Retrieved from www.nia.nih.gov/alzheimers/publication/alzheimers-disease-medications-fact-sheet?utm_source=20140825_ADmeds&utm_medium=email&utm_campaign=ealert

NIA (2014b). Brain health resource. Retrieved from www.nia.nih.gov/health/publication/brain-health-resource?utm_source=20140922_brainhealthresource&utm_medium=email&utm_campaign=ealert#handouts

Pimplikar, S. J. (2010). Alzheimer's isn't up to the test. *New York Times,* July 19 Opinion Section. Retrieved from www.nytimes.com/2010/07/70/opinion/20pimplikar.html

U.S. Department of Health and Human Services (2014). National plan to address Alzheimer's disease: 2014 update. Retrieved from http://aspe.hhs.gov/daltcp/napa/NatlPlan2014.shtml

Waite, L. (2012). Dementia: An international crisis?: *Perspectives in Public Health, 132*(4), 154–155. doi: 10.1177/1757913912450648

Whitlatch, C. J., Judge, K., Zarit, S. H., & Femia, E. (2006). Dyadic intervention for family caregivers and care receivers in early-stage dementia. *The Gerontologist, 46*(5), 688–694.

WHO (World Health Organization) Alzheimer's Disease International (2012). *Dementia: a public health priority.* Geneva: World Health Organization.

Woods, B. & Clare, L. (2008). *Handbook of the clinical psychology of aging.* Chichester: John Wiley & Sons.

Chapter 22

The future of end-of-life care

As palliative care gains momentum, what is the future of hospice?

Michelle K. Brooks and Judith L. M. McCoyd

Context

The Palliative Care movement is rooted in the hospice philosophy of care, which seeks to ameliorate the physical, emotional, and spiritual suffering associated with life-threatening, and typically terminal, illness. All hospice care is palliative (ameliorating pain and suffering), but not all palliative care is hospice. Palliative Care (when capitalized it refers to the way it is organized and funded within medical institutions, not as a philosophy of care) is an adjunct to other medical treatment that allows for curative treatments to continue. Hospice developed first as a way of delivering palliative services, including both pain relief and psycho-social-spiritual support, at the point where a physician determined that a patient was expected to live less than six months. Hospice generally allows individuals to remain in their home and receive all care and services there.

At the outset, palliative care grew from hospice's focus on ameliorating suffering of all types, including pain from medical treatments. As hospice became more widely accepted, individuals receiving curative treatments for cancer and other illnesses wanted access to the pain amelioration for which hospice was known. Palliative Care teams began to be a consulting service within hospitals to help manage pain and suffering while patients were being treated for their conditions. It was assumed that the development of Palliative Care teams would create a natural bridge to help move individuals into hospice care when that became appropriate. Hospice is appropriate when the focus of care changes from the pursuit of cure to assuring symptom management and comfort during final life stages, including psychosocial and spiritual support (Caregiver's Library, 2015). Palliative Care and hospice share a focus on symptom management that has greatly improved patients' experience of illness and disease treatment. Although sometimes difficult to distinguish from each other in practice, they differ in that hospice is defined by Medicare regulations to include social work and chaplaincy supports (not ongoing curative care), and promotes a unified care team of services within the patient's home; Palliative Care is covered under the patient's insurance plan as an adjunctive, consultative service (usually hospital-based) focused on pain management and generally not covering many psychosocial services. Both Palliative Care and hospice are associated with reducing unnecessary intensive care, emergency room, and other high-cost care at the end of life (Abernethy et al., 2013; Wang, Piet, Kenworthy, & Dy, 2015).

Research indicates that when referral to hospice comes from a Palliative Care team, hospice length of service (LOS) is typically longer, enabling more psychosocial support and better bereavement care for the family in the comfort of their home (Scheffey et al., 2014). Even so, Wang et al. (2015) note that there seem to be two different patient groups: those for whom Palliative Care is the transition to accepting hospice services and those who will not accept a hospice referral but who wish for symptom palliation. This creates a group of people who may move into the dying phase without the benefit of broader hospice services.

As a manager for our mid-size Hospice and Home Care service (including palliative care services), supervising the social work, chaplaincy, and other allied health caregivers, I (MB) am in the position to see some of the most challenging aspects of the transition from home care to Palliative Care to hospice. I am also quite aware that Palliative Care teams differ; some focus mostly on keeping patients involved with hopes for curative care and helping them manage pain and other side effects of treatment, whereas others work actively to help patients recognize the point at which hospice will best help them live a quality life until death. As someone who helps train and supervise our social work staff, I am acutely aware of the social work role in helping patients recognize when hospice will be more helpful to them. I am also aware of the personal, insurance coverage, and medical culture issues that keep patients grasping at curative and Palliative Care. Remaining in curative treatment rather than transitioning to hospice often means that families are unsupported in their adjustment to the patient's impending death, the patient has little psycho-social-spiritual support around end-of-life issues, and survivors have no bereavement services. A key intervention for identifying the time to transition to hospice is the "goals of care" conversation, during which the goal changes from "cure" to "comfort."

Policy

In 1971, President Richard Nixon declared "War on Cancer," investing US$1.5 billion into the research and development of cancer treatments (Nixon, 1971). Some 40 plus years plus later, there are many more options for patients diagnosed with cancer. Cure is sometimes possible and care at the end of life has become more humane. Many of the options, such as palliative radiation and palliative chemotherapy, did not exist when the concept of hospice was introduced to this country in 1973. The hospice movement started with Dame Cicely Saunders in the United Kingdom as she provided care for the dying in the late 1940s and into the following decades. In 1967, she established St. Christopher's Hospice in London, and when Florence Wald came to visit on sabbatical from Yale University, she brought the concepts and perspectives of hospice back to the United States in 1969. This coincided with the publicity Elisabeth Kubler-Ross was receiving for her work with the dying, and in 1974 Wald established the Connecticut Hospice (NHPCO, 2015). Although the initial legislation to provide hospice services in the United States was initiated in 1974, and the Department of Health Education and Welfare supported the idea by 1978, it was 1982 before Congress supported a hospice benefit within Medicare and 1986 before it was made permanent. Today, Medicare certification and regulation are tightly tied to reimbursement (NHPCO, 2015). Although widely accepted initially, by the late 1990s, hospice LOS began to decrease, indicating that referral to hospice was delayed until just days prior to death. Yet, research indicates that people who receive timely hospice referral live 29 days longer on average than those who do not (matched for diagnosis) and reduce costs of care (NHPCO, 2015). Still, patients often resist hospice referral until it is too late for them to make use of its benefits.

Hospice care is funded differently from traditional medical care; it is based on a set rate of care provided to dying patients (a physician must certify that the patient is not expected to live longer than six months) that ensures that their medical care will be delivered in their home (though some free-standing hospices have evolved for respite and for patients with unstable living circumstances). Once on hospice, patients do not travel to medical providers or hospitals but receive all care, medications, and support services in their homes. This can mean that treatments done for palliation via radiation or chemotherapy to shrink painful lesions may not be utilized. Palliative Care is funded like any other medical consultation team (neurology, hematology) and patients are expected to continue their medical treatments in hospital or other medical environments and therefore can access palliative treatments such as radiation that are only offered in hospitals. As the patient does not move to a "hospice benefit" when using Palliative Care, psychosocial and other supportive services are covered meagerly and generally for very few visits – only those related directly to the medical condition (not for the existential issues individuals may struggle with as they grasp their own mortality).

Initially envisioned as a way to help inpatients with painful treatments become acquainted with palliative treatment to reduce suffering and as a bridge toward hospice care where appropriate, the use of Palliative Care teams spread rapidly during the first decade of the millennium (NHPCO, 2001, 2015). As medicine has developed more technologies for aggressively fighting life-threatening illness, Palliative Care services came into being and referrals to hospice were no longer the only way to access medical care that would manage the suffering of treatment- and disease-related symptoms. Medicare defines the scope of hospice services and generally provides needed comfort care, homemaker services, nurses, social workers, chaplains, respite, and sometimes music, art, movement, and other therapies in the patient's home to enable the patient to enhance the quality and comfort of their life until natural death; it includes an automatic bereavement benefit for family members for over a year after the patient's death (Centers for Medicare and Medicaid Services, 2015). Although Palliative Care initially provided few of these services other than symptom management, their enlarged scope and movement into home-care settings has changed the earlier trajectories of care. Under Palliative Care, no assertion of a likely death within six months is made (and patients do not have to accept that possibility). Symptoms are palliated, but the focus of hospice on psychosocial support and work with the family within the home does not inform typical Palliative Care practice.

Technology

Technologies for diagnosis and treatment of life-threatening disease expand and become more complex each year. Radiological, chemotherapeutic, and now personalized genetic medicine have all expanded treatment options and often interact with the technological imperative to pursue any treatment at all costs (Fuchs, 1972). Despite widespread awareness that high use of technology at the end of life adds emotional and financial costs that families and caregivers do not like (Pattison, Carr, Turnock, & Dolan, 2013), physicians nevertheless remain trained and primed to deploy such advanced technologies in the guise of maintaining "hope," even in the face of knowledge that the care is futile if the goal is cure (Mattes & Sloane, 2015).

One technology for social workers in collaboration with medical team members includes "goals of care" conversations, during which the patient and family are helped to identify what goals they have for their care, often most specifically, whether comfort is a primary goal or whether pursuit of a cure is the primary goal. Just as we include therapeutic modalities as a form of social work technology (as well as intervention), goals of care conversations are a "technology" focused and structured to help patients articulate their preferred goal(s). When the futility of aggressive medical technologies for cure is recognized, patients and

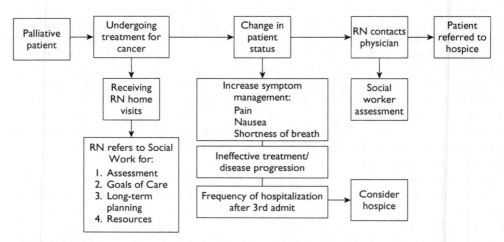

Figure 22.1 Pathway oncology patient – Palliative Care to hospice

their families often come to recognize that comfort is a preferred goal of care over continued surveillance and intervention by medical (hospital-based) teams. Movement to hospice care with its home-based palliative approach to symptom management and psycho-social-spiritual approaches to building on family relationships, addressing existentialist questions, and help with preparing for death and anticipating its impacts can promote comfort throughout the entire family (Bentur, Resnizky, Balicer, & Eilat-Tsanani, 2014). In short, social workers can help patients and their families begin to transition their "hope" from cure to hope for deeper relationships with family, comfort care, and a peaceful, reconciled death. See Figure 22.1 for an example of the typical pathways a patient travels from palliative care to hospice.

Organization

In our organization, Palliative Care teams are available within many parts of the organization – as consultants for inpatients, within the outpatient clinics, on the unit where respite is offered for hospice patients and others with life-threatening illness, and as part of the home-care team. We have an active research agenda with a recently ended grant-funded program to examine the trajectory of cancer patients starting in-home care services. The grant-funded program allowed more psychosocial support to be delivered as a part of the Palliative Care team's work. Some academic groups are examining the way decisions are made at end of life (University of Pennsylvania, 2012), while a coalition of hospices is allowing us to examine how to best provide care at the end of life (Choice Hospices, 2015). The structures of Palliative Care teams and their interactions and referrals to hospice remain somewhat idiosyncratic from one medical system to the next. For many patients, continued hope for cure and the associated aggressive treatment that goes with it (and subsequent decision to use Palliative Care) outweighs the ability to stay in one's home and avoid lots of medical visits and focus on comfort and quality of life at home (hospice).

Some aggressive Palliative Care teams now consist of physicians, nurse practitioners, nurses, social workers, and even chaplains. The professional structure of many Palliative Care teams is ever-more similar to the structure of a hospice team, with the exception of the bereavement component (a 13-month support program) which remains unique to hospice care. Indeed, there is a movement to institutionalize Palliative Care units in hospitals rather than have them just be a consultative service. In a large research-based comparison, inpatient Palliative Care units were found to be superior in survivors' ratings of the patient's last month of life and the only way that the consultation teams were rated superior was in their more consistent use of "goals of care" discussions (Casarett, Johnson, Smith, & Richardson, 2011). Institutionalized Palliative Care teams within the hospital blur the boundaries between Palliative Care and hospice for many patients and can complicate the referral process that moves patients from Palliative Care to hospice care. This slows the hospice referral and means that patients often come onto the hospice service when there is no time to work with them longer term to preserve their quality of life, engage in promoting family relationship-building, provide spiritual support in their homes, and access the bereavement services that are part of the hospice benefit.

Description of typical clients

It is difficult to describe typical clients as they may be middle aged or aging, may have aggressive lung cancer or slow-moving dementia, may be resolved about their prognosis or may be fighting it with every ounce of their being. This is why our care teams need to be flexible in meeting the client/patient where he or she is, working quickly to get to know them, building trust, and helping to understand and articulate the priorities they have for their life, for their level of care, and for their ultimate deaths. Many of our patients start in-home care in earlier hospitalizations and move through Palliative Care while they are in treatment, and move to hospice at the point where they are ready to embrace comfort rather than cure and high-level compassionate care rather than high-tech intervention.

Decisions about practice

Definition of the client

Lisa is a 60-year-old White female diagnosed nearly a year ago with metastatic lung cancer. Lisa is a practicing Roman Catholic whose faith grew stronger after the loss of a child nearly three decades ago. Lisa told her social worker that the death of this child was the beginning of the problems in her first marriage. She and her first spouse had three more children before the marriage dissolved. Lisa has three living adult sons aged 25–35 years, three young grandchildren, and currently is in the process of a "messy" divorce with her second spouse. Prior to her illness, Lisa held a professional position at a local college, was an active volunteer serving on the board of large non-profit, health-related charity, and was involved in her church. She has one sister, Margo, who is also her Power of Attorney (POA).

Lisa has been actively involved in pursuing curative treatment since her diagnosis. She became a patient of the Palliative home-care program six months into her treatment. During the last five months, with the support of frequent home nursing and social work visits, Lisa has remained out of the hospital. She goes to great lengths to hide her symptoms from her family and her physicians. Although her illness has progressed to the point where she expresses fears about "suffocating to death," she remains a full code (desires resuscitation) and continues to state that she "wants more time." She is reluctant to disclose these symptoms to her oncology team and has not been honest with her family members about her level of discomfort either.

Lisa believes that continuing treatments aimed at a cure will provide her with more time, a conviction she feels has been supported by members of her oncology team. After a reasonable course of radiation and chemotherapy, an oncology team member shared his belief that the treatment was slowing down, if not stopping, the tumor growth. Lisa's oncology team fills her with hope. For Lisa, hope means a long life, which is not likely given the extent of her disease. She is therefore being a good patient, working hard to tolerate the side effects, and underreporting the symptoms to ensure that she is in line for more treatment and clinical trial opportunities. Lisa believes that if she tells her physician how difficult the symptoms have become, they (the medical team) will "give up" on her.

Lisa desires, needs, more time. She is engaged in several conflicts and issues with her immediate family. Lisa believes that many of these conflicts are directly connected to her illness. First, neither her son, Chuck, nor her sister, Margo, has engaged with her since she disclosed her diagnosis nearly a year ago. Margo was someone Lisa had always felt close to, but the sisters have only seen each other a few times since Lisa's diagnosis. Lisa misses Margo, but assures the social worker that she understands that her sister is busy with her family and grandchildren. She misses both Chuck's and Margo's roles in her life but has also done little to try to re-engage them. It is unclear whether she keeps them held at a distance (as seems characteristic of her) or whether they became fearful after her illness disclosure and pulled away themselves. One of her sons, Tim, has a long history of mental health and substance abuse problems and has moved home with her several times. Lisa struggles to create boundaries for Tim while also trying to help him. Lisa's relationship with Tim is judged by other family members as enabling, and she believes it drives other family members away. Her other son, Eddie, is married, has three small children, and recently moved into the home of his recently widowed mother-in-law. Eddie is a "good son," but Lisa says she is worried that she is creating trauma for her grandchildren who are upset that she is using a walker and wheelchair. Lisa is envious of the new relationship developing between the children and their maternal grandmother. "I feel like she is taking my grandchildren from me when I have so little time." In short, Lisa is isolated and lonely. The social work visits seem to be the only opportunity for her to explore her feelings and her struggles.

Goals, contracting, and objectives

The goal of Palliative Care social work is to support the patient through the process of treatment, while continually exploring for shifts in a patient's goal(s) of care. The therapeutic relationship is what is most critical to this work. The social worker supports the patient but is always open and ready to explore the barriers that may be inhibiting the patient from potentially transitioning to care that might enable a higher quality of end of life. This is challenging with Lisa, who has been stymied by her focus on the family relationships and dilemmas. In addition, Lisa's ever-increasing anxiety seems to be connected with her declining health and isolation, leading to a lack of movement in her psychosocial care. When she first met the social worker, Lisa reassured her that she was not afraid of dying, but as her health declines Lisa's death anxiety seems to be increasing.

The social worker has an implicit goal for her work with Lisa: she hopes to help her resolve some of the family conflicts so that she can begin to focus on her own care and comfort. She has contracted with Lisa to help her to establish healthier boundaries with Tim, and she has also helped to motivate Lisa to write a letter to her oldest son. These explicit goals are part of the implicit goal to help Lisa get to a place where she can focus more readily on her own health and well-being. But Lisa now feels disappointed that Chuck has not responded to her letter and worries that Tim might attempt suicide. Lisa needs intensive intervention from her social worker to help her family understand the state of Lisa's health and to try to engage them more fully in supporting Lisa. Instead, Lisa hides her illness from them in the hope that she can support them.

All of Lisa's physical symptoms indicate that her disease is progressing, but she remains interested in any treatment the oncology team has to offer. She is open to any and all interventions and asserts that she will continue with treatments until it is deemed hopeless by the medical team. The team (Palliative home-care RN and SW) have discussed the care option of hospice, but for Lisa that means "giving up." She reminds the team that she wants more time; she needs to get her family back on track. This has been a challenging case for the Palliative home-care team. The work is compromised because of Lisa's belief that aggressive treatment will give her more time, even though the treatments have not been successful and have escalated many of her symptoms. The social worker believes that if she could help Lisa navigate the conflicts with her family, the patient may be ready for a higher level of care such as hospice. The challenge is magnified by a relentless oncology care team who are trying to follow Lisa's lead (to give her "hope"). Yet the oncology team does not know of the increased burdens Lisa is experiencing because of the treatment; they are not even aware of her treatment side effects. They certainly have not prioritized having honest conversations with family members to try to help them see Lisa's need for their support rather than her expending limited energy with ongoing attempts to pretend all is fine.

Several weeks ago, the oncology team told Lisa that they were running out of treatment options and that the clinical trial they were considering was no longer an option. This news has been crushing for Lisa. She says she wants to try to get a little healthier with hopes that something (meaning more treatment) will become available. As the weeks have gone by, Lisa is not feeling healthier – in fact she feels much weaker and more anxious. For the first time, she is considering hospice but seems fearful about broaching this with her family and oncology team. The social worker is poised to help with goals of care discussions and to help Lisa think about how to talk with her family. The home-care team has played an important role in Lisa's life. They have seen her disease progress, and each of them sees clearly that the patient would benefit from hospice care, but in many ways the patient is getting this support from the Palliative care team. The team is aware that they were able to provide hospice-level services because of the research-grant-funded palliation program, but the grant has ended. We will not be able to continue that level of service unless Lisa is ready to move to hospice care. We all hope to be able to help her continue to manage her physical symptoms, provide emotional support, help her manage her anxiety, and help her engage her family in her care. We want her to be able to hold onto the hope of improved health and well-being that hospice may be able to provide until her disease takes her life. We are ready to help her with a family meeting to help her share her prognosis and decisions about goals of care, and to enlist family support.

Meeting place/use of time

Our social work protocol is to meet with each patient at least twice a month and Lisa and her social worker have been doing that since service began in February. This frequent visit pattern was enabled due to the grant-funded Palliative Care program that allowed additional social supports for oncology patients. This grant concluded at the end of June 2015, and visits are now determined by the patient's insurer, which tends to view social work interventions with a great deal of scrutiny. We hope to continue to meet with Lisa in her home. If she is not yet ready for transition to hospice, we will work diligently using more phone intervention and occasional home visits to try to help her process the pros and cons of hospice. We will help her consider the benefits (and risks) of honestly addressing her health situation with her family members.

Strategies and interventions

Supportive counseling with gentle confrontation and deliberation, along with typical problem-solving, are the main strategies and tools of the home-care social worker as well as the social worker in Palliative Care and hospice roles. Although home care is fast-paced and often more information and referral oriented, Palliative Care and hospice roles involve the ability to slow down and be fully with the patient as they grapple with the changes in their health and with the existential questions that are related to dying. Often, family situations that were already complex become more problematic, possibly even escalating to crisis. Our use of crisis intervention, helping patients foresee ramifications of actions, and using psychoeducation to help them understand the benefits of honesty and transparency in regards to their health situations are all interventions we deploy regularly. Even so, we are aware that these family dynamics are of long-standing, and in hospice especially, we have little time to change patterns that are enduring. We understand that we are not there to do therapy, but to use our therapeutic skills to help find the most feasible ways of engaging the family in support of their dying family member. We sometimes ask clients to describe how they are feeling in their bodies as a way of opening honest conversations. If they respond with defensiveness or upset, we can gently reflect "Wow, it's really hard for you to talk about that." It is amazing how often this gentle observation can lead to open discussion. Likewise, a quiet observation that this is a difficult time and that everyone handles it differently, followed by "I wonder what feels most scary for you in all of this" allows the patient to be seen as an individual with his or her own fears and strengths. Opening these conversations is the critical skill for social workers in Palliative and hospice care.

Stance of the social worker

As indicated above, the stance is one of "being with," although this requires the ability to sit quietly and calmly at some times and to gently raise issues or question values or decisions more actively at other times. With Lisa, after we have explored her understanding of her health status, her prognosis, and her fears and hopes about her future, it may involve doing role-play to help her practice talking with her sons about her prognosis, fears for their futures, and desires for her death and aftermath of her death. Much of the stance of the worker is determined by the needs of the client and the stage where they are in the dying process. We cultivate a relationship of openness, honesty, and willingness to grapple with "non-polite" conversation. At some point, the patient often becomes withdrawn (as the work of dying brings inward focus) and much of the work is with the family as they adjust to providing care and comfort to the loved one with the knowledge that there is little time left to resolve prior tensions in relationships.

Use of resources outside the helping relationship

Although services such as home health, durable medical equipment, and chaplaincy are used, the world of the hospice patient often becomes comfortably smaller. These services tend to be part of the hospice agency and family members are helped to access caregiver supports as well. Yet, one major benefit of hospice is that it allows services to come into the home and patients are not stressed to go out to access services.

Reassessment and evaluation/case conclusion

Eleven months have passed since Lisa received her cancer diagnosis. The cancer continues to progress, and she remains a patient of the Palliative Care team. A CT scan several weeks ago indicated that the cancer was progressing, but the oncology team believed that the chemotherapy has been effective in slowing the disease growth. Lisa continues to "want more time," and prepares to have a chest wall port placed for her next round of chemotherapy. The social worker continues to reach out to the patient, but most phone calls are not returned. The nurse case manager reports that Lisa continues to lose weight, has increased episodes of shortness of breath, and reports elevated pain at the cancer sites. Efforts continue to support Lisa in communicating with her family, but there has been little movement or progress. Lisa's energy is low; she continues to underreport symptoms for fear that the next treatment will not be offered. As her energy decreases, she becomes more isolated and less willing to engage in working to engage with her family. It is hard to say if Lisa will ever consider hospice care as an option or a choice; she certainly will not do so as long as the oncology team continues to offer next steps. For Lisa, the treatments represent hope and proof that she "is not giving up." The team has been working with Lisa for over six months and, to date, has yet to meet the family members.

Differential discussion

If there were less of a sharp distinction (especially in the funding stream) between Palliative Care and hospice, we might have more success in helping patients to be willing to receive palliative, intensive, compassionate care such as hospice can provide. One barrier is physicians. Physicians who are not ready to acknowledge that patients are within the last part of their lives have a difficult time making the referral to hospice and so Palliative Care teams allow for palliation of symptoms, but without the intensive home-care and support personnel that hospice enables. We strongly suspect that allowing hospice social workers and Palliative Care social workers to have access to patients earlier in the treatment process will help set the stage for patients to understand the goal of comfort as likely to enable longer, more quality life than chasing the next chemotherapy or radiation treatment. Regardless of our knowledge that hospice is likely to improve clients' lives, we nevertheless respect clients' right to refuse care as a form of acknowledging their right to self-determination. We gently keep working to provide information and ask questions to help Lisa continue to consider hospice without forcing it on her.

The "open access hospice," whereby the physicians offering palliative treatments work directly with the hospice care staff, is one option. The American Society of Clinical Oncology (2008) supports open-access hospice as a way to avoid having to make a decision to accept hospice but lose access to palliative treatments that may be directed to the disease on one level (to shrink a tumor for instance) but are being done for comfort reasons rather than for cure. This model allows gradual transition from focus on cure to focus on comfort and quality of life while also accessing supportive services that hospice can offer to focus on the whole of life. One problem with the model is that these treatments are expensive and the hospice benefit cannot cover the expenses of such care as it currently stands (American Society of Clinical Oncology, 2008). Perhaps, this could lead to improving the final days of these very sick patients.

As I (MB) am writing this, I am thinking of another patient, a 40-year-old man admitted to hospice late one Thursday afternoon; he died Saturday morning. For this family, hospice was a last choice at a moment when they felt like they had no choice. The Palliative Care team managed his physical symptoms, but the existential work was left undone. He may have enjoyed more time and conversation with his family had he come onto the hospice service earlier, before treatments had debilitated him and sapped the last of his energy.

Open-access hospice could expand the current hospice benefit and could allow palliative end-of-life technology to coexist with end-of-life care. The pathway would allow for patients and families to be cared for by end-of-life clinicians while winding down final treatments, thus beginning the process of working with the whole person rather than with the disease. There are a multitude of reasons to consider open-access hospice during palliative treatments, but none are more compelling than supporting individuals and families at the end stage of their life.

Discussion questions

1   What are your beliefs about the pros and cons for Palliative Care versus hospice care? How might your thoughts be influenced about those pros and cons when deciding for yourself versus for your parent versus for your child?
2   Consider a client like Lisa who wants to still "have hope" and not to "give up." How might you reframe these phrases to help her come to accept that hospice may provide the hope of managing family relationships, care, and comfort?

References

Abernethy, A. P., Bull, J., Whitten, E., Shelby, R., Wheeler, J. L., & Taylor, J. H. (2013). Targeted investment improves access to hospice and palliative care. *Journal of Pain and Symptom Management, 46*, 629–639. doi: 10.1016/j.jpainsymman.2012.12.012

American Society of Clinical Oncology (ASCO) (2008). The debate in hospice care. *Journal of Oncology Practice, 4*(30), 153–157. Retrieved from http://jop.ascopubs.org/content/4/3/153.full. doi: 10.1200/JOP.0838503

Bentur, N., Resnizky, S., Balicer, R., & Eilat-Tsanani, T. (2014). CLINICAL: Quality of end-of-life care for cancer patients: Does home hospice care matter? *American Journal of Managed Care, 20*(12), 988–992. www.ajmc.com/journals/issue/2014/2014-v0120-n12/Quality-of-End-of-Life-Care-for-Cancer-Patients-Does-Home-Hospice-Care-Matter

Caregiver's Library (2015). Hospice vs. Palliative Care. Retrieved from www.caregiverslibrary.org/caregivers-resources/grp-end-of-life-issues/hsgrp-hospice/hospice-vs-palliative-care-article.aspx

Casarett, D., Johnson, M., Smith, D., & Richardson, D. (2011). The optimal delivery of palliative care: A national comparison of the outcomes of consultation teams vs inpatient units. *Archives of Internal Medicine, 171*(7), 649–655. doi: 10.1001/archinternmed.2011.87

Centers for Medicare and Medicaid Services (2015). Medicare Hospice Benefits. Retrieved from https://www.medicare.gov/Pubs/pdf/02154.pdf

Choice Hospices (2015). Retrieved from www.choicehospices.org/

Fuchs, V. R. (Ed.) (1972). *Essays in the economics of health and medical care.* New York: Columbia University Press.

Mattes, M. D. & Sloane, M. A. (2015). Reflections on hope and its implications for end-of-life care. *Journal of the American Geriatrics Society, 63*, 993–996. doi: 10.1111/jgs.13392

NHPCO (National Hospice and Palliative Care Organization) (2001). *Hospital–hospice partnerships in palliative care: creating a continuum of care.* Retrieved from www.nhpco.org/sites/default/files/public/NHPCO-CAPCreport.pdf

NHPCO (2015). History of hospice care. Retrieved from www.nhpco.org/history-hospice-care

Nixon, R. M. (1971). Signing of the National Cancer Act, December 23, 1971. Retrieved from https://www.youtube.com/watch?v=qX8d1vOI818

Pattison, N., Carr, S. M., Turnock, C., & Dolan, S. (2013). 'Viewing in slow motion': patients', families', nurses' and doctors' perspectives on end-of-life care in critical care. *Journal of Clinical Nursing, 22*(9/10), 1442–1454. doi: 10.1111/jocn.12095

Scheffey, C., Kestenbaum, M. G., Wachterman, M. W., Connor, S. R., Fine, P. G., Davis, M. S., & Muir, J. C. (2014). Clinic-based outpatient palliative care before hospice is associated with longer hospice length of service. *Journal of Pain and Symptom Management, 48*, 532–539. doi: 10.1016/j.jpainsymman.2013.10.017

University of Pennsylvania (2012). Video excerpt Scott Halpern. Retrieved from http://ldi.upenn.edu/about/news/2012/09/23/video-excerpt-scott-halpern-at-penn-cmu-roybal-retreat

Wang, L., Piet, L., Kenworthy, C. M., & Dy, S. M. (2015). Association between palliative case management and utilization of inpatient, intensive care unit, emergency department, and hospice in Medicaid beneficiaries. *The American Journal of Hospice & Palliative Care, 32*(2), 216–220. doi: 10.1177/1049909113520067

Resources

American Cancer Society, www.cancer.org/treatment/findingandpayingfortreatment/choosingyour treatmentteam/hospicecare/index

National Caregivers' Library, www.caregiverslibrary.org/home.aspx

National Hospice and Palliative Care Organization (NHPCO), www.nhpco.org/

Social work and public health

Chapter 23

Public health social work primer

Toba Schwaber Kerson and Jessica Euna Lee

Context

Policy and organization

Social workers have been involved in public health activities since the founding of the Children's Bureau in 1912. During the Progressive Era, social workers used informal risk analysis to promote early intervention among vulnerable groups. Recruited primarily from the ranks of hospital social work, they began to play important roles in helping to track infectious diseases and locate those who had been badly disabled as a result of these illnesses (Kerson, 1981). One sees their work in settlement houses, in tuberculosis and syphilis clinics, and in response to major incidents such as the influenza epidemic of 1918, several polio epidemics, World Wars I and II and the Coconut Grove Fire of 1942 (Kerson, 1980; Margolis & Kotch, 2013). Public health social work's responsiveness to the needs of patients and the government resonates in the following quote from Ida Cannon's 1918 address to the American Hospital Association about the Division of Venereal Disease of the Public Health Service. This service was created through the passage of the Chamberlain–Kahn Act because of rising proportions of the population (about 10%) who were infected with syphilis, gonorrhea, and chancroid. Cannon said:

> I know of nothing in the realm of medicine that more clearly reflects the influence of sociology on medical science than the changing attitude towards our responsibility for the care of patients with syphilis and gonorrhea. I say changing because we have only begun to see how much rests upon us in the promotion of the government's program.

Public health social work is distinguished by its reliance on epidemiological information and its focus on structural interventions, often at the primary care level, and on population health (NASW, 2005; Social Work Policy Institute, 2007). Its goals are to avoid risk, prevent illness, promote healthy behaviors, and enhance the environment. Public health social workers think, strategize, and practice beyond the individual level in order to advocate for vulnerable populations and engage in political action (Congress, 2013; Hurdle, 2004). They are, by nature, boundary spanners, keeping in mind that clients at every level are representative of populations who need advocates, strategists, and interveners to expand the reach of their roles, becoming forces in and across systems and levels of government (Kerson, 2002).

Lately, there is much discussion in the literature about the differences between public health and population health. Although there are many similarities and we will use both terms in this chapter, the following is a brief discussion of the differences between the two terms (Kindig, 2015). Traditionally, public health has dealt with state and local health department functions through encouraging healthy behaviors, preventing epidemics, and containing environmental hazards. Now, the Institute of Medicine is urging new intersectoral partnerships, drawing on and actively engaging diverse communities' resources and perspectives for health action (Institute of Medicine, 2003). Much of the work that the Institute of Medicine calls for and the resources required are outside of the purview of traditional public health authority and the authority of particular states and communities. To those of us who define public health as "the health of the public," there is little difference between population health and public health except to define a particular population more precisely. In time, it may be that all of public health will be called population health, but for our purposes, the terms will be interchangeable.

The model in Figure 23.1 illustrates the multi-systemic factors involved in public health social work and, indeed, all of public health. In this diagram, Kindig demonstrates that policies and programs influence health determinants or factors, which produce the health outcomes in the left-hand box (Kindig, 2015).

Much of this work is carried out under governmental auspices because of the states' responsibilities for the health, education, and welfare of their citizenry. In recent times, the federal government has become increasingly involved in health care through the funding of Medicare and Medicaid, as it collaborates with the states to provide health care for the poor and to eventually see that every U.S. citizen has health insurance. Thus, population health, the health of a state's population or a certain category of citizens, such as mothers and young children or the elderly, can be best understood by thinking about a large category of people about whom a state or local government or the federal government is concerned. In fact, the health problems of that particular category are of concern to a state or a local government

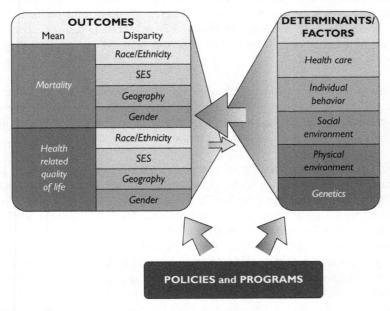

Figure 23.1 Influences on public health of demographics.

Source: From Kindig (2015)

because they pose a threat to its entire population. Examples include HIV/AIDS and Ebola virus, the recent outbreak of measles in many states in the United States, the health threats to New Orleans and other related areas by Hurricane Katrina, the growth of the elderly population and the high levels of dementia in that population, veterans returning home with post-traumatic stress disorder and/or severe bodily injury. Once one subscribes to these notions of population health, one can understand why HIV/AIDS, child and elder treatment, acute and chronic health services, disaster preparedness, and maternal and child health are important subjects for public health social work (Ruth & Sisco, 2008).

The effects of health disparities on health outcomes

The effects of particular policies, institutions, organizations, and social forces are observable in the morbidity and mortality of unequally positioned populations in the United States. Such effects, particularly in the arena of health disparities, are of special concern to public health (Keefe, 2010; Roux & Mair, 2010). These are the great disparities found in health status, outcomes, and the delivery of health care in the United States and around the world (Barr, 2014). Thus, mitigating health disparities and inequalities is a crucial focus of public health social work and reflects the profession's commitment to social justice (Kerson & Lee, 2014).

Simply put, a disparity is a state of being unequal. One can think about health disparities in three ways: (1) health status – how healthy people are; (2) access to and utilization of health care – whether people have entrée to health services and then use them; (3) social determinants of health – how much of people's health is determined by social factors such as socio-economic status, educational level, sex, race/ethnicity, sex, income, and geographic location (Jonsen-Reid, Drake, & Zhou, 2013; Mensah & Glover, 2011). Thus, a disparity can occur in access to the kind of environment (food, air, water, safe living spaces) that supports health, to health care at all decision levels (who is referred, who self-refers, who is chosen for which interventions), and to healthy outcomes. For example, within health and mental health systems, disparities limiting access to necessary services perpetuate poor health outcomes, and race is a factor in health disparities even when controlling for income (Fong, Dettlaff, James, & Rodriguez, 2015). These and other disparities are seen in inequitable and discriminatory health care distribution (Keefe & Evans, 2013). They are perpetuated by systems including governments, social norms, services, and built environments.

The ways in which political and organizational structures affect health disparities are often invisible to most people. One example is Medicaid, whose purpose is to assure the health of the impoverished but whose policies, as interpreted and adopted by individual states, determine who among the poor in the United States has access to health insurance and through health insurance to particular institutions, professionals, and other caregivers. Thus, public health social workers must understand the political, cultural, and organizational structures that affect clients' health and be able to act as advocates for structural change.

Healthy People 2020 and health disparities focus areas

Seven health disparities focus areas that are emphasized in the literature and on the websites of government agencies are heart disease and stroke; cancer; HIV/AIDS; respiratory diseases; diabetes; maternal, infant, and child health; and mental health. The reduction or eradication of health problems in these areas is the goal of "Healthy People," a federal effort towards improving the health of the United States population that sets science-based measureable objectives in 10-year cycles. The goals for Healthy People 2020 are: (1) to attain high-quality, longer lives free of preventable disease, disability, injury, and premature death, (2) to achieve health equity, eliminate disparities, and improve the health of all groups, (3) to create social and physical environments that promote good health for all, and (4) to promote quality of life, healthy development, and healthy behaviors across all life stages (Healthy People 2020, 2015). In addition to goals, Healthy People 2020 lists leading health indicators including physical activity, overweight and obesity, tobacco use, substance abuse, responsible sexual behavior, mental health, injury and violence, environmental quality, immunization, and health care access.

Healthy People 2020 contains 42 topic areas and over 1,000 objectives. Here, we list the Healthy People 2020 Leading Health Indicators to communicate high-priority health issues and actions that can be taken to address them: (1) Access to Health Services; (2) Clinical Preventive Services; (3) Environmental Quality; (4) Injury and Violence; (5) Maternal, Infant, and Child Health; (6) Mental Health; (7) Nutrition, Physical Activity, and Obesity; (8) Oral Health; (9) Reproductive and Sexual Health; (10) Social Determinants; (11) Substance Abuse; and (12) Tobacco. What is important to note for this primer is that these objectives are measureable. Such pointed behavioral work is important in addressing critical public health issues facing the United States. For example, the United States has the highest infant mortality rates of the 27 Organisation for Economic Co-operation and Development (OECD) countries behind Mexico, Chile, and Turkey, with an estimated 6.1 infant deaths per 1,000 live births (OECD, 2015). To these ends, Healthy People 2020 discusses the knowledge and skills needed for collaborative community and organizational efforts including assessment, intervention, evaluation, networking, and interpersonal skills. Examples of specific capacities include distributive leadership, facilitation, participatory problem/priority identification, decision-making, team building, communication, conflict resolution, management of individual and task groups, budgeting, and fundraising.

Technology – epidemiology

The primary area of technology that distinguishes public health social work is epidemiology – the science that studies the patterns, causes, and effects of health and disease conditions in defined populations. According to the Institute of Medicine, the heart of public health is organized community effort directed at health promotion and disease prevention with links to many disciplines and a scientific core of epidemiology (Institute of Medicine, 2003). Identifying targets for preventive care and risk factors for disease informs evidence-based practice and policymaking (Brownson, Fielding, & Maylahn, 2009). Public health social workers use epidemiological information to conceptualize interventions for issues such as homelessness, chronic illness, substance abuse, urban health, violence, and maternal and child health.

Over time, the focus of the specialization of social work in public health has changed somewhat as has the focus of public health itself. That is, many communicable diseases have become treatable and/or curable (e.g., polio) while the numbers of people affected by chronic non-communicable disease have grown and, in many cases, can be tied to health behaviors. Now, public health social workers are likely to be directing their efforts towards helping individual clients and populations to improve their health by addressing their own behaviors. This epidemiological transition is a world-wide phenomenon. New health issues have continued to emerge or reemerge, such as AIDS, substance abuse, child abuse, violence, community-level trauma, and terrorism. Of course, many additional dimensions of technology are important in public health social work, including changes in surveillance, medical interventions on all levels, electronic record keeping, on-line treatment, and e-health (see Chapter 16 for discussion of the way the Department of Veterans Affairs is using e-health).

Organization

Organizations in which public health social work occurs incorporate primary, secondary, and tertiary prevention efforts. The roles of public health social workers include: provider of direct services, researcher, administrator, consultant, program planner, evaluator, and policymaker (NASW, 2005). No matter what their roles or settings, public health social workers think in terms of populations and how different systems interact with each other.

Some organizations with which public health social work interacts

Professional organizations including the American Public Health Association (APHA) Social Work Section, Association of State and Territorial Public Health Social Workers, Group for Public Health Social Work Initiatives, and National Association of Social Workers (NASW) foster social work in public health. Governmental commitment and support varies and shifts in response to contextual changes (sociopolitical and economic circumstances) and to the level of threat experienced by governments and populations. The state at whatever governmental level is deemed responsible sets priorities and determines interventions and the participation of public health social workers.

Most useful to public health social workers are the standards and competencies developed by key organizations that focus on public health social workers' comportment, knowledge, and skills in assessment and intervention in diverse practices. A Standards Working Group of the Public Health Social Work section of the American Public Health Association, in consultation with the Centers for Disease Control and Prevention (CDC), public health social work departments, practitioners, and social work educators, developed 14 professional standards and five core competencies for public health social workers (APHA, 2005). The core competencies listed by the Standards Working Group include: the theoretical base, methodological and analytical process, leadership and communication, policy and advocacy, and values and ethics. Both professional standards and core competencies are informed by APHA's and NASW's codes of ethics.

Standards 1–4 use social epidemiology principles to assess social problems that affect health and social functioning, identify factors that promote health, measure social factors associated with ill-health, and evaluate interventions. Thus, the standards help to assess and monitor social problems affecting the health status and social functioning of at-risk populations within the context of family, community, and culture; identify and assess the factors associated with resiliency, strengths, and assets that promote optimal health; identify, measure, and assess the social factors contributing to health issues, health hazards, and stress associated with ill-health and evaluate the effectiveness, accessibility, and quality of individual, family, and population-based health interventions.

Standards 5–10 use planning, development, and marketing for public health education to empower participants to address public health concerns, enforce laws related to public health, hold the public accountable for population well-being, and develop primary prevention strategies that promote health and alleviate health concerns. More fully, these standards use social planning, community organizational development, and social marketing principles to inform and educate individuals, families, and communities about public health issues. They empower and mobilize individuals, families, and communities to become active participants in identifying and addressing public health concerns to improve individual, family, and societal well-being. The standards also promote and enforce legal requirements that protect the health and safety of individuals, families, and communities; they assure public accountability for the well-being of all, with an emphasis on vulnerable and underserved populations. Additionally, the standards develop primary prevention strategies that promote the health and well-being of individuals, families, and communities as well as develop secondary and tertiary prevention strategies to alleviate health and related social and economic concerns.

Standards 11 and 12 say that public health social work provides leadership and advocacy to assure the elimination of health and social disparities wherever they exist, such as, but not limited to, those based on community, race, age, gender, ethnicity, culture, or disability. The standards call for the promotion of policy development for providing quality and comprehensive public health services within a cultural, community, and family context. According to Standard 13, public health social work supports and conducts data collection, research, and evaluation, and Standard 14 states that public health social work assures the competency of its practice to address the issues of public health effectively through a core body of social work knowledge, philosophy, code of ethics, and standards. Such standards and competencies mobilize social workers for action. By seeing clients as representatives of a population, public health social workers move from individual health issues to population problems to policy change.

Decisions about practice

While many public health social workers work on individual and family levels, every practice decision that they make with individual clients carries overarching notions of population, threats to population health, epidemiological information, and structural interventions. These decisions are all set within context (policy, technology, and organization). Policies determine population parameters and where governments perceive threats. They are administered through governmental and other organizations, and technological advances make it possible to intervene and address these threats. Thus, when one thinks of the definition of the client, it is with an understanding that the population to which the client belongs has been determined by some level of government to require intervention by social workers and others. Within that broad definition of the client, programs and then individual professionals make decisions about who the client is, whether an individual, a dyad, a family, or a group.

Similarly, the conditions of goals, outcomes, and contracting, use of time, meeting place, strategies and interventions, and case or care management are often set by what the federal or state government or state has determined will best address the threat that it has identified and the interventions that it is willing to fund. Public health social workers continue to advocate for clients and to span boundaries to have more flexibility in terms of stance and use of resources, but they maintain a commitment to these two broad notions of the client; that is, the client is both the population and the individual or other small unit with whom they are actively intervening.

Structural interventions

Thus, public health social workers are committed to intervening with clients at individual, family, and small group levels while also being concerned about structural interventions.

A broader definition of structural interventions as efforts that promote health by altering the structural context within which health is produced and maintained aligns with the Practice in Context framework. Thus, such interventions for public health social work target multiple systems from individuals as parts of populations to community, state, and federal levels. Generally, these prevention interventions include physical, social, cultural, organization, community, economic, legal, and policy factors. At times, structural approaches view public health problems as being the result of social causation. Thus, structural approaches "locate the cause of public health problems in contextual or environmental factors that influence risk behavior, or other determinants of infection or morbidity" instead of locating the cause in characteristics of individuals (Blankenship, Friedman, Dworkin, & Mantell, 2006, p. 59). Always contextual, structural interventions shape an individual's risk of illness through indirect mechanisms (Pronyk, Schaefer, Somers, & Heise, 2013). What seems like an increasing emphasis on structural approaches and interventions to public health problems is not an innovation but a return to public health social work's early roots as a movement to improve public health through environmental approaches and social reform (Colgrove, Fairchild, & Rosner, 2013).

The most developed discourse on structural interventions appears in the public health literature on HIV/AIDS. Such interventions have received the most attention as a strategy because they have proven effective for HIV/AIDS prevention (Bloom & Cohen, 2007). A working group at the CDC developed a framework of nine systems to describe structural interventions in relation to HIV prevention and four levels of barriers or facilitators for HIV prevention. The systems include: governments, service organizations, business, workforce organizations, faith communities, justice systems, media organizations, education systems, and health care systems. The levels include: economic resources, policy supports, societal attitudes, and organizational structures (Bloom & Cohen, 2007). Blankenship and colleagues highlight four types of effective structural interventions for HIV/AIDS: community mobilization, integration of HIV services, contingent funding, and economic and educational interventions (Blankenship et al., 2006). Structural interventions require a longer time frame than other interventions; however, researchers expect that structural interventions will be better sustained over time because they target the structural root of problems (Pronyk et al., 2013). Effective structural interventions can be used to intervene on macro levels, such as where there are suicide hotspots (Pirkis et al., 2013). They are complex, involve multiple interacting components, often cannot be randomly assigned, and the behaviors of those involved can affect the intervention and outcomes. In order for public health social workers to promote structural interventions, it is important for them to develop tools for assessment, policy development, and assurance.

Throughout this book, there are many examples of structural interventions. Some are included in the public health social work section while others are included in the sections following the first primer because they focus more on individual relationships than work at the population level. For instance, community health programs could be considered structural interventions under this broader definition, as is discussed in the chapter about Bhutanese refugee health access and the community-grown initiative, the Bhutanese American Organization-Philadelphia (see Chapter 31). But this would be true also for the chapter on social work practice in settings where the work is with undocumented immigrants (see Chapter 17). Other examples of structural/population work found in the Part 1 include Birmingham et al.'s chapter on work with HIV-positive children (see Chapter 6), Wilkenfeld's chapter on work with children with disabilities (see Chapter 8), and Moulton's chapter on Woman to Woman, a hospital-based support program for women with gynecological cancer and their families (see Chapter 14). Indeed, many of those chapters include focus on the population (veterans, transgender, gerontology), just as many of the chapters in this public health section include individual and family work (see Ciporen on type 2 diabetes in children in Chapter 26, Barker on work with homeless populations in Chapter 29, etc.). Many of the chapters in each section include modifying the social environment, an intervention that includes modifying social norms, the level of safety or violence, and the social connection and networks among neighbors. The focus of the practitioner on the individual/family or on the population/structure varies and provides a rationale for why chapters are placed within each section: nonetheless, the way many chapters could fit in either section is testament to how good social work practitioners function always by considering micro, mezzo, and macro implications of their work and interventions.

Available on-line are some chapters from the third edition of this book that are vibrant examples of public health social work. They include "Advocacy and compensation programs for radiation exposure claimants" (Dawson & Madsen, 2010) and "Fighting cancer in India: Implementing cancer control strategies at a national level" (Naik, 2010). Another example, "YOUR blessed health: A faith-based, community-based participatory research project to reduce the incidence of HIV/AIDS and sexually transmitted infections" (Robinson, Campbell, & Campbell, 2010) describes systematic social observation where public health social workers enter environments to gather key information that cannot be obtained otherwise. In each of these chapters, social workers acted to make structural changes that addressed health disparities and changed health outcomes. Public health social workers are also working in child neglect (Jonson-Reid et al., 2013) and intimate partner violence (Dichter & Rhodes, 2011), homelessness among female veterans (Byrne, Montgomery, & Dichter, 2013), and in coalition capacity-building (Shapiro, Oesterle, & Hawkins, 2015). Approaches include space–time analysis that considers where a population resides and the location of daily activities. For example, health workers implemented police trainings in order to improve police relations and to reduce interference in syringe exchange programs, with such programs having been shown to be an effective structural intervention in reducing the injection-related transmission rates of HIV (Beletsky, Grau, White, Bowman, & Heimer, 2011) or help in implementing condom-availability programs in urban high schools in order to prevent HIV and STI transmission (De Rosa et al., 2012). Other approaches use surveys and questionnaires to gather information from large numbers of individuals in order to understand stakeholder attitudes towards topics of interest or geographic information systems (GIS) that can measure neighborhood density (Keefe, 2013) as well as the built and social environments (e.g., mapping neighborhood whose houses contain lead-based paint).

Conclusion

In conclusion, public health social work can be understood using the Practice in Context framework. It differs from some other types of social work in health care because public health social workers often work directly with clients while focusing on a population to which those clients belong. It is the same as all other types of social work in that it, too, relies on the relational skills of the social worker. For the work to progress, it is necessary for social workers to develop trusting relationships with clients and to use those relationships to help clients to reach their goals within context (Kerson, 2002; Kerson & McCoyd, 2013, 2014; McCoyd & Kerson, 2013).

Public health social workers are charged also to think in terms of structural interventions and the organizational and policy changes that are necessary to carry out such interventions. Public health social work is critical to the future of social work in health care. It changes the world view of the social worker from focus on the individual as a unique entity to larger structural/population changes. The world view for public health says that there is a whole population whose problems have been confounded and magnified because of society's views, and that the problem source is not the individual, but societal disparities. While individuals have to be held accountable for their behavior, thinking of ways to address problems community by community, and population by population, will develop structural interventions that will benefit the larger population as a whole. Public health social workers may work on a small scale as they move from client to client, but in the best of the boundary-spanning tradition in social work, they think and act as often as possible on a larger scale, addressing the needs of populations.

References

APHA (American Public Health Association) (2005). Practice Standards Development Committee, Beyond Year 2010: *Public health social work standards and competencies*. Retrieved from http://nciph.sph.unc.edu/cetac/phswcompetencies_may05.pdf

Barr, D. A. (2014). *Health disparities in the U.S: Social class, race, ethnicity, and health* (2nd edn.). Baltimore, MD: Johns Hopkins University Press.

Beletsky, L., Grau, L. E., White, E., Bowman, S., & Heimer, R. (2011). Prevalence, characteristics, and predictors of police training initiatives by US SEPs: Building an evidence base for structural interventions. *Drug and Alcohol Dependence, 119*, 145–149. doi: 10.1016/j.drugalcdep.2011.05.034

Blankenship, K. M., Friedman, S. R., Dworkin, S., & Mantell, J. E. (2006). Structural interventions: Concepts, challenges and opportunities for research. *Journal of Urban Health, 83*, 59–72. doi: 10.1007/s11524-005-9007-4

Bloom, F. R. & Cohen, D. A. (2007). Structural interventions. In S. O. Aral & J. M. Douglas (Eds.), *Behavioral interventions for prevention and control of sexual transmitted disease* (pp. 125–141). New York: Springer.

Brownson, R. C., Fielding, J. E., & Maylahn, C. M. (2009). Evidence-based public health: A fundamental concept for public health practice. *Annual Review of Public Health, 30*(1), 175–201.

Byrne, T., Montgomery, A. E., & Dichter, M. E. (2013). Homelessness among female veterans: A systematic review of the literature. *Women & Health, 53*(6), 572–596.

Cannon, I. M. (1918). Speech at the 20th annual convention. American Hospital Association, Atlantic City, New Jersey.

Colgrove, J., Fairchild, A., & Rosner, D. (2013). The history of structural approaches in public health. In M. Sommer & R. Parker (Eds.), *Structural approaches in public health* (pp. 17–27). New York: Routledge.

Congress, E. (2013). Ethics for public health social workers. In Social Work Section of the American Public Health Association (Ed.), *Handbook for public health social work* (pp. 21–40). New York: Springer.

Dawson, S. E. & Madsen, G. E. (2010). Advocacy and compensation programs for radiation exposure claimants. In T. S. Kerson & J. L. M. McCoyd, *Social work in health settings: Practice in Context* (3rd edn., pp. 363–373). New York: Routledge.

De Rosa, C. J., Jeffries, R., Afifi, A. A., Cumberland, W, Chung, E., et al. (2012). Improving the implementation of a condom availability program in urban high schools. *Journal of Adolescent Health, 51*(6), 572–579. doi: 10.1016/j.jadohealth.2012.03.010

Dichter, M. & Rhodes, K. V. (2011). Intimate partner violence survivors' unmet social service needs. *Journal of Social Service Research, 37*, 481–489. doi: 10.1080/01488376.2011.587747

Fong, R., Dettlaff, A., James, J., & Rodriguez, C. (2015). *Addressing racial disproportionality and disparities in human services: Multisystemic approaches*. New York: Columbia University Press.

Healthy People 2020 (2015). Retrieved from www.healthypeople.gov

Hurdle, D. (2004). Qualitative research: Cancer Prevention in older women. In A. R. Roberts & K. R. Yeager (Eds.), *Evidence-based practice manual: Research and outcome measures in health and human services* (pp. 713–720). Oxford, UK: Oxford University Press.

Institute of Medicine (2003). *The future of the public's health in the 21st century*. Washington, DC: The National Academies Press.

Jonson-Reid, M. Drake, B., & Zhou. (2013). Neglected subtypes, race, and poverty: Individual, family and service characteristics. *Child Maltreatment, 18*(1), 30–44. doi: 10.1177/1077559512462452

Keefe, R. H. (2010). Health disparities: A primer for public health social work. *Social Work in Public Health, 25*, 237–257. doi: 10.1080/19371910903240589

Keefe, R. H. (2013). Neighborhoods and health. In Social Work Section of the American Public Health Association (Ed.), *Handbook for public health social work* (pp. 273–286). New York: Springer.

Keefe, R. H. & Evans, T. A. (2013). Introduction to public health social work. In Social Work Section of the American Public Health Association (Ed.), *Handbook for public health social work* (pp. 3–20). New York: Springer.

Kerson, T. S. (1980). Eleven Medical Social Work Interviews, Archives, Simmons College School of Social Work and Social Welfare Archives, University of Minnesota.

Kerson, T. S. (1981). *Medical social work: The pre-professional paradox*. New York: Irvington.

Kerson, T. S. (2002). *Boundary spanning: An ecological reinterpretation of social work practice in health and mental health systems*. New York: Columbia University Press.

Kerson, T. S. & Lee, J. E. (2014). Global public health (entry). In *Encyclopedia of Social Work* (21st edn.). Washington, DC: NASW Press.

Kerson, T. S. & McCoyd, J. L. M. (2013). In response to need: An analysis of social work roles over time. *Social Work, 58*, 333–343. doi: 10.1093/sw/swt035

Kerson, T. S. & McCoyd, J. L. M. (2014). In response to need: An analysis of social work roles over time. (2014, October 27). InSocialWork Podcast Series. Episode 154 [Audio Podcast]. Retrieved from www.insocialwork.org/episode.asp?ep=154

Kindig, D. A. (2015). *Improving population health*. Retrieved from www.improvingpopulationhealth. org/blog/what-is-population-health.html

Margolis, L. & Kotch, J. B. (2013). Tracing the historical foundations of maternal and child health to contemporary times. In J. B. Kotch (Ed.), *Maternal and child health: Programs, problems, and policy in public health* (3rd edn., pp. 11–34). Burlington, VT: Jones & Bartlett.

McCoyd, J. L. M. & Kerson, T. S. (2013). Teaching reflective social work practice in health care: Promoting best practices. *Journal of Social Work Education, 49*(4), 674–688. doi: 10.1080/10437797.2013.812892

Mensah, G. A. & Glover, V. J. (2011). Epidemiologic profiles of racial and ethnic disparities in health and health care. In R. A. Williams (Ed.), *Healthcare disparities at the crossroads with healthcare reform* (pp. 23–39). New York: Springer. doi: 10.1007/978–4436–4_3

Naik, N. (2010). Fighting cancer in India: Implementing cancer control strategies. In T. S. Kerson & J. L. M. McCoyd (Eds.), *Social work in health settings: Practice in Context* (3rd edn., pp. 374–384). New York: Routledge.

NASW (National Association of Social Workers) (2005). NASW standards for social work practice in health care settings. Retrieved from www.socialworkers.org/practice/standards/naswhealthcar-estandards.pdf

OECD (Organisation for Economic Co-operation and Development) (2015). Retrieved from http://stats.oecd.org/

Pirkis, J., Spittal, M. J., Cox, G., Robinson, J., Cheung, Y. T. D., & Studdert, D. (2013). The effectiveness of structural interventions at suicide hotspots: A meta-analysis. *International Journal of Epidemiology, 42*(2), 541–548. doi: 10.1093/ije/dyt021

Pronyk, P., Schaefer, J., Somers, M. A., & Heise, L. (2013). Evaluating structural interventions in public health: Challenges, options and global best-practices. In M. Sommer & R. Parker (Eds.), *Structural approaches in public health* (pp. 187–205). New York: Routledge.

Robinson, K. J., Campbell, B., & Campbell, T. (2010). YOUR blessed health: A faith-based, community-based participatory research project to reduce the incidence of HIV/AIDS and sexually transmitted infections. In T. S. Kerson & J. L. M. McCoyd (Eds.), *Social work in health settings*: *Practice in Context* (3rd edn., pp. 340–350). New York: Routledge.

Roux, A. & Mair, C. (2010). Neighborhoods and health. *Annals of the New York Academy of Sciences, Biology of Disadvantage*: *Socioeconomic status and health, 1186*, 125–145. doi: 10.1111/j.1749-6632.2009.05333.x

Ruth, B. & Sisco, S. (2008). Public health social work. In T. Mizrahi & L. E. Davis (Eds.), *Encyclopedia of Social Work* (20th edn.). New York: Oxford University Press.

Shapiro, V., Oesterle, S., & Hawkins, J. (2015). Relating coalition capacity to the adoption of service-based prevention in communities that care. *American Journal of Community Psychology, 55*, 1–12. doi: 10.1007/s10464-014-9684-9

Social Work Policy Institute (2007). Public Health Social Work. Retrieved from www.social workpolicy.org/research/public-health-social-work.html

Work with special populations

Chapter 24

Social work practice in an adolescent parenting program

Traci Wike, Kathleen Rounds, and Helen Dombalis

Context

The last 20 years have seen a consistent decline in the rates of adolescent pregnancies in the United States. From 1990 to 2008, rates of pregnancy among adolescents aged 15–19 years dropped from an all-time high of 11.6% (1990) to 6.98% (2008), representing a 40% overall reduction in the number of pregnancies experienced by adolescents in the United States (Ventura, Abma, Mosher, & Henshaw, 2008). Although the birth rate for adolescents aged 15–19 increased 3% in 2006 for the first time since 1991 (Martin et al., 2009), it reached historic lows in 2013, decreasing 10% from 2012 to 2013 and decreasing 38% since 2007 (Hamilton, Martin, Osterman, & Curtin, 2014). The stable decline in teen pregnancy and birth rates is good news. However, the long-term social and economic consequences associated with adolescent childbearing continue to be pressing societal concerns.

The social and economic costs of teen childbearing are high. The National Campaign to Prevent Teen Pregnancy (2013) reports that in 2010, the cost related to adolescent pregnancy and parenting was estimated at 9.4 billion dollars. This includes costs associated with health care, child welfare, public assistance, and criminal justice (National Campaign to Prevent Teen Pregnancy, 2013). Costs experienced by young women who bear children in adolescence include: decreased educational attainment, decreased marital stability, higher rates of depression, and increased financial stress (Koleva & Stuart, 2014). Children of adolescents are less likely to be on par with their peers at school entry in the areas of cognition and knowledge, language and communication, emotional well-being and social skills, and physical well-being and motor skill development (Hoffman & Maynard, 2008; Terry-Humen, Manlove, & Moore, 2005), and are more likely to be poor, experience abuse and neglect, and enter the child welfare system (Hoffman, 2006).

The intergenerational impact of teen childbearing is particularly concerning as daughters of teen mothers are more likely to become teen mothers themselves. Approximately one-third of female adolescents born to a teenage mother became teen mothers themselves, compared to 11% of those whose mothers were age 20–21 at the time of their first birth (Hoffman, 2006). Additionally, adolescents who give birth before age 15 are more likely to experience a second pregnancy during adolescence than those who give birth to their first child later in adolescence (Boardman, Allsworth, Phipps, & Lapane, 2006). Thus, it becomes important to not only work toward preventing a first pregnancy, but also to support adolescents who do become parents in preventing a second pregnancy and avoid perpetuating the cycle of intergenerational childbearing.

This chapter focuses on social work services provided to pregnant and parenting adolescents under the auspices of the North Carolina's Adolescent Parenting Program (APP), a program that aims to prevent repeat pregnancies during adolescence and to promote high school graduation among adolescent parents. North Carolina's birth rate for adolescents aged 15–19 years was 31.8 births per 1,000 teens (Martin et al., 2012), ranking it 30th in the nation, with 50 being the highest (National Campaign to Prevent Teen and Unplanned Pregnancy, 2013). In 2013, 24.3% of adolescent pregnancies in North Carolina were repeat pregnancies, making a program such as the Adolescent Parenting Program critically important in preventing subsequent pregnancies in adolescence (Adolescent Pregnancy Prevention of North Carolina [APPNC], 2014).

Description of the setting

The North Carolina Adolescent Parenting Program (APP) is a pregnancy-prevention program that has served pregnant and parenting teens in North Carolina for over 25 years. It involves a two-part state-wide initiative: the North Carolina Teen Pregnancy Prevention Initiative (TPPI), which aims to reduce the high state-wide teen pregnancy rate, and the Adolescent Pregnancy Prevention Program (APPP) that focuses on primary prevention of teen pregnancy. The APP is a program partially funded by a federal initiative, administered and funded at the state level by the North Carolina Department of Health and Human Services, and implemented at the local level. The program is designed to provide services at the county level in various agency settings, such as public health departments, mental health centers, schools, departments of social services, and private non-profit agencies. Currently, there are 22 local APP programs operating in 21 of North Carolina's 100 counties (North Carolina Department of Health and Human Services, 2014). Each local APP offers case management and other services to participants with the primary goal of preventing a second pregnancy during adolescence while helping pregnant and parenting teens achieve personal self-sufficiency and economic self-support. The local APP described in this chapter is located in a school in a county that is a mix of both rural and small town residents.

Policy

Federal legislation to reduce the incidence of teen pregnancies historically focused on efforts to prevent a first pregnancy rather than preventing a second pregnancy. From 1981 to 2009, efforts primarily took the form of abstinence-only-until-marriage education interventions funded heavily through programs such as Community-Based Abstinence Education (CBAE) and Title V of the 1996 Welfare Reform Law. Federal policies impacting youth who were already pregnant and parenting included Temporary Assistance to Needy Families (TANF) and Title XX of the Public Health Service Act, the Adolescent Family Life Act (AFLA).

As part of the 1996 welfare reform, TANF includes special provisions specifically addressing minor parents. First, minor parents are required to live with a parent, caregiver, or in an adult-supervised setting. Second, minor parents are required to participate in education leading to a high school diploma or its equivalent (Hummel & Levin-Epstein, 2005). TANF legislation limits the amount of time one can receive federal aid and mandates work requirements in order to discourage chronic dependence on government assistance (Levin-Epstein & Hutchins, 2003). By specifically including minor parents, TANF intends to address and break the cycle of intergenerational teen childbearing. A 2007 report by the National Campaign to Prevent Teen and Unplanned Pregnancy indicated that none of the welfare reform legislation directed at adults has shown any positive effects on preventing children from becoming teen parents (Kirby, 2007). However, these studies did not evaluate the legislation directly affecting minor parents, and effects for minor parents are unknown (Kirby, 2007).

Enacted in 1981, the AFLA contained a prevention component supporting abstinence-based education, with a lesser component supporting comprehensive health, education, and social services to pregnant and parenting adolescents, their children, family members, and young fathers. In 2010, reacting to substantial evidence for comprehensive education approaches in preventing adolescent pregnancy, the Obama administration eliminated two-thirds of federal funding for abstinence-only programs in support of more comprehensive health and evidence-based prevention approaches (Sexuality Information and Education Council of the United States [SIECUS], 2010). This initiative, the Consolidated Appropriations Act of 2010, is administered under the newly-created Office of Adolescent Health (OAH). In addition, the Affordable Care Act, signed into law in 2010, includes provisions for the Personal Responsibility Education Program (PREP) that provides grant funding for innovative, evidence-based comprehensive education programs (SIECUS, 2010). Yet, reauthorization of the Title V State Abstinence Education Grant Program continues funding for abstinence-focused programs (SIECUS, 2010).

This legislation provides states more flexibility in choosing abstinence-only and comprehensive approaches, and leaves the design and implementation of such programs to the discretion of state and local authorities. North Carolina's APP programs are funded through a combination of federal, state, and local dollars. Because many of the program's participants are minors and most do not have private insurance, the programs are able to bill Medicaid for many of the case management and psychosocial counseling services.

School-based policies can significantly impact pregnant and parenting teens' ability to achieve the goal of finishing high school, which will ultimately affect their self-sufficiency and economic stability. For example, offering an evening class schedule or GED (General Educational Development) classes for adolescent parents who find it difficult to attend during the regular school day, or having an on-site daycare option for students who need help with childcare while they attend classes can make a difference in an adolescent completing high school. Flexible school attendance policies for pregnant and parenting teens can greatly impact their chances at school success.

Technology

Advances in information technology and management information systems have significantly improved social work practitioners' abilities to document and track their work with clients. This includes tracking the type of and amount of services provided to clients as well as clients' progress toward meeting program goals, an important component in determining the efficacy and effectiveness of program services. With the shift to evidence-based practice and a tight funding climate that often depends on providing evidence of program effectiveness, it is now more necessary to provide accurate data on how well a program is serving its clients and on the degree to which the program is meeting its goals.

To this end, the North Carolina TPPI currently utilizes a web-based data entry system called EZTPPI (www.eztppi.org/northcarolina). The coordinators of the local APP programs are required to enter data on clients using a client intake form, individual service forms, group activity forms, goal plan forms (initial, periodic update, and review), and case closure forms. The system was developed so that the state agency could monitor local programs as well as track service delivery across all the local programs. Training is provided to all program coordinators on how to use the database for tracking and evaluation purposes. With the use of web-based meeting technology, the state TPPI program staff can also hold meetings with local program coordinators across the state to disseminate new guidelines and best practices. Local program coordinators can use this format in addition to listserves and social networking sites for sharing information on strategies that work in their programs.

In addition to using the internet for data entry, the APP programs utilize a range of internet health information resources. For example, several national websites provide helpful information for professionals as well as lay consumers that coordinators use to strengthen their own health education knowledge and skills as well as sources of information for teens. These include the March of Dimes (www.marchofdimes.org), the Maternal and Child Health Bureau (http://mchb.hrsa.gov), and the National Campaign to Prevent Teen and Unplanned Pregnancy (http://thenationalcampaign.org).

Organization

The TPPI provides the overall state-wide administration and funding for the 22 local APP programs. Each local program is under the auspices of a health and human service organization such as a public health department, local non-profit agency, department of social services (DSS), or school system. The sponsoring organization applies to TPPI for a 5-year annually renewable grant to support the program, provides matching community funds, and physical space for the program, and hires and supervises the program coordinator. Under this arrangement, each local APP coordinator reports to the sponsoring agency and to the state TPPI director who establishes guidelines regarding participant eligibility, case load sizes, mandated services, data collection requirements, and community advisory council. State-level TPPI program staff support local program coordinators through regular state-wide meetings and conferences about best practices and an annual graduation conference for clients and staff of the programs. The organizational culture of each program is heavily determined by its physical location and sponsoring agency. For example, an APP located in a DSS office has a different organizational culture than one located in a high school.

A full-time coordinator (often a master's level social worker) administers each county APP program and provides direct services to program clients. In addition, local APP coordinators engage in planning, implementing, and evaluating the program; recruiting, training, and supervising volunteer mentors; developing and maintaining agency partnerships; conducting community outreach and education; and advocating for services for pregnancy prevention and parenting teens. Each coordinator is required to organize a community advisory council that meets at least four times per year. This advisory council is made up of representatives from agencies and community groups that will support the program in developing linkages that the coordinator can tap into for client services, fundraising, and marketing the program. The overall goal of the community advisory council is to promote pregnancy prevention education and empower youth to make healthy life choices.

In the role of direct service provider, coordinators conduct an initial individual assessment with each client, work with the client to set goals and objectives and develop a plan to reach those goals, provide home visiting services utilizing an evidence-based curriculum, and organize peer education and support groups. Other services may include community education and outreach, classroom presentations, peer leadership activities, teen and parent workshops, counseling and referrals, and developing and researching educational and informational materials. Coordinators carry a case load of 15–25 clients. In order to increase the impact of the program, APP coordinators match volunteer mentors with participants to serve as role models and to help them navigate the social service, health care, and school systems.

Decisions about practice

Definition and description of the client

Pregnant and parenting teens, female or male, are able to receive TPPI program services if they are age 19 or younger and do not experience an additional pregnancy while participating in the program. Teachers, guidance counselors, and Maternity Care Coordinators at local public health departments typically refer teens to the program. In addition, friends and/or siblings who are current or former participants of the program refer teens. Adolescent parents are not considered emancipated minors in North Carolina, so although program participation is voluntary, parental consent is required for all minor participants.

Tanya Smith is a 17-year-old White female in the 11th grade. She is the mother of 2-year-old Sean. Tanya and Sean live in a small two-bedroom apartment with Tanya's mother Danielle, who is 33 and employed at a local fast-food restaurant. Tanya is a high school student who enjoys learning and performed well academically and was a cheerleader prior to her pregnancy. While Tanya is at school and Danielle is at work, Sean spends the day at a family-home daycare near Tanya's school.

A teacher referred Tanya to the APP when she discovered that Tanya was pregnant at age 15; Tanya was afraid to tell her mother about her pregnancy. She wanted to enroll in the program but could not do so without parental consent. Tanya and the APP coordinator, Liz, conducted a role-play in which Tanya practiced telling her mother about her pregnancy and prepared herself for her mother's possible responses. Ultimately, Tanya chose not to tell her mother in person but left a handwritten letter on her pillow before leaving the house one morning for school. Danielle was initially upset, deeply disappointed, yet supportive. She became a teenage mother at 16 when she gave birth to Tanya and had always hoped that Tanya would at least finish high school before becoming a parent.

After completing enrollment paperwork for the program, Tanya and Liz discussed Tanya's options: parenting, adoption, and termination of the pregnancy. When Tanya chose to continue with the pregnancy and parent, Tanya's boyfriend – Sean's father – quickly ended the relationship with Tanya. Tanya's mother Danielle and Liz became her primary supports throughout her pregnancy. Meeting with both Tanya and her mother helped Liz better understand the cultural context of this family and why Tanya had decided to go ahead with the pregnancy and parenting at such an young age. In accordance with her family's religious beliefs, Tanya would not have terminated the pregnancy. Tanya was part of a large extended family in which teen parenting was not unusual and in which family members supported teens in raising their children. As Danielle expressed, "This is not how I would have had it for Tanya. But, we will make the best of this."

As Tanya's pregnancy progressed, she became embarrassed to be in school surrounded by classmates who frequently commented on her changing body. Her grades suffered as she neared Sean's birth. A week before her due date, Tanya went on homebound status, requiring a teacher to provide assignments and tutoring at home. Following Sean's birth, Tanya remained on homebound status for six weeks, the maximum time allowed by her school.

Upon her return to school, her world rapidly changed. Tanya's typically high grades gradually worsened because she had less time available for studying and assignment completion;

she was severely sleep deprived for the first five months post-partum. During her pregnancy, Tanya dropped off the cheerleading squad and because of parenting responsibilities after school, she could not return to cheerleading or any extracurricular activities. Tanya observed that her friends spent their evenings doing homework, talking on the phone, and watching television; Tanya spent her evenings feeding and bathing Sean and putting him to bed. Fortunately, in the first eight months of Sean's life, Danielle assisted with these tasks. For the first year of Sean's life, Tanya was an active participant in the APP. Both the program and her mother helped Tanya as she learned to juggle school and parenting. Although she faced challenges and her grades fluctuated, Tanya used program resources effectively for support.

As Tanya moved through high school, Danielle's perception of Tanya changed from that of a teenager needing help to that of an adult fully capable of independently raising a child and running a household. Danielle increased her hours at work into evening hours, and Tanya became responsible not only for caring for her son but also for housework; she cooks, cleans, shops, and pays bills. Meanwhile, Danielle became less involved in her family's life and more involved in her relationship with her boyfriend who stays overnight at the apartment several nights a week, offering less time and support for Tanya. Recently the household responsibilities have overwhelmed Tanya. Her grades are plummeting. Tanya's relationship with Danielle continues to worsen. Tanya reports that when she asks her mother for help or explains that her responsibilities are more than she can handle, she is told to "grow up" and to "act your age." Tanya feels that her mother and her mother's boyfriend criticize her constantly and do not understand how overwhelmed she feels.

For the past six months, Tanya has had a boyfriend who is a senior at her school. He is attentive to Tanya and her son. He is not Sean's father, so he cannot officially enroll in the program and cannot receive APP services, but he can and does attend peer group meetings when invited by Tanya. Few of the other participants in her program are in relationships and even fewer have their boyfriend's support at meetings. Tanya reports that she is struggling to find time to be with her boyfriend.

Despite fluctuations in her grades and parental support, Tanya's participation in the program has rarely wavered. She visits Liz's office a couple of times per week for counseling on life management; they discuss such issues as Tanya's arguments with her mother, financial hardships, frustrations with teachers, and poor grades. She also attends the monthly peer group meetings, which provide an opportunity for all program participants to socialize and to learn information and skills from presenters on topics including parenting, stress management, children's development, and adolescent advocacy. See Figure 24.1 for an ecomap showing Tanya's social context.

Goals

The primary aim of APP is to increase the likelihood that young parents will obtain self-sufficiency and be better able to provide a positive, stable foundation for their child. Coordinators are mandated to focus on two primary goals with participants: (1) increasing the self-sufficiency outcomes for APP participants by increasing the delay of a subsequent pregnancy and increasing graduation from high school with diploma or completion of the GED; and (2) improving child welfare and school readiness outcomes for the children of APP parents by increasing incidence of positive parenting to support the child's cognitive development and mental health and increasing incidence of child's physical well-being by establishing the child's medical home and creating a safe home environment (North Carolina Department of Health and Human Services, 2014). APP coordinators are required to use the evidence-based

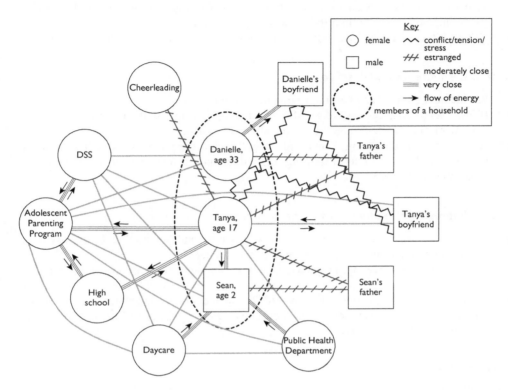

Figure 24.1 Ecomap for Tanya Smith

practice of motivational interviewing (MI), a guidance technique that elicits and strengthens motivation for change. Using MI, coordinators develop individualized goal plans with each participant. The goal plan is reviewed monthly during the scheduled home visit. During this monthly visit, program participants work with their coordinator to develop additional goals or revise current goals based on individual situations and needs.

Contract and objectives

Upon entering the program, Tanya met with Liz to develop an individual plan which includes goals, objectives, and activities to meet these goals which they review monthly. This process is similar to a contracting process in that Liz and Tanya plan how and when they will accomplish goals and objectives. The following is an example of the objectives for three goals that Tanya and Liz established in their most recent meeting.

Goal 1: Delay a subsequent pregnancy

- Tanya will participate in the next peer group session on birth control methods; she will invite her boyfriend to this meeting.
- At a subsequent session, Tanya and Liz will role-play how to negotiate condom use with her boyfriend.

- Tanya will schedule a doctor's appointment to discuss getting an intrauterine device (IUD) implanted. She will notify Liz when she does this.
- Tanya will consistently use condoms in addition to her other chosen birth control method.

Goal 2: Graduate from high school

- For the next month Tanya will have no unexcused absences.
- If an absence is necessary, (e.g., MD appointment), Tanya will submit the necessary paperwork (i.e., doctor's note) to get the absence excused.
- At each scheduled meeting, Tanya and Liz will review her progress and will discuss any need for academic support or tutoring. Liz will contact Tanya's teachers to obtain their assessment of her progress.

Goal 3: Improve her relationship with her mother

- Liz will schedule a counseling session with Tanya and her mother to discuss their relationship and Tanya's sense of being overburdened.
- To prepare for this meeting, Tanya will keep a week long daily log of how she is spending her time.
- Prior to the session, Liz will role-play with Tanya about how she will tell her mother her feelings of being overburdened with household responsibilities and her desire to have more time with her mother.

Meeting place

The APP discussed in this case is located in a high school, which makes it ideal for frequent contact between the coordinator and the participants. Tanya regularly drops in to see Liz, and Liz has easy access to Tanya's teachers. Liz is able to use a school classroom for after school peer group meetings. Thus, the group meetings are much more accessible to participants as they are already at school. Liz is mandated to meet with Tanya in her home at least 8 out of the 12 monthly required formal visits. The volunteer mentor, who is assigned to Tanya, frequently picks her up after school for activities or to take her to appointments.

Use of time

Tanya and Liz meet three to five times per month. One of these meetings is a formal, scheduled meeting of about an hour for review of Tanya's progress in meeting goals. Many meetings occur informally when Tanya drops in to talk with Liz; some are scheduled as needed when Tanya is having a problem at school or at home. Liz spends a fair amount of her time checking in with service providers such as the day care and the public health department who are providing services to Tanya and Sean.

Strategies and interventions

Liz uses various interventions in her work with clients including crisis intervention, case management, case level advocacy, group work using a psychoeducational approach, motivational interviewing, and brief solution-focused work by developing "short-term goals and contracting within a long-term relationship" (Kerson, 2002, p. 323). The primary goal of these interventions is to educate, support, and empower teens to manage their lives and effectively solve problems as they arise. She uses her knowledge of adolescent development and a risk and resiliency framework (Fraser, 2004; Rounds, 2004) to adapt interventions to the cognitive, psychological, and social capabilities of her clients and to the context of their lives. In addition, Liz engages in advocacy, both at the case level (e.g., advocating with the school for a change in class sections for a student) as well as at the class level. Liz also engages in macrolevel social work interventions such as class level advocacy (e.g., participating in a legislative action day to increase funding for adolescent pregnancy prevention), community outreach, and collaborating with other community agencies.

Stance of the social worker

Liz uses a problem-solving and empowerment approach. Through modeling, she teaches Tanya how to seek help and advocate for herself and her son. Liz focuses on relationship building and collaboration with staff from other agencies. She is very skilled at developing a network of helping agencies that she can call on when APP clients need resources and when she needs community support for the program.

Uses of resources outside of the relationship

In order for the APP to be successful and for the coordinator to secure needed resources for the teens in the program, the coordinator is heavily dependent upon collaborative working relationships with staff of local agencies, including the sponsoring agency. Because the program is located in a school and due to the emphasis on school success for program participants, Liz meets frequently with school counselors and individual teachers. One of her key responsibilities is to develop a network within the community to support the program and individual clients. She frequently calls on members of the advisory council to help her develop and maintain these relationships. Additionally, Liz has developed an active volunteer mentoring program to extend the program's services. To network with community groups, she serves on a local community board that is composed of representatives from social services, mental health, public health, and other key community agencies. Her participation on this board provides her with invaluable insight into the workings of various community agencies and she uses these meetings to promote awareness of the APP and the problems of teen pregnancy. Liz also enlists community speakers, leaders, and trainers to conduct educational sessions at the peer group meetings on topics such as early child development, how to protect oneself from sexually transmitted infections, and how to complete a job application.

Reassessment and evaluation

Liz participates in reassessment at two different levels: the individual client level and the program level. As noted earlier, she and Tanya meet monthly to formally review and update Tanya's goal plan. To evaluate the program, Liz also asks program participants to complete an evaluation form on the educational component of each peer group meeting. She uses this feedback on speakers and content to assist with planning of future meetings. In addition, at the quarterly advisory council meetings she asks members to provide feedback and to assess program performance and development. Finally, as mandated by the state, she enters client level and program data into the web-based data entry system (EZTPPI) that is used by the state to formally evaluate her program and the other 22 programs across the state and the overall TPPI.

Transfer or termination

Tanya can stay in the program until she graduates from high school or completes her GED, as long as she does not become pregnant again. She has been an active program participant, and Liz hopes that she will continue in the program and develop into one of the role models and leaders. During Tanya's senior year, she and Liz will focus their work on preparing Tanya for the transition to employment or further education, ensuring that adequate support is in place for this transition. Her graduation from the program will be marked by a state-wide graduation celebration.

Differential discussion

In reviewing her work with Tanya, Liz realized that she has learned much from working with Tanya. At first she was dismayed when Tanya came in to the program at age 15; she had not worked with a pregnant teen who was so young; all of the other program participants were 17- to 19-year-olds. In order to be effective, she needed to quickly update her knowledge of development of young teens and locate additional resources to address the issues for this age group.

Looking back, as additional younger teens entered the program, she wonders if she should have developed separate peer group meetings for the younger girls in the program. Because she did not have the resources to run separate groups, she tried to ensure that issues concerning the younger teens were addressed and that they felt they could speak up in the group meetings. Liz plans to use her network of other APP coordinators to learn how others are addressing the increase in pregnancy among very young teens.

Because the APP is located in the local high school and not in the middle school, Liz did not have the same relationships with, and access to, teachers and the school counselor that she has at the high school. Liz realizes that she needs to foster closer relationships to the middle school as she is receiving more referrals of middle school age girls. She plans to raise this challenge with her Advisory Council at their next meeting to get their input. Liz would like to open a satellite office at the middle school, but realizes that this is a politically and culturally sensitive issue and would need the support of the school board, the middle school staff and teachers, and the parents.

Liz also realized how important it is to fully engage a young teen early on in the program and to work on retention issues, including pregnancy prevention and school success. She feels that she has been successful with Tanya because they developed a close relationship early on in the process, and she has been able to match Tanya with an excellent volunteer mentor who has made a long-term commitment to working with Tanya. She was not as successful with two of the other young clients who left the program after their second year; one became pregnant and the other dropped out of school.

Finally, reviewing her work with Tanya has made Liz realize how important the teen's relationship is with her family. While she spent a great deal of time with both Tanya and Danielle during the first year or so of Tanya's time in the program, over the last year her focus has shifted to helping Tanya finish high school and prepare for employment or additional education. While this is appropriate, she wishes that she had also paid more attention to Tanya's relationship with her mother. Tanya is only 17 and although a parent herself, is developmentally an adolescent and still needs and wants the involvement of and guidance from her mother. In looking forward to Tanya's eventual graduation from the program and transition to becoming more independent, Liz realizes that Tanya's relationship with her mother will be critical.

Discussion questions

1   If the organization within which you are working has a policy that you must discharge someone who "fails" (in this case, teenagers who become pregnant again; in other cases, those who have a relapse of some sort), what do you believe your duties to the client are? What do you believe your advocacy role entails?
2   When teenagers become pregnant, relatives frequently view them as having chosen to accept adult roles and therefore needing to fulfill them. If you were working with Tanya and her mother, how might you help them understand the continuing need Tanya has for her mother while also supporting Tanya's need to take responsibility?
3   Liz was able to develop a mentoring program to help support the teenagers in her program. How might you use community resources to assist the populations with whom you work?

Acknowledgments

The authors would like to acknowledge Caitlin Georgas and Kristen Carroll for their help in preparing this manuscript.

References

Adolescent Pregnancy Prevention of North Carolina (2014). North Carolina repeat pregnancies, ages 15–19. Retrieved from www.shiftnc.org/data/map/northcarolina

Boardman, L. A., Allsworth, J., Phipps, M. G., & Lapane, K. L. (2006). Risk factors for unintended versus intended rapid repeat pregnancies among adolescents. *Journal of Adolescent Health, 39*(4), 597.

Fraser, M. W. (Ed.). (2004). *Risk and resilience in childhood: An ecological perspective.* Washington, DC: NASW Press.

Hamilton, B. E., Martin, J. A., Osterman, M. J. K., & Curtin, S. C. (2014). Births: Preliminary data for 2013. *National Vital Statistics Reports, 63*(2), 1–18.

Hoffman, S. (2006). By the numbers: The public costs of teen childbearing. National Campaign to Prevent Teen Pregnancy. Retrieved from www.teenpregnancy.org/costs/default.htm

Hoffman, S. D. & Maynard, R. A. (Eds.). (2008). *Kids having kids: Economic costs and social consequences of teen pregnancy* (2nd edn.). Washington, DC: Urban Institute Press.

Hummel, L. & Levin-Epstein, J. (2005). *A needed transition: Lessons from Illinois about teen parent TANF rules.* Retrieved from www.clasp.org

Kerson, T. S. (2002). *Boundary spanning: An ecological reinterpretation of social work practice in health and mental health systems.* New York: Columbia University Press.

Kirby, D. (2007). *Emerging answers 2007: Research findings on programs to reduce teen pregnancy and sexually transmitted diseases.* Washington, DC: National Campaign to Prevent Teen and Unplanned Pregnancy.

Koleva, H. & Stuart, S. (2014). Risk factors for depressive symptoms in adolescent pregnancy in a late-teen subsample. *Archives of Women's Mental Health, 17,* 155–158.

Levin-Epstein, J. & Hutchins, J. (2003). *Teens and TANF: How adolescents fare under the nation's welfare program.* Retrieved from www.clasp.org

Martin, J. A., Hamilton, B. E., Osterman, M. J. K., Curtin, S. C., & Mathews, T. J. (2012). Births: Final data for 2012. *National Vital Statistics Reports, 62*(9), 1–68.

Martin, J. A., Hamilton, B. E., Sutton, P. D., Ventura, S. J., Menacker, F., Kirmeyer, S. & Mathews, M. S. (2009). Births: Final data for 2006. *National Vital Statistics Reports, 57*(7), 1–102.

National Campaign to Prevent Teen and Unplanned Pregnancy (2013). Counting it up. The public costs of teen childbearing: Key data. Washington, DC. Retrieved from www.teenpregnancy.org/costs/default.htm

National Campaign to Prevent Teen and Unplanned Pregnancy (2015). Teen birth rate comparison, 2013. Retrieved March 27, 2015 from https://thenationalcampaign.org/data/compare/1701

North Carolina Department of Health and Human Services (2014). *Teen pregnancy prevention initiatives.* Retrieved March 24, 2015, from www.teenpregnancy.ncdhhs.gov/app.htm

Rounds, K. A. (2004). Preventing sexually transmitted infections among adolescents. In M. W. Fraser (Ed.), *Risk and resilience in childhood: An ecological perspective* (pp. 251–279). Washington, DC: NASW Press.

SIECUS (Sexuality Information and Education Council of the United States) (2010). A brief history of federal funding for sex education and related programs. Retrieved from www.siecus.org

Terry-Humen, E., Manlove, J., & Moore, K. A. (2005). *Playing catch up: How children born to teen mothers fare.* Washington, DC: National Campaign to Prevent Teen Pregnancy.

Ventura, S. J., Abma, J. C., Mosher, W. D., & Henshaw, S. K. (2008). Estimated pregnancy rates by outcome for the United States, 1990–2004. *National Vital Statistics Reports, 56*(15), 1–26.

Websites

March of Dimes, www.marchofdimes.com

Maternal and Child Health Bureau, http://mchb.hrsa.gov

Chapter 25

Screening for perinatal depression in an inner-city prenatal setting

Laudy Burgos

Context

Perinatal depression is one of the most common complications of pregnancy and a well-known public health concern (Association of State and Territorial Health Officials, 2005). Perinatal depression refers to major and minor depressive episodes that occur during pregnancy or in the first year following delivery. The *DSM-5* defines it as the onset of a major depressive disorder that begins during pregnancy and/or within the first four weeks postpartum (American Psychiatric Association, 2013). Perinatal depression is estimated to affect 10–14% of pregnant women and 10–20% during the postpartum period (Gjerdingen & Yawn, 2007). Rates are higher among inner-city women of low socioeconomic status (Goodman, 2009). It disproportionately affects U.S. ethnic minorities, African American women, and Latinas in particular (Meltzer-Brody, 2011).

Perinatal depression is associated with a higher risk of adverse pregnancy outcomes such as prematurity, fetal distress, neonatal behavioral differences, along with an increased risk for postpartum depression (Freeman, 2007). It can compromise a woman's health and the health of her unborn baby through decreasing her capacity to care for herself; affected women often have inadequate nutrition, increased drug or alcohol use, and inconsistent clinic attendance. Although perinatal depression can cause adverse pregnancy outcomes, the U.S. Department of Health and Human Services estimated that about half of women with postpartum depression do not receive any kind of mental health assessment and treatment; and only 23% of women diagnosed with prenatal depression received mental health services prenatally (Le, Perry, & Stuart, 2011). Legislation has increasingly focused on identification and treatment of postpartum depression. Pregnancy and the postpartum period characterize ideal points during which consistent contact with the health care system will allow women at risk to be identified and treated (American College of Obstetricians and Gynecologists Committee Opinion No. 453, 2010). While 4–6 weeks post partum is the optimal and recommended time for screening, women can and should be screened whenever they present in obstetrical, pediatric, or primary care visits during the first year after giving birth. However perinatal depression may be missed during routine prenatal visits, emphasizing the need for better screening in obstetrical.

Screening for perinatal depression is feasible using valid, reliable, free, and easy-to-administer measures, such as the Edinburgh Postnatal Depression Scale (EPDS) and Patient Health Questionnaires (PHQ-9 and PHQ-2). The EPDS measures current mood disturbance for women in the perinatal period and consists of 10 statements with four possible responses and is rated on a 4-point scale. The patient chooses the response that is closest to how she has felt in the past 7 days. The EPDS is a screening, not diagnostic tool and is validated for pregnant and parenting women. Scores above the specified threshold indicate the person may be depressed and further investigation is recommended (Cox & Holden, 2003). The PHQ-9 is another screening tool; the 9-item questionnaire is based on *DSM-IV* diagnostic criteria. Women rate items about loss of interest, depressed mood, sleep disruption, fatigue, changes in appetite, guilt, feelings of worthlessness, changes in concentration, psychomotor retardation/agitation, and frequency of thoughts of suicide within the past two weeks (Davis, Pearlstein, Stuart, O'Hara, & Zlotnick, 2013). The 2-item PHQ-2 is another screening tool that can be used, especially in busy clinics where time is limited. The PHQ-2 contains the first two questions from the PHQ-9 and asks about the frequency of depressed mood and anhedonia over the past two weeks (Kroenke, Spitzer, & Williams, 2003).

Even when there are barriers to screening, it is important to provide support and resources during pregnancy in the form of psychoeducation and/or psychotherapy because these interventions may reduce positive screenings as well as postpartum depression. In a recent randomized controlled trial conducted at Mount Sinai Hospital, newly delivered African American and Latina mothers volunteered and were assigned to either a behavioral educational intervention by a master's level social worker or a control group. The mothers in the intervention group were educated about modifiable factors associated with symptoms of postpartum depression (physical symptoms, low social support, etc.). These mothers were helped to identify and manage potential issues in the postpartum period that may trigger depressive symptoms and encouraged to use community resources for social support and services. The results showed that mothers who received the intervention were less likely to screen positive for depression than mothers in the control group: at three weeks (8% compared with 15.3% respectively) and at three months (8.4% compared with 13.7% respectively) (Howell et al., 2012).

Description of the setting

The Obstetrics and Gynecology (OB/GYN) Ambulatory Practice comprises the ambulatory clinics of Mount Sinai Hospital's Women and Children's Division. The patient population reflects a diversity of socioeconomic, racial, and ethnic groups. Continuity of care is provided by physicians, physician assistants, midwives, nurses, and social workers. The OB/GYN Ambulatory Practice has a renowned high-risk obstetrical and gynecological oncology service and a very active midwife and physician assistant program. Many of the women who seek care in this area are non-English speaking, medically high risk, have a history of multiple psychosocial stressors, are uninsured, undocumented, and lack adequate social support. Pregnant women who report symptoms of anxiety and depression at their initial prenatal visit are followed throughout their pregnancy by one of the licensed master's prepared social workers in the clinic.

Policy

Policymakers and advocates for women's health would like to see an increase in the number of women screened for depression, with appropriate linkage to treatment (Price, Corder-Mabe, & Austin, 2012). Screening for perinatal mood disorders in the United States is not standardized. Several state screening initiatives have passed as the public health effects of perinatal depression are recognized as detrimental to both maternal and child health. For example,

Texas legislation mandates that women who give birth must receive educational materials regarding postpartum depression prior to discharge (Shivakumar, Brandon, Johnson, & Freeman, 2014). New Jersey became the first state to require postpartum depression screening of women with recent births in 2006. The New Jersey Postpartum Depression Act mandates that health care professionals educate women and their families about postpartum depression, before and after delivery. The law requires that licensed health care professionals caring for women after they deliver must screen women before they are discharged from the hospital and then during the initial postpartum follow-up visits (New Jersey Assembly, 2006). In 2008, Illinois enacted the Perinatal Mental Health Disorders Prevention and Treatment Act. This act requires several state agencies to develop appropriate educational programs for women and their families, provide screening questionnaires for use during prenatal and pediatric visits, and review the questionnaire in accordance with recommendations of the American College of Obstetricians and Gynecologists (Rhodes & Segre, 2013). In April 2009, the Uniform Maternal Screening Act passed in West Virginia that requires education and screening of perinatal women and requires women entering prenatal care to be assessed for their risk for depression (Rhodes & Segre, 2013). In the same year, the National Research Council (NRC) and the Institute of Medicine (IOM) reaffirmed the significant linkages between parenting and mental health, calling for improved screening and intervention efforts during the prenatal period (National Research Council and Institute of Medicine, 2009).

At the federal level, the Melanie Blocker Stokes MOTHERS Act was passed along with the U.S. Senate version of the Patient Protection and Affordable Care Act in January 2010. While it does not mandate screening, it encourages broader services, education, public awareness research, and concrete services to assist new mothers to access treatment.

New York state's (where the OB/GYN Ambulatory Practice is located) health care system currently has no system-wide screening and referral procedure for postpartum depression. The Maternal Depression Bill (S. 7234B/A. 9610B) passed in 2014 provides educational services and promotes screening and treatment for maternal depression. It is intended to ensure that New Yorkers are informed of the public health services that will help them understand, identify, and treat maternal depression (Krueger, 2014).

Technology

Several years ago, Mount Sinai Hospital began using electronic documentation, which has been quite helpful. Not only is it more secure but it also allows us to easily access client records and track them. We must be mindful of the language we use in social work documentation of women experiencing perinatal depression. Technologies such as computers, smartphones, and tablets enable professionals to network and learn about perinatal depression through webinars and access to academic journals and books. New research teaches providers about evidence-based interventions. Clients also have access to these technologies that allow them to do research, obtain support, and learn to advocate for themselves.

The internet provides access to a wealth of resources for women affected by perinatal depression. Websites provide resources, online chats, events, and referral information. Some include online support groups to address the needs of women who do not have access to a support group in their area. There is increasing use of non-traditional social work interventions to engage clients. For example, Text4baby is a free text messaging program for pregnant women and new moms. Mothers can receive weekly messages, free of charge, on their cell phone to help them through their pregnancy and their baby's first year. Additionally, iPads are distributed in inpatient units so that clients can communicate with their loved ones during antepartum stays. These technologies promote social support, an influential factor in perinatal mood disorders.

Organization

The Mount Sinai Hospital OB/GYN Ambulatory Practice provides medical, nutrition, and social work services to pregnant patients. During the initial visit, all patients receive a social work screening to identify any psychosocial risk factors, including but not limited to child protection involvement, past psychiatric history, substance abuse, domestic violence, and homelessness. The 2-item PHQ-2 screening tool is also used. Should a patient identify any current concerns or if they have a positive PHQ-2 screen, they receive social work intervention throughout their pregnancy. Depending on the needs, the social worker will provide case management services, mental health treatment, or both. In their third trimester, regardless of whether or not they have been working with a social worker, all patients are screened for depression again by a nurse using the PHQ-2. Women who score positive are then referred to social work for a full assessment and treatment. This provides an opportunity to identify those patients who may not have initially experienced symptoms. Patients are also screened with the EPDS at their six-week postpartum visit and are referred to the social worker if they score 9 or above. The social worker completes a comprehensive assessment and with the patient's permission, makes a mental health referral to a community agency, preferably close to the patient's home. See Figure 25.1 for a flow chart of how the screening and intervention process works.

Description of typical clients

The clients seen in the OB/GYN Ambulatory Practice are generally single, minority women residing in poor neighborhoods in New York City, predominantly Manhattan and the Bronx. Most are eligible for Medicaid, unemployed, and receive food stamps and public assistance. The social worker may also work with the father of the baby, or another relative who is significantly involved with the pregnancy. Additionally, typically community referrals are made for preventive services, parenting classes and baby supplies, and home visiting programs.

Most clients with current psychosocial concerns are identified during their initial visit. Those who are not identified early on will eventually be referred by the medical provider or nurse if a concern arises.

Decisions about practice

Description of the client

Denise Garcia, a 30-year old Hispanic single woman, is the mother of three children ages 8 years, 6 years, and 3 months. I began meeting with Ms. Garcia early in her pregnancy with her now 3-month-old. They reside in public housing in Manhattan, NY. She is a high school graduate with some college credits, and works part time in a clothing store. Her low income entitles her to food stamps and Medicaid. Her mother, her primary support, resides in the Bronx, NY, and assists with childcare and emotional support.

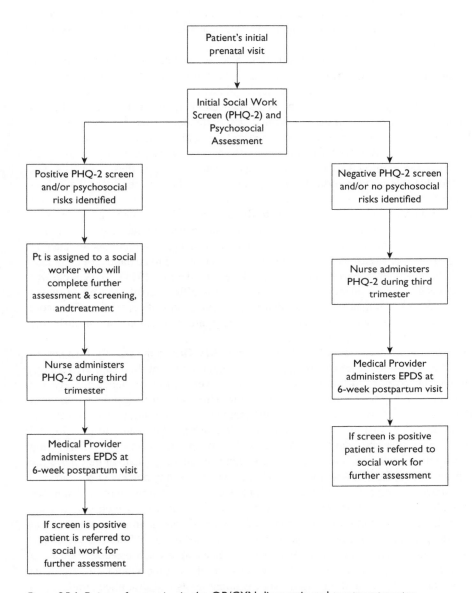

Figure 25.1 Points of screening in the OB/GYN diagnostic and treatment center

Ms. Garcia began prenatal care at the OB/GYN Ambulatory Practice at 11 weeks ges-tational age (not quite three months pregnant) feeling happy and excited about pregnancy with her partner of six months, Juan. She received the routine initial social work screen-ing and disclosed that she had been the victim of domestic violence. She reported many instances of abuse by the father of her 6-year-old daughter. This relationship affected her self-esteem and caused her to feel depressed. Ms. Garcia did not seek mental health treat-ment at the time because her primary concern at that time was leaving the relationship, and she subsequently entered the NYC shelter system. About a year later, she got public housing. Aside from feeling depressed at that time, Ms. Garcia denied a history of depression as a child or adolescent.

During the social work assessment, Ms. Garcia also noted that she had some concerns about her relationship with her current boyfriend, Juan, with whom she had planned this pregnancy. She believed that he was not as happy about the pregnancy as she was. She reported that he was not providing any financial assistance to her, despite the fact that he was staying with her frequently and eating two meals a day in the home. She expressed growing concern that her daughters were growing attached to him, and worried that if he left, they would be emotionally upset. Given the concerns that she shared, Ms. Garcia was assigned to a social worker for additional support during the pregnancy. Despite these concerns, Ms. Garcia asserted that this was a good relationship for her and she was confident that things would get better.

I initially met with Ms. Garcia a few times to discuss strategies to improve her communication with Juan. During these visits she was stressed and frustrated but denied symptoms of depression. Women who experience perinatal mood disorders are sometimes reluctant to report symptoms for many reasons. They assume they are supposed to be happy, but feel lack of motivation, fatigue, and embarrassment (Ribowsky & Henderson, 2011). Ms. Garcia was about five months into her pregnancy when she arrived at my office tearful about an argument with Juan. I decided to administer the EPDS to assess for symptoms of depression. The score indicated that Ms. Garcia was experiencing both anxiety and depression, having difficulty sleeping, in short feeling sad and miserable.

Once these symptoms were identified, I explained to Ms. Garcia the risk for postpartum depression and urged her to agree to ongoing mental health treatment. In a supportive, non-judgmental manner I explained that it was common for women to experience anxiety and depression during pregnancy and that she was not alone. This was a turning point in our work as she was now able to freely discuss the stressors that were contributing to her symptoms.

Ms. Garcia admitted for the first time that the relationship with Juan had deteriorated and she wondered if it was beyond repair. She expressed deep sadness that her unborn baby would be born into a broken relationship. She also reported feeling ashamed that her three children had different fathers and was worried about how others may perceive her.

As our sessions progressed, her relationship worsened. Juan withdrew emotional support, increased his alcohol use, did not come home at night, and was very secretive about his activities. Ms. Garcia began expressing feelings of anger and confusion about the fact that they planned the pregnancy together, yet he was now unsupportive of it. She was not able to sleep well due to her worries about Juan's whereabouts. She had low self-esteem, was crying frequently, and increasingly anxious about how her current situation would affect parenting their baby and her other children. As we set treatment goals and discussed strategies to decrease her depression and anxiety, Ms. Garcia became more engaged in her treatment. We explored her social support system; aside from her mother Ms. Garcia had not identified anyone else who could provide support and assistance. She had mentioned her sister but stated that they were not close and her interactions with her were stressful. She also shared that she did not have close friends and that she did not relate well to her mother's family. However, she did report that she had cousins on her father's side with whom she had lost touch as they grew due to conflict between her mother and her paternal aunts.

We addressed Ms. Garcia's tendency to be dependent on a partner in order to define who she was and to feel content. She acknowledged being quite sexually active as a teenager, and disclosed that she could not remember a time when she was on her own for more than a few weeks. She used sex as a way to obtain gifts and financial assistance from men and later felt angry at herself when these men had expectations of a long-term relationship.

Through our work, Ms. Garcia became aware that she was very possessive and jealous, causing problems in the relationship due to her difficulty trusting men. She admitted that when Juan stayed out, she would text and call him constantly, occasionally even showing up at his job. As the relationship deteriorated, there was constant arguing and Juan decided to move out. Nevertheless, he would show up drunk in the middle of the night, they would engage in sex, and he would stay through the night, always leaving early in the morning without any mention of when he would return. Ms. Garcia felt used and devalued as a result, but struggled to set limits with him. Ms. Garcia realized that the situation was causing so much stress that she was not giving her daughters proper attention and stimulation. She was so upset that she could not enjoy activities with them, causing tremendous guilt.

Goals, objectives, and outcome measures

Developing clear goals and objectives can significantly facilitate the helping process. The primary goals were for Ms. Garcia's mood to improve so that she could successfully parent her daughters and her unborn baby, and to regain a sense of control over her life. The mutually agreed upon objectives were:

- To focus on specific activities that would make her feel happy and accomplished:

  o Ms. Garcia would engage in an activity with her daughters;
  o Ms. Garcia would start going to the gym;
  o Ms. Garcia would visit her mother more often as she enjoyed spending time with her.

- To increase her social support network:

  o Ms. Garcia would attend a pregnancy support group;
  o Ms. Garcia would reach out to her paternal cousins and schedule visits with them;
  o Ms. Garcia would accept invitations from two co-workers with whom she could form friendships;
  o Ms. Garcia would accept referral to the Prenatal Partnership Program (program designed to pair patient with a medical student who will accompany client to appointments and be present when client delivers).

- To develop better boundaries and set firm limits with Juan:

  o Ms. Garcia would not contact him (to create some space to grieve the break-up);
  o Ms. Garcia would not allow him into her home when he showed up unannounced;
  o when Juan did call, Ms. Garcia would focus conversation on how they planned to co-parent, rather than argue about their past relationship.

- To begin to prepare for new baby without Juan's support:

  o Ms. Garcia would accept referral to agency providing baby supplies;
  o Ms. Garcia would create a budget to set aside funds to purchase basic baby items.

- To engage in services to address her relationship with her daughters:

  o Ms. Garcia would accept referral to preventive service agency in the community.

Contracting

Ms. Garcia actively participated in establishing treatment goals and exploring how they would be met as I emphasized the need for goals to be measurable so that we could track her progress. Objectives were identified recognizing the realities of her current situation and the potential for benefitting her and her family. The goals were reviewed every session to track progress. Ms. Garcia was aware that these goals were recorded in her medical chart and would guide my interventions. At every session, we selected two objectives that she would focus on for the week. She reported on her progress at the following session.

Meeting place

Social work sessions take place in a private office located in the OB/GYN Ambulatory Practice. This setting provides a quiet area where client's confidentiality can be ensured and we are able to work without any interruptions. A study conducted a few years ago found that a large number of pregnant women reported that they preferred to receive mental health treatment in the obstetric clinic as opposed to a mental health clinic or psychiatry site. The reasons for this preference included immediacy of help, familiarity with clinic and staff, and the convenience of receiving treatment in the same building, on the same day as their obstetrics appointment (Flynn, Henshaw, O'Mahen, & Forman, 2010). This treatment preference has important implications suggesting that adequate OB/GYN care includes prenatal care, support, and mental health treatment in one site. Between weekly sessions, Ms. Garcia sometimes called me on the telephone if she felt she was in crisis, and I provided crisis intervention counseling to alleviate symptoms.

Use of time

The duration of work with a pregnant woman is determined by the client's entry into prenatal care at different gestational stages. Ms. Garcia began care early in her pregnancy so we had ample time to establish a strong therapeutic relationship and work on most of her goals. We can continue to work together postpartum for a few weeks to a few months, depending on the individual needs. Sessions are scheduled once weekly for 45 minutes and can be coordinated with the client's medical appointments.

Interventions

Both psychosocial and psychological interventions have been found effective in reducing perinatal depression symptoms. Cognitive behavioral therapy (CBT) and interpersonal therapy (IPT) are found to be helpful in significantly reducing perinatal depression symptoms. CBT is based on the theory that one's thoughts influence one's feelings and actions; if thoughts can be modified, then feelings and behaviors will change as a result. With IPT, the emphasis is on identifying issues and problems in interpersonal relationships and learning ways to address and resolve problems while improving relationships.

My main intervention with Ms. Garcia was supportive therapy including elements of CBT and IPT. Supportive therapy often leads to improvement in adaptation and interpersonal functioning by fortifying the client's strengths and providing encouragement and direction (Kleiman, 2008). Through supportive therapy, clinicians help patients learn how to move forward and make decisions or changes as they adjust to an important change. These changes may be acute, including a break-up or distressing event, or chronic situations, such as an illness (physical or emotional). Often, before adaptation can be accomplished, clients need to be given the opportunity to express their feelings and thoughts about the issues.

During the treatment phase, I gathered information regarding the frequency and duration of Ms. Garcia's depressive symptoms. As I assessed how she viewed her current situation, we confronted her negative thoughts regarding her pregnancy, worked on her role transition to mother of three children, focused on her broken relationship, and helped her to focus on positive thoughts and actions. She was encouraged to improve her communication with Juan in an effort to discuss how they would co-parent and at the same time accept the end of their romantic relationship and move forward.

Techniques used in supportive counseling such as praising, clarification, confrontation, and interpretation helped her identify areas of change, establish boundaries, and create more balance in her perception of her roles while evaluating and modifying expectations that may have been unrealistic. She set new priorities that would give her a sense of control and stability. When appropriate, I gently confronted her about dysfunctional behavior, such as her continued sexual relationship with Juan despite knowing that he no longer wanted a relationship and was seeing other women.

Stance of the social worker

Work with depressed pregnant women requires that the social worker allow clients to speak freely about their histories, their concerns, and their fears about their pregnancy. Pregnancy, childbirth, and motherhood are easily one of the most significant and stressful times in a woman's life. There are societal pressures to value these moments and be happy, expectations that force many women to suffer in silence. Additionally, I must intervene in a compassionate and non-judgmental manner because women affected by perinatal depression are often afraid to share their feelings and behaviors. They fear their children could be taken away (by Child Protective Services), that they will be asked to take psychiatric medication, or even the widespread stigma that persists about mental health treatment. I need to be comfortable hearing women describe how they may not be parenting optimally due to their symptoms, and reassure them that with symptom relief they can become nurturing parents.

I also work with the medical providers to encourage them to involve social workers as early as possible when clients report any symptoms of depression. Some medical providers attribute depressive symptoms to hormonal changes during pregnancy and dismiss the client's concerns. With enough time for intervention, we can assist women in managing their symptoms and avoid deterioration of their social situations. Helping to educate our colleagues about the importance of early intervention for perinatal depression is another important role.

Reassessment

Pregnant women with perinatal depression experience many physical and emotional changes through the gestational period. Medical issues may arise that create emotional distress for the client. Relationships with family members and significant others may change, affecting a client's overall functioning and emotional well-being. Many of our clients break up with, or are abandoned by, the fathers of their babies. Clients' housing situations change as well. Many of our clients reside in substandard or overcrowded housing and are forced to enter the NYC shelter system. The chaos and uncertainty of shelter living causes tremendous stress and hopelessness. Clients often have difficulties related to work as they may have to stop working earlier than expected, or deal with the fact that they will lose income while on maternity leave. These issues have to be addressed at every visit, to evaluate whether goals need to change so that the client does not feel overwhelmed. Clients' needs must be assessed and re-prioritized at each visit.

Case conclusion

Ms. Garcia is a capable, articulate, and responsible woman who demonstrated self-awareness and insight into her mental health concerns. She consistently attended both medical and mental health appointments and always came prepared to address her efforts toward meeting her goals. She discussed any impediments that kept her from accomplishing our mutually agreed upon objectives. Because we were able to identify symptoms of depression early on and work on strategies to alleviate these symptoms, Ms. Garcia was well prepared for her baby both physically and emotionally. Despite feelings of loss and abandonment by Juan, by late in the pregnancy she had recognized that he would not be very involved in their baby's life. Although Juan was present at the time of delivery, Ms. Garcia's mother and prenatal partners were also available to provide support. She was prepared for the baby and felt confident that she had what she needed for her daughter. Ms. Garcia also established relationships with some members of her paternal family and knew to call on them for support on days when she felt sad and hopeless. Ms. Garcia was diligent about keeping her mental health appointments post partum. At her six-week visit, I administered the EPDS and her score was not very high, confirming my observation of improvement. She was also exclusively breastfeeding and I was impressed to see how nurturing and bonded she was with her baby. Three weeks after that visit, we terminated treatment.

Differential discussion

Reflecting on my work with Ms. Garcia, I realize that I learned valuable lessons about work with women with perinatal depression. I had read a lot and received training about postpartum depression. Although symptoms of depression are the same across categories, a woman with postpartum depression experiences these symptoms much more strongly and can be impaired to the point where she is unable to do the things she needs to do every day. It is difficult to be responsible for another life when one is experiencing sleep deprivation, hormonal fluctuations, and needing to adjust to new roles.

An important lesson learned was that many women are depressed even before their child's birth and intervening early can have positive outcomes for the client's emotional health and for the mother–child relationship. If the client receives mental health treatment during the pregnancy, there will be some symptom relief. This means that by the time of childbirth, those negative feelings are not experienced as intensely. The importance of screening for perinatal depression at different points in the pregnancy with standardized tools (scales) is also clear. This helps us conduct a more comprehensive assessment and allows us to identify clients who may not voluntarily discuss their symptoms of depression.

After becoming aware of how isolated Ms. Garcia was during her pregnancy, I realized that having an on-site support group for women like her, who are experiencing symptoms of depression, would have been quite helpful. After I terminated treatment with Ms. Garcia I, with the help of a social work intern, started a support group in the clinic. Support groups can be a fruitful intervention for reaching more women in need, while allowing them to form ongoing support networks that may outlive their group involvement. Our clinic, like many others, lacks on-site psychiatric services for patients. Luckily, Ms. Garcia responded to therapy. However several clients in our clinic have histories of psychiatric illness, often with medication regimens, and they need a more comprehensive assessment by a psychiatrist for medication evaluation and management. The social work manager in the clinic continues to advocate to get this service for our clients. This case highlights the need to intervene early among mothers with perinatal depression, to provide follow-up evaluation, tailored referrals, and treatment. Screening must be a routine part of prenatal and postpartum care as there are effective treatments available that can prevent unnecessary suffering.

Discussion questions

1   Why should obstetric services have screening for perinatal depression throughout an entire pregnancy and postpartum course? What happens when screening shows a natural response to difficult circumstances?
2   What does social support have to do with perinatal depression? How does a social worker help isolated people find useful social support?
3   Explain the kind of work social workers can do with women with perinatal depression.

References

American College of Obstetricians and Gynecologists Committee Opinion No. 453 (2010). Screening for depression during and after pregnancy. *Obstetrics & Gynecology, 115*, 394–395.

American Psychiatric Association. (2013). *Diagnostic and statistical manual of mental disorders (5th edn.).* Arlington, VA: American Psychiatric Publishing.

Association of State and Territorial Health Officials (2005). Maternal and child health fact sheet. Retrieved from www.nashp.org/sites/default/files/abcd/abcd.perinataldepressionfs.pdf

Cox, J. & Holden, J. (2003). *Perinatal mental health*: *A guide to the Edinburgh Postnatal Depression Scale (EPDS).* London: Gaskell.

Davis, K., Pearlstein, T., Stuart, S., O'Hara, M., & Zlotnick, C. (2013). Analysis of brief screening tools for the detection of postpartum depression: Comparisons of the PRAMS 6-item instrument, PHQ-9, and structured interviews. *Archives of Women's Mental Health, 16*(4), 271–277. doi: 10.1007/s00737-013-0345-z

Flynn, H. A., Henshaw, E., O'Mahen, H., & Forman, J. (2010). Patient perspectives on improving the depression referral processes in obstetrics settings: A qualitative study. *General Hospital Psychiatry, 32*(1), 9–16. doi: 10.1016/j.genhosppsych.2009.07.005

Freeman, M. P. (2007). Antenatal depression: navigating the treatment dilemmas. *American Journal of Psychiatry, 164*(8), 1162–1165. doi: 10.1176/appi.ajp.2007.07020341

Gjerdingen, D. K. & Yawn, B. P. (2007). Postpartum depression screening: Importance, methods, barriers, and recommendations for practice. *Journal of the American Board of Family Medicine, 20*(3), 280–288. doi: 10.3122/jabfm.2007.03.060171

Goodman, J. H. (2009) Women's attitudes, preferences, and perceived barriers to treatment for perinatal depression. *Birth, 36*(1), 60–69. doi: 10.1111/j.1523-536X.2008.00296.x

Howell, E.A., Balbierz, A., Wang, J., Parides, M., Zlotnick, C., & Leventhal, H. (2012). Reducing postpartum depressive symptoms among black and Latina mothers. *Obstetrics and Gynecology, 119*(5), 942–949. doi: 10.1097/AOG.0b013e318250ba48

Kleiman, K. (2008). *Therapy and the postpartum woman.* New York: Routledge.

Kroenke, K., Spitzer, R., & Williams, J. (2003). The Patient Health Questionnaire-2 Validity of a two-item depression screener. *Medical Care, 41*(11), 1284–1292.

Krueger, L. (2014). Gottfried-Kruger Maternal Depression legislation. Retrieved from www.nysenate. gov/press-release/gottfried-krueger-maternal-depression-legislation-passes-both-houses-will-help-new-mot

Le, H. L., Perry, D. F., & Stuart, E. A. (2011). Randomized controlled trial of a preventive intervention for perinatal depression in high-risk Latinas. *Journal of Consulting and Clinical Psychology, 79*(2), 135–141. doi: 10.1037/a0022492

Meltzer-Brody, S. (2011). New insights into perinatal depression: Pathogenesis and treatment during pregnancy and postpartum. *Dialogues in Clinical Neuroscience, 13*(1), 89–100. Retrieved from www.ncbi.nlm.nih.gov/pmc/articles/PMC3181972/

National Research Council and Institute of Medicine (2009). *Depression in parents, parenting, and children: Opportunities to improve identification, treatment, and prevention.* Washington, DC: National Academies Press.

New Jersey Assembly (2006). An act concerning postpartum depression and amending P.L.2000, c.167 (C.26:2 -176). Retrieved from www.njleg.state.nj.us/2006/Bills/PL06/12_.HTM

Price, S.K., Corder-Mabe, J., & Austin, K. (2012). Perinatal depression screening and intervention: Enhancing health provider involvement. *Journal of Women's Health, 21*(4), 447–455. doi: 10.1089/jwh.2011.3172

Ribowsky, J. & Henderson, C. (2011). Probing postpartum depression. *Clinician Reviews, 21*(2), 29–34. Retrieved from www.clinicianreviews.com/index.php?id=31613&type=98&tx_ttnews[tt_news]=231369&cHash=da03e20e36

Rhodes, A. & Segre, L. (2013). Perinatal depression: a review of U.S legislation and law. *Archives of Women's Mental Health, 16*(4), 259–270. doi: 10.1007/s00737-013-0359-6

Shivakumar, G., Brandon, A. R., Johnson, N. L., and Freeman, M. P. (2014). Screening to treatment: obstacles and predictors in perinatal depression (STOP-PPD) in the Dallas Healthy Start Program. *Archives of Women's Mental Health, 17*(6), 575–578. doi: 10.1007/s00737-014-0438-3

Websites for support and information

New York State Department of Health, Screening for Material Depression, www.health.ny.gov/community/pregnancy/health_care/perinatal/maternal_depression/providers/screening.htm

Postpartum Progress, The Symptoms of Postpartum Depression & Anxiety (in Plain Mama English), www.postpartumprogress.com/the-symptoms-of-postpartum-depression-anxiety-in-plain-mama-english

Postpartum Support International, www.postpartum.net/

Chapter 26

Social work in the pediatric endocrinology and diabetes setting

Fighting the new epidemic of type 2 diabetes in children

Helaine Ciporen

Context

Epidemic levels of type 2 diabetes mellitus (T2DM) are now evident in children (Caprio et al., 2008). Once called adult-onset diabetes, T2DM was renamed to reflect the growing number of children affected (CDC, 2014). While this type of diabetes is associated with a genetic predisposition, the single trigger that activates the gene during childhood is obesity. A complex web of environmental, economic, political, cultural, genetic, and psychological factors have changed our lifestyle into one that promotes obesity (Bowen, Barrington, & Beresford, 2015). Currently, one third of all children in the United States, from birth through 19, are overweight or obese (CDC, 2014). This statistic foreshadows disastrous repercussions for affected children as well as potential economic havoc for our health care and insurance systems. Responses to the epidemic appear to be gaining momentum. As a result, the prevalence of childhood obesity, which had increased in the 1980s and 1990s, showed no significant change between 1999 and 2008 (Ogden, Carroll, Kit, & Flegan, 2012). Society, when motivated, can act effectively to stop this needless epidemic, especially in children (Dabelea, 2009).

While T2DM is currently more prevalent in certain ethnic, economic, and regional groups, it crosses all boundaries. Emerging first in the United States, this epidemic is now a worldwide concern. The number of people with diabetes mellitus has more than doubled globally during the past 30 years (Chen, Magliana, & Zimmet, 2012). In the U.S. health care system, racial and ethnic minorities are treated differently from White populations. The great availability of fast foods, cutbacks in physical education programs at school, trading active play time for TV and computer time, and the lack of access to fresh fruits and vegetables in certain neighborhoods, are a few of the factors contributing to the problem (Chow, Foster, Gonzalez, & LaShawn, 2012). Agricultural policy may be another force driving the proliferation of junk foods, with three subsidized crops – wheat, corn, and soybeans – being the main ingredients in processed packaged foods (Goran, Stanley, Ulijaszek, & Ventura, 2013). Meaningful lifestyle changes through individual, family, group, and outreach educational approaches can address the maladaptive behavioral, family system and psychological issues that support the epidemic (Kobel et al., 2014). Increasingly, hospitals have been called on to help. Here, social workers, as educators, advocates, and therapists, have a unique, creative opportunity to play a role in the battle (Ciporen, 2012). Credit for the deceleration of obesity in youth and the subsequent downshift of new cases of T2DM can be given in part to Michelle Obama's Let's Move program and the Robert Wood Johnson Foundation. These initiatives have spawned many local programs that have improved school menus, fitness options, and other factors that affect the health of children.

In 2006, the Hall Family Clinic for Pediatric Endocrinology and Diabetes was established as a new facility at the Mount Sinai Medical Center, a major, urban hospital complex. This specialty has always existed as a distinct service within pediatrics, serving patients with a variety of hormonal disorders, primarily type 1 diabetes, but also hyperthyroidism, premature or delayed puberty, and growth issues. Now many are seen for the prevention and/or treatment of T2DM. Typically they are between 10 and 18 years of age, but they can be as young as 5. The area served by the hospital and its immediate neighborhood has one of the highest prevalence rates of T2DM in the city and state. The population in this neighborhood is mainly Hispanic, from many nations, or African American and living at or below the poverty level. This mirrors the national profile of children most affected by T2DM (Pulgaron & Demamater, 2014).

An explanation of T2DM

The hormone insulin is required to break down carbohydrates. It is produced as needed, by the pancreas, in proportion to the amount and type of foods we ingest. T2DM occurs when the body develops a resistance to insulin and no longer uses it properly. As the need for insulin rises, the pancreas gradually loses its ability to produce sufficient amounts needed to regulate the blood sugar. Although T2DM is associated with a genetic predisposition, it will only manifest in youngsters when triggered by obesity, which puts undue stress on the pancreas. Formerly known as "old age onset" diabetes, T2DM occurs when the body's organs, including the pancreas, are naturally diminished in their functions. People began to develop T2DM at younger ages as excessive weight gain made it difficult for the pancreas to keep up with increased demands for insulin. Despite genetic predisposition, T2DM is not activated at a young age if an appropriate weight is maintained. Once T2DM is established, the persistence of obesity interferes with the response to treatment; therefore, regulating weight remains an important goal (Lawrence et al., 2008).

T2DM is generally diagnosed through presentation of clinical symptoms, including excessive thirst (polydipsia), excessive urination (polyuria), and hunger (polyphagia). In addition, when blood sugars reach very high levels, symptoms commonly mistaken for flu, such as stomach-ache, vomiting, and weight loss may occur. Acanthosis nigrocans, a darkening of the skin, typically around the neck, is another common indicator. Diagnosis is confirmed through blood glucose testing. An elevated C-peptide level signals a resistance to insulin, indicating a higher risk for developing T2DM.

Obesity trends in children show that the number of 6- to 11-year-olds at the 95th percentile of BMI (body mass index, a ratio of height and weight) was 7% in 1980 and 17.7% in 2012. Children aged 12–19 with a BMI in the 95th percentile rose from 5% in 1980 to 20.5% in 2012 (Dabelea et al., 2014). In New York City, in 1996, almost 20% of third-grade children and more than 20% of sixth-grade children were found to be overweight; in 2003, an estimated 43% of public elementary school students were overweight, and 24% of those students were obese. Currently, due to the success of various interventions, the prevalence of obesity in grades K–8 decreased 5.5%, from 21.9% in 2006–2007 to 20.7% in 2010–2011. Among children in all age groups, socioeconomic and racial/ethnic populations, the decrease was smaller among Black (1.9%) and Hispanic (3.4%) children than among Asian/Pacific Islander (7.6%) and White (12.5%) children (CDC, 2011). Children who are overweight are at risk for a multitude of related medical problems, including heart and kidney disease, sleep apnea, exacerbation of asthma, and cardiovascular problems leading to blindness and amputation (Kaufman, 2002).

Government bodies are beginning to address the T2DM epidemic, yet to date, no coherent national policy has emerged. New York City is a leader in establishing aggressive health policies. Trans fats have been banned as an ingredient in prepared foods, calorie counts are mandated to be listed on menus, school menus are being revamped, and fruit and vegetable selling green carts have opened in neighborhoods designated as food deserts. On the state level, a tax on sugared soda had been considered but proved highly unpopular with consumers. Much like the cigarette tax, this new "obesity tax" was intended to reduce the consumption of highly caloric drinks while raising money for health programs (Chan, 2008). Health insurers are considering new policies as well, as they try to limit their costs of care per subscriber. Like auto insurers who offer incentives for good driving records, health insurers may someday tie rates to healthy, or lowered, BMIs. In the private sector, the Robert Wood Johnson Foundation devoted itself to abolishing obesity in children by the year 2015, offering a wide range of grant support to creative initiatives and research throughout the country. While they have not met this goal, they have certainly raised awareness and helped to foster a successful variety of programs nationwide. Despite its chronic nature, T2DM is not considered a disability and therefore those who have it do not qualify for SSI or other supplemental entitlements or benefits.

Technology

Developments in pharmacological, technological, and surgical interventions mean that we know far more about the management of diabetes than we did, even 10 years ago. Theoretically, no one need suffer the devastating side effects, such as blindness or amputation of lower limbs that were viewed as inevitable just a generation ago. The development of long- and short-acting insulin makes the careful regulation of blood possible and Glucophage, the only oral agent approved for pediatric use, may suffice as the only necessary medication. With improved technology one gets nearly instant blood glucose level readings from a tiny drop of blood. These readings are stored within the meter, so personal trends can be monitored, insulin needs calibrated, and medication levels adjusted for more accurate control. Patients now have a choice of insulin delivery systems, such as ports or pumps inserted on the abdomen or thigh, that only need to be changed every other day, replacing multiple daily injections.

When lifestyle changes or pharmacological interventions fail to produce the desired results, various bariatric surgical interventions, such as gastric bypass or gastric banding, can be considered to control obesity. This surgery has been used successfully with adults, but is considered a last resort for teens who suffer multiple complications related to T2DM. There are stringent guidelines for both the medical team and the teenage patient, including six months of lifestyle modification and a psychosocial evaluation to ensure appropriate family support and medical adherence after surgery (Endocrine Society, 2015). This intervention has various risks and side effects, and is in the early stages of being offered to older teens.

Ironically, low-tech interventions and simple lifestyle changes prove to be the safest, least costly, and most effective interventions, but lifestyle change is elusive. Yet it is here, in the "low-tech" solution, that social workers can be most effective. Social workers can explore the psychosocial factors that impede treatment and develop pragmatic plans to overcome them. Social workers are trained to address the psychological and motivational issues that are too often overlooked. I have successfully used individual psychotherapeutic work with children, psychoeducational work with families, group work, and outreach education events as interventions to meet these goals.

Organization

Patients are generally referred to this specialty clinic by their pediatrician or pediatric emergency room. A multi-disciplinary team of endocrinologists, nurse practitioner, nutritionist, and social worker meet with patients and their families to develop appropriate treatment plans for prevention or management of diabetes. Social work clinical practice in endocrinology and diabetes requires a working knowledge of current medical practice, features of various treatment options and technologies, and access to local resources in order to facilitate the family's decision making process. It also requires strong clinical skills, especially in understanding the effects of chronic illness on the patient and family.

Decisions about practice

John, a 12-year-old Hispanic boy, was referred to the clinic by his pediatrician for evaluation of obesity and risk for T2DM. He lives near the hospital with his parents, two younger sisters, and paternal grandmother. There is a strong family history of T2DM, with his father and grandmother affected among others. John presented with a BMI in the 92nd percentile and acanthosis nigricans, a skin disorder characterized by dark, thick velvety skin in body folds and creases, visible around his neck.

Definition of the client

In a pediatric setting, because patients are minors, they are accompanied by their caregivers, most often their mothers, but also other family members or guardians. Teens returning for routine follow-up may arrive independently. The child and primary caregiver are thought of as a unit. When this dyad is part of a larger unit, the entire family is considered the patient. It is likely that the lifestyle modifications being called for will, to some extent, affect all family members. It is also likely that other family members are overweight and at risk for T2DM, but may not recognize this in themselves. This is true for John's family, where his father, paternal grandmother, and two younger sisters are all overweight.

There is often a multi-generational awareness of T2DM because it is genetically linked. It is important to explore the family's preconceptions about T2DM because members' experiences and possible idiosyncratic misconceptions may exist as hidden barriers to treatment. Family members may have varying points of view on how to treat illness. These opinions may differ between generations or between the main decision-makers, the parents. Consideration must be given to the family's cultural and religious background, as well as their economic and educational status in developing effective plans. John's mother was very worried about her children getting T2DM. She saw its devastating effects on her husband and mother-in-law and was motivated to help her children in any way she could. However, John's father had not taken an active stance in controlling his own weight or blood sugars, considering T2DM inevitable. John's grandmother was depressed by the complications she had already suffered. This sense of hopelessness was perceived by the children and may have triggered a level of anxiety they then attempted to quell by overeating.

In the pediatric setting, responsibility for executing treatment plans falls to the parents or caregivers, and educational efforts are largely aimed towards them. Caregivers are also the ones who buy, prepare, and serve the family meals. They can be empowered to make needed changes by reminding them that, in the same manner they have taught their children to brush their teeth and cross the street safely, they are also teaching them how to make diet and exercise choices, either directly or by example. Establishing the right habits early in life is the best prevention for a host of future health problems related to or exacerbated by obesity.

Receiving a diagnosis of T2DM is life altering, and can be traumatic for parents who may feel guilt about transferring a condition with a genetic component. Children's reactions are often cued by parents' response to the diagnosis, therefore helping parents cope by providing the "permission" they need to attend to their own needs can also be beneficial in mediating the child's adjustment process. Type 2 diabetes, once contracted, becomes a lifelong consideration; so prevention or forestalling of onset is well worth the effort. By informing John's parents of the latest developments in diabetes care, I was able to motivate his mother and pique his father's interest in exploring lifestyle changes that could benefit the whole family.

A family's coping style may be shaped by cultural or religious heritage. For instance, one family had a heightened need for confidentiality because they felt their child's future prospects for marriage would be compromised if the child's condition was known within their community. Another family initially rejected pharmacological solutions due to religious teachings, another due to their cultural preference for herbal remedies. Ethnicity also plays a large role in foods the family cooks and eats, creating resistance to change and making this topic difficult to discuss. When John's mother met with our nutritionist, they made slight adjustments to treasured family recipes, reducing the fat content and increasing the quantity of vegetables. The family was also encouraged to switch, first to 2% milk, then later to 1%, so the taste difference would hardly be noticed. Making one small change at a time is a surer routine to lasting lifestyle changes than is crash dieting, which eventually wears out one's willpower, leading only to frustration and failure.

Poverty, lack of disposable income, educational status, poor access to resources, and chaotic family life can pose serious obstacles to making fitness changes. Many creative options can be considered, including free activities sponsored by the local parks department, sports leagues, volunteering for gardening or dog walking duties, or simple family walks after dinner. Other economic considerations include access to and cost of food. Many poor neighborhoods are food deserts, do not have adequate supermarkets, and rely on small shops where choices are limited to expensive prepared foods. Access to farmer's markets may be limited or families may not be familiar with the array of fruits and vegetables available there. John's mother was introduced to the hospital's newly established farmer's market and was motivated to use it when she learned of the acceptance of food vouchers, additional discount coupons, and available recipes. A family may run out of food vouchers before the end of the month and fall back on a diet of less-expensive high-carbohydrate foods, such as rice and beans. Education on alternative food options and assistance in planning family menus can be a helpful solution.

The effects of poverty can be far reaching on very personal levels. For instance, our staff were concerned that the daughters of one family, headed by a single mother, were watching too much TV and therefore not getting enough physical activity. The mother did not attempt to hide her contempt when she explained why she was happy to know her girls were safe at home. She had lost her teenage son to the lures of the street and gang violence and had no intention of allowing the girls to stray. She felt misunderstood and frustrated in resolving her daughters' health issues, which seemed less important than other potential dangers they faced. Now she also felt abandoned by our staff. In letting her know that her circumstances were understood and helping her prioritize and deal with other issues, such as her daughter's school placements, I established a better partnership with her and devised a more reasonable health plan with them.

Strategies and intervention

I employ four distinct forms of intervention: working individually with children, working with the family unit, group work, and outreach education efforts (Figure 26.1). I will address the

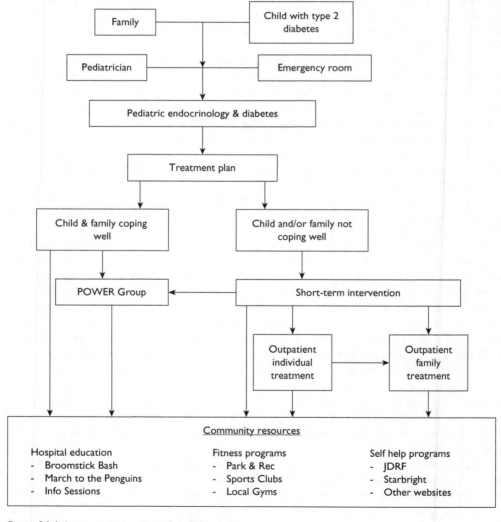

Figure 26.1 Intervention options for diabetes care

goals, contracting, meeting place, use of time and resources, social work stance, reassessment, and transfer needs that are unique to each interventional forms.

Common to all is a family-centered approach because a family is a natural "team." It follows that family-based weight management works best; it takes advantage of a pre-existing, cohesive support network. Recommendations on food and fitness are beneficial to all family members. I avoid singling out overweight children here because doing so could make them feel deprived or judged as a result of their health needs. It is recommended that the families eat together, eat the same healthy foods, and exercise together whenever possible.

Working individually with children

The decision to work therapeutically with children is made based on their adjustment to the diagnosis and their coping ability. The need for intervention will usually manifest in a variety of acting out behaviors, such as a change in school performance or peer relationships, tearfulness, volatility, or loss of interest in their usual activities. They may experience a loss of their age appropriate sense of invulnerability and feel they are now "broken." There are several goals in working with children individually: facilitate adjustment to the diagnosis, uncover and address any psychological issues that would impede adherence to medical treatment, enlist the child's active participation in developing and executing the treatment plan. A parent's permission and cooperation must be obtained before intervening with a child and it is best to meet with parents at regular intervals to ensure continuity of care. Children's participation is key to the success of the treatment plan and, more importantly, to their future well-being. This is a "teaching moment" when positive attitudes and good habits can be established. Motivational interviewing and play therapy can be especially effective in eliciting a child's active involvement.

Among attitudes and concerns to be explored are: the effect of the diagnosis on self-image, the understanding of the diagnosis and the treatment needs, the relationship to family members, especially parents, communication styles within the family, needs for privacy, and plans to share information with others. Children often feel they are limited to "eavesdropping" on their parents in order to learn about their medical condition. Encouraging children to ask questions and express their feelings helps to illuminate issues and misconceptions.

Children can be very concrete in their thinking. John, upon hearing that he was now at risk for T2DM, began to cry inconsolably. With further support, he was able to articulate his fear of imminent death; "Why else would they call it 'die'-abetes?" This level of thinking must be considered at any age. For instance, in devising a weekly exercise or snack plan, a child will be familiar with the concept of a "week," but not necessarily know that it consists of seven days. It is safest to provide a calendar or other age-appropriate, concrete, or visual supports.

I consider the full range of child therapy interventions in devising a treatment plan, and I assess the child's maturational, as well as chronological age, interests, and skill levels. Keeping a diary, for instance, may be a good tool for a teenage girl, but not for one who has a reading disability and/or is disinterested in writing. Teaching hypnotherapy or relaxation techniques can be effective in assisting the child in managing the fear or pain of injections and finger pricks.

Children see themselves as members of a family system, identifying with their culture, religion, and other family traits. While this is often positive, it can sometimes work in a negative way. In John's case, mirroring an attitude expressed by his father, he assumed T2DM was his unavoidable fate. He was terrified because he had seen his grandmother's complications, including amputation of lower limbs. I explained that these side effects are now avoidable, and his relief was palpable when his misconceptions were addressed. John had no underlying psychopathology and needed only short-term intervention. In partnership with our medical team, he learned to forestall the onset of T2DM by making healthier decisions. John transformed from a belligerent resister who quelled his anxieties with food, to a full partner, enlisting his mother's and our support in the plan he helped devise to stay healthy.

It is important to help children think through their attitudes towards privacy. Even the child who seems to be adjusting well and wants to share information about their diabetes with friends may not be prepared for the variety of responses they may encounter. For instance, some friends may fear that diabetes is contagious, some may be repulsed by the possible need for daily injections, while others may consider it heroic. It is best to prepare the child, in advance, for these types of questions and reactions. Unanticipated overexposure to public scrutiny may interfere with the child's adherence to treatment. They may become reluctant to go to the school nurse before lunch time or consume inappropriate snacks along with their friends after school in an effort to conceal their medical needs.

The relationship between child and clinic generally lasts many years. I begin to make plans for transfer to an adult service a year prior to children's aging out of pediatrics at 21. We discuss the transition of disengaging from a trusted, long-term relationship with our staff to reengaging with a new support team who will expect them to behave as autonomous adults. This new expectation accounts for the major differences in adult and pediatric treatment style.

Working with the family

The medical team views the parent as the adult responsible for overseeing adherence to the treatment plan. My goal is to ease parents through the first stage of coping with the new diagnosis and then help them integrate the demands of the treatment plan into the family's existing routine. A non-judgmental and pragmatic approach, framing a series of desired adjustments as small, manageable steps, helps to diminish their feelings of being overwhelmed. Children are still growing and should not be on restrictive diets which may trigger an eating disorder. Instead, establishing moderation and healthy choices should be fostered. Often, the objective is simply for the child to not gain additional weight. As they grow taller, their BMI will automatically be reduced. Small changes, such as switching to 1% milk, giving up sugared drinks, or adding 15 extra minutes of daily physical activity may be all that is needed.

Meetings with individuals or families take place in my office. The clinic itself is a new facility offering a pleasant and cheerful atmosphere for children and families, but the hospital is a large, imposing building and often associated with health crises and stressful times for families. An individual session will be between 30 minutes and an hour. Patients are scheduled for routine follow-up clinic visits four times per year, but more frequent visits will occur as required, especially after a new diagnosis. At this time or during crises, I may see patients as often as once or twice per week. Patients are free to see the social worker during any clinic visit, and I use each encounter to reassess the family's needs and make appropriate adjustments or interventions.

In family work, I am often the families' and medical staff's "go-between." As I explore what has transpired, I reword medical explanations to be more easily understood, and I urge the family to bring any questions to the appropriate team professional. I explained to John, in terms he could understand, how high blood glucose levels contribute to circulatory problems and in turn, provoke the consequences his grandmother suffered. He could understand that these problems were avoidable if he utilized the technology available to him today to keep his blood sugars stable. I advise the staff of these conversations, both in patient chart notes and during our twice-weekly medical rounds, so they can be better prepared for their next patient encounters.

In our urban community, we have a variety of resources. I keep lists, including local playgrounds and parks, their classes and other activities, important informational web sites, low-calorie snack recipes, self-help groups, etc., and distribute them. John eventually decided to pursue his interest in soccer, and I directed him to a local league and secured a waiver for his fees and uniform. His father enjoys watching John's games and may become involved with the league himself. I also make in-house referrals to the Adolescent Health Center, child psychiatry, and other specialty clinics. Referrals often include social, legal, employment, education, housing, and other services. Thus, I build a partnership with the family. As other possibly more pressing family stressors are relieved or resolved, there is more capacity to focus on health issues.

Working with groups – the POWER Program

The POWER Group (Parent Power Over Weight, Eating Right) was established to empower parents to protect their families from the avoidable health risks associated with obesity, including T2DM. In addition to information about nutrition and fitness, we discuss the behavioral, environmental, and motivational issues the families face. The twice monthly program is free and open to any parent or caregiver who wants to attend. The mix of participants varies in each session. Members of the group are mostly mothers of clinic families from the neighborhood who are able to attend on weekdays. Randomly, the group may or may not be cohesive in its ethnic, economic, or geographical make-up, but the uniting factor is members' concern for their children. This is a powerful bond, allowing seemingly disparate parties to communicate effectively. Those who have attended six or more sessions seem to benefit most in adapting and implementing new approaches to their family's health needs.

My stance in group work is to promote a level of comfort by introducing the participants, helping them identify a subject or theme, and taking a back seat to their spontaneous discussion, intervening only when needed. I always learn something new which often leads to ideas for more effective interventions. In this setting, John's mother explored behavioral issues that were undermining her efforts to improve the family's health. Excessive TV and snacking are common concerns. Mothers encouraged each other to set time limits on TV viewing, and together we devised a multi-stepped plan of first switching to healthier snacks, then limiting portions, and finally substituting some TV time with family activities such as preparing healthy snacks together. Synergistically, I addressed John's TV habits with him in our individual sessions and enlisted his cooperation in limiting his viewing time. As his fear of diabetes subsided and his sense of mastery grew, his need to quell his anxiety through overeating also diminished.

Outreach education

The goal of outreach education is to raise awareness of preferred nutritional and physical fitness habits. The Broomstick Bash, a candy-less Halloween party, and March to the Penguins, a family exercise experience, are enjoyable ways to learn about health.

Events have experiential and interactive learning components. These high "entertainment value" events have proven to be an effective means of reaching people, attracting as many as 800 participants at a time. Children with type 1 diabetes or T2DM are invited. To encourage prevention, the events are also advertised through diabetes organizations and to the public.

The Broomstick Bash takes place in the large public lobby of a main campus building, festively decorated for the occasion. Children are rewarded with non-edible treats, such as stretchy skeletons, day-glo bracelets, and vampire teeth as they complete each activity. Family goody bags that include educational resource materials, farmer's market food coupons, recipes, free gym passes, and other pertinent gifts are distributed. Families are gathered in small groups and escorted through the event by a trained "team host." Each group is led through three educational stations: "Freaky Foods" to investigate healthier food choices, "Monster Moves" to explore incorporating fitness into one's daily routine, and "Pumpkin Pledges" to activate their motivation and set goals for themselves. Members of our clinic staff use an interactive approach, engaging the children directly in games and conversation about the given subject. Appealing and engaging visual aids are used to support the interaction. An inclusive "good, better, best" approach is employed to encourage children and families to examine current practices and take small steps towards developing better habits. For instance, one game "swaps" fast foods options to make healthier choices. Trading large for regular-size French fries, eliminating cheese from a hamburger or adding a salad are all small, realistic decisions that result in better outcomes. Lessons are graphic, concrete, and appropriate for a range of ages. For instance, faced with a table set with many small cups filled with one tablespoon of sugar each, children appear startled to discover how many tablespoons (8 or more) are in drinks like soda. They develop a more concrete understanding of the hidden calories they are consuming and can make smarter choices. John, who had come to this event with his sisters and a few classmates, was overheard debating with them about their food choices and who had guessed correctly in some of the games they played. My hope is that this sort of healthy competition will be reactivated at school and will nudge them into choosing healthier snacks. After participants complete all three educational stations, additional activities include Monster Mash dance exercises (led by local youth karate instructors), broomstick and mask decorating, and face painting. Children are eligible for additional raffle prizes when they drink and submit their emptied water bottle, received earlier at the "hydration station." There is a vegetable soup making demonstration and tasting. Children are surprised to learn they actually do like vegetables. Families are encouraged to repeat this at home; they receive the recipe and food coupons to spend at the local farmer's market.

The spring event, March to the Penguins, has a similar format, but with an emphasis on exercise. Families are gathered in small groups and led through the three educational stations to explore food, exercise, and goal-setting options. Then, they are outfitted with a penguin logo backpack filled with lunch, water bottle, educational materials, and a pedometer. Taking advantage of the hospital's geographic location, the experiential segment of this event consists of each group walking, parade style, through Central Park to its zoo, where families gain free entry. The walk is broken into four 15-minute segments, with a short session of exercises, such as jumping jacks, at each stop. At the last stop, we eat our picnic lunch and participate in a final round of group exercise, using fitness bands that participants keep as motivational awards. Upon reaching the zoo, families are free to enjoy the rest of the afternoon on their own.

Differential discussion

Is it possible to change a culture? Is it possible to alter a lifestyle that makes fast food and other time-saving conveniences a necessity but leaves no time for cooking nutritious meals or exercise? In a word, yes. We have good examples of society making major, previously unimaginable shifts in cigarette smoking, driving while intoxicated, and wearing seat-belts. While none of these problems has been completely eradicated, they reveal our societal ability to reverse harmful, unhealthy trends. Unfortunately, these efforts have succeeded less well in marginalized segments of our society where social workers have a critical role to play in improving social justice. It is essential to not ghettoize a health issue as important as obesity. The food industry has been adroit in adapting to and exploiting the latest trends, as there is a clear economic advantage for them to provide newly packaged "lite" foods. Likewise, television, with shows like "Biggest Loser," is keen to capitalize on trends of interest to its viewers. Governmental agencies and legislators tend to enact change at a slower pace, but The Affordable Care Act has fomented a major shift in focus for the medical sector. Previously remunerated for curing illness, now there is financial reward for preventing it. A constellation of broad measures, from all sectors, public, private, and personal, will be needed to reverse this trend. With programs like Let's Move, national attitudes appear to be changing. The deceleration of children's obesity rates indicates the "tipping point" for significant change may be near.

Discussion questions

1   Many T2DM issues have to do with a combination of the built environment and health behaviors. Although it is very difficult to help people to change their health behaviors, change can happen with the social worker's help. How about the built environment? How can social workers exert their influence in this regard?
2   This chapter is distinguished by the range of interventions that the social worker uses. Should we expect all social workers in health care to have that range of skill sets? Why or why not?
3   The family about whom the case chapter is written is considered Hispanic (although the word Hispanic only refers to being Spanish speaking). Does that categorization help social workers to make practice decisions with their clients? Why or why not?

References and resources

Bowen, D. J., Barrington, W. E., & Beresford, S. A. (2015). Identifying the effects of environmental and policy change interventions on healthy eating. *Annual Review of Public Health, 36*, 289–306. doi: 10.1146/annurev-publhealth-032013-182516

Caprio, S., Daniels, J. R., Drewnowski, A., Kaufman, F. R., Palinkas, L. A., Rosenbloom, A. L., & Schwimmer, J. B. (2008). Influences of race, ethnicity and culture on childhood obesity: Implications for prevention and treatment: consensus statement of shaping America's health and the obesity society. *Diabetes Care, 31*, 2211–2221. doi: 10.2337/dc08-9024

CDC (Centers for Disease Control) (2011, December 16). Obesity in K-8 Students New York City, 2006–07 to 2010–11 school years. *Morbidity and Mortality Weekly Report (MMWR), 2011/60*(49), 1673–1678.

CDC (2014). *National diabetes statistics report*. Retrieved from www.cdc.gov/diabetes/pubs/statsreport14/national-diabetes-report-web.pdf

Chan, S. (2008, December 17). Tax on many soft drinks sets off a spirited debate. *New York Times*, p. A 36.

Chen, L, Magliana, D. J., & Zimmet, P. Z. (2012). The worldwide epidemiology of type 2 diabetes mellitus – present and future perspectives. *Nature Reviews Endocrinology, 8*, 228–236. doi: 10.1038/nrend0.2011.183

Chow, E. A., Foster, H. F., Gonzalez, V., & LaShawn, M., (2012). The disparate impact of diabetes in racial/ethnic minority populations, *Clinical Diabetes, 30*, 130–133. doi: 10.2337/diaclin.30.3.130

Ciporen, H. (2012). Social workers' role in combating the new epidemic of type 2 diabetes in children: Clinical interventions at the Hall Family Center for pediatric endocrinology and diabetes. *Social Work in Health Care, 51*, 22–35. doi: 10.1080/00981389.2011.622634

Dabelea, D. (2009). The accelerating epidemic of childhood diabetes. *The Lancet, 373*(9680), 1999–2000.

Dabelea, D., Mayer-Davis, E. J., Saydah, S., Imperatore, G., Linder, B., Divers, J., et al. (2014). Prevalence of type 1 and type 2 diabetes among children and adolescents from 2001 to 2009. *Journal of the American Medical Association, 311*, 1778–1786. doi: 10.1001/jama.2014.3201

Endocrine Society (2015). *Prevention and treatment of pediatric obesity: Clinical practice guideline based on expert opinion.* Retrieved from https://www.endocrine.org/education-and-practice-management/clinical-practice-guidelines

Goran, M. L., Stanley, L., Ulijaszek, J., & Ventura, E. J. (2013). High fructose corn syrup and diabetes prevalence: A global perspective. *Global Public Health, 8*, 55–64. doi:10.1080/17441692.2012.736257

Kaufman, F. R. (2002). Type 2 diabetes in children and young adults: A "New Epidemic". *Clinical Diabetes, 20*, 217–218. doi: 10.2337/diaclin.20.4.217

Kobel, S., Wirt, T., Schreiber, A., Kesztyus, D., Kettner, S., Etkelenz, N., et al. (2014). Intervention effects of a school-based health promotion programme on obesity related behavioural outcomes. *Journal of Obesity, Article ID 476230*, 8 pages. doi: 10.1155/2014/476230

Lawrence, J. M., Liese, A. D., Lui, L., Dabelea, D., Anderson, A., Imperatore, G., & Bell, R. (2008). Weight-loss practices and weight-related issues among youth with Type 1 or Type 2 diabetes. *Diabetes Care, 31*, 2251–2257.

Ogden, C. L., Carroll, M. D., Kit, B. K., & Flegan, K. M. (2012). Prevalence of obesity and trends in body mass index among US children and adolescents, 1999–2010. *Journal of the American Medical Association, 307*(5), 483–490. doi: 10.1001/jama.2012.40

Pulgaron, E. R. & Demamater, A. M. (2014). Obesity and type 2 diabetes in children: Epidemiology and treatment. *Current Diabetes Reports, 14*, 508. doi: 10.1007/s11892-014-0508-y

Helpful websites

American Diabetes Association, www.diabetes.org
International Diabetes Federation, www.idf.org
Juvenile Diabetes Research Foundation, www.jdrf.org
Let's Move, www.letsmove.gov
Robert Wood Johnson Foundation, www.rwjf.org
Search for Diabetes in Youth, www.searchfordiabetes.org

Managing asthma from a social work perspective in a center for children with special health needs

Laura Boyd and Toba Schwaber Kerson

Context

Policy and technology

According to the American Lung Association, asthma is an inflammatory condition of the bronchial airways. These changes produce airway obstruction, chest tightness, coughing, and wheezing. If severe, this can cause severe shortness of breath and low blood oxygen. Each individual suffers a different level of severity. Virtually all children with asthma, however, do enjoy a reversal of symptoms until something triggers the next episode (American Lung Association, 2015).

National policies affecting the care of children with asthma are related to the Maternal and Child Health Bureau (a section of the Health Resources and Services Administration), the State Children's Health Program, Medicaid, the Affordable Care Act, and Individualized Education Plans (IEPs) that are mandated through the Individuals with Disabilities Act. Since each of these policies is described elsewhere in this volume, I will only name them here. Suffice to say that, especially among the urban poor and members of minority groups, childhood asthma is a growing problem. In the United States, the prevalence of asthma increased 12.3% from 7.3% (20.3 million persons) in 2001 to 8.2% (24.6 million persons) in 2009. Among those less than 18 years old, the prevalence was 9.6%, highest among poor children (13.5%) and among non-Hispanic Black children (17.0%) (Vital Signs, 2011). Currently, about 8.7 million children ages 5–17 years old have asthma (American Lung Association, 2012). Asthma's impact on the health care system is extraordinary, accounting for 500,000 hospitalizations, 13.9 million outpatient visits, two million Emergency Department visits, and 5,000 deaths annually (Ur-Rehman Malik, Kumar, & Frieri, 2012). More uninsured persons with asthma than insured could not afford to buy prescription medications (40.3% versus 11.5%), and fewer uninsured persons reported seeing or talking with a primary care physician (58.8% versus 85.6%) or specialist (19.5% versus 36.9%) (Vital Signs, 2011). For a pediatric social worker, the impact of asthma on a child's development and behavior, ability to participate in both school and other activities, and on the family is critical.

In 1991, The National Cooperative Inner-City Asthma Study (NCIAS) received funding and, in 2000, the Inner-City Asthma Intervention (ICAI) was awarded additional funding to develop a coordinated, focused, evidence-based intervention program for children with asthma (Findley et al., 2011; Spiegel et al., 2006). Uniquely, this program focused on both medical and social interventions with its primary purpose being prevention. With other team members, they developed a finely tuned, comprehensive approach that allows families to effectively create environments in which their children's asthma can be best managed outside of the medical setting (American Academy of Pediatrics, 2015). Project results show that while families face challenges, a multi-faceted approach is often successful. My role on the team was to weave medical management into patients' everyday lives.

If asthma can be largely controlled, why does it profoundly affect children, preventing them from enjoying typical activities, interfering with their education, and resulting in so many hospitalizations? For example, asthma is one of the most common causes of school absenteeism (CDC, 2015). Families with asthmatic children report higher incidences of ADHD, anxiety, depression, and learning disabilities (Imami et al., 2014; Terre, 2011). This added stress can negatively affect families' and children's abilities to develop positive coping strategies and manage the illness. Social workers are crucial parts of this puzzle linking children and families with appropriate medical, social, and behavioral services to minimize the negative impact of asthma.

Due to medical advances, asthma can largely be controlled with preventive medications, specialized treatments for exacerbations, and lifestyle and environmental changes. With these advances in technology and improved understanding of asthma triggers, children's asthma can be better managed. Other changes in technology relate to internet access and record-keeping. Electronic medical records (EMR) enable pediatricians to track admissions, prescriptions, and specialists' reports within a hospital system. Furthermore, increased internet access provides additional education and allows parents and children to communicate with others struggling with asthma.

Organization

José, the child who is the focus of this case study, is a patient of the Center for Children with Special Health Care Needs at St. Christopher's Hospital for Children. The hospital is located in an impoverished area that is considered a "food desert" and the third hungriest district in the United States. The neighborhoods surrounding the Hospital are made up of a population that is multi-ethnic, mostly poor, working class White, Hispanic/Latino, African American, and Asian with a growing number from the Middle East. The disproportionate rates of asthma among inner-city impoverished communities and members of minority groups is concerning because the insufficient resources and educational opportunities in such areas contribute to a rising public health concern (Bryant-Stephens et al., 2012; Clark, 2012). The best way to rectify this inequity is through a multi-faceted, systems approach specifically tailored to the needs of the family, an approach so often at the core of social work.

When the Center began, professional staff consisted of two primary care physicians specializing in children with special needs, a nurse care coordinator, and a social worker. The Center provides a medical home for children and adolescents who must learn to manage chronic conditions such as asthma, obesity, mental and behavioral issues, or poor oral health. The Center's mission is to reinforce recommended medical management for at-risk children and to support stability within the family by providing resources, coordination, health education, and intensive follow-up. Frequently, the lack of family stability causes caregivers to struggle to manage their children's medical needs, resulting in increased emergency room visits and hospitalizations. It can be challenging to remember a child's medication schedule and specialist appointments, and to recognize symptoms before the child is in crisis. It can be increasingly challenging to coordinate all of the above when the caregiver struggles with social issues such as inappropriate housing, domestic violence, neighborhood violence, mental health issues, and substance use within the family. Often, preventive medical care goes by the wayside.

Typical clients and situations

As you can surmise from the description of our surroundings and the problems that families must manage, our typical clients are impoverished, living in very poor housing with few neighborhood amenities, and often dealing with domestic violence, lack of adequate employment, and mental health issues. They all have chronic medical diagnoses.

Decisions about practice

Description of the client situation

José, 11 years old and Hispanic, is diagnosed with severe, persistent asthma and a learning disability, both of which severely affect his home and school life. He lives with his mother, Evelyn, and his 9-year-old sister, Sara, and has a 21-year-old transient brother, Carlos. When Carlos was living at home, he stayed out very late, bringing home friends involved in the drug trade who were often under the influence, loud, and occasionally violent. Carlos had been incarcerated in the past. Evelyn became so worried about Carlos's safety that she would sometimes leave both of her younger children alone sleeping at home to follow Carlos through the streets of their high crime area in order to protect him. This often left Evelyn tired, angry, and depressed the following day and meant that she did not consistently have the patience necessary for her other children, their school meetings, and medical appointments.

Evelyn left her husband, the father of her three children, about 5 years ago after enduring years of physical violence, emotional turmoil, and financial control as well as the roller coaster ride of living with a crack cocaine user. After she left, her husband never again physically hurt Evelyn or the children, but his threats felt very real, and Evelyn feared bumping into him in their neighborhood. She has few people whom she trusts and who help her. Still, to avoid further threats and harassment, Evelyn agreed that their father could see José and Sara on the weekends without court involvement.

Unfortunately, José's father's lifestyle is not conducive to the consistency needed to raise children, especially a child with a learning disability and chronic medical condition. His father rarely remembered José's medication, and both parents believed that an 11 year old should be able to manage his own medication often saying: "He's old enough to figure it out and to deal with the consequences if he doesn't. It's his problem." Both parents have asthma and it seemed normal to them that José's asthma prevented him from many outdoor activities and being a carefree child. José's parents saw his asthma as an inevitable part of life rather than a manageable condition that should not prevent him from age-appropriate activities.

The prevalence of asthma in Philadelphia is extremely high, with approximately 22% of Philadelphia children under 18 diagnosed with asthma – nearly double the national rate (Philadelphia Allies Against Asthma, 2015). This extremely high rate of asthma could make it appear that asthma is commonplace and not serious. Research has shown that asthma has particular links with urban centers and poverty due to substandard housing conditions, early exposure to high levels of mite allergen (in dust), and life stressors linked with poverty that pose challenges to consistent coordinated medical care (Imami, 2011). In addition, José's learning disability meant that he spent half of his school day in special education core academic classes. Managing asthma is an enormous responsibility for any child but more so for a child with José's limited abilities and supports.

Sadly, due to many other issues occurring at his mother's and his father's homes as well as a lax attitude towards the severity and controllability of asthma, many preventive measures were ignored. José did not regularly take medication at home, his parents did not create an asthma action plan, and recommended routine medical appointments with his pulmonologist did not occur. Much of José's medical management came during an asthma attack when he was already in a health crisis. The family often ended up in the emergency room, and José was hospitalized on several occasions including twice in intensive care.

When José came to us, he said frequently that he was not feeling well, he was failing in school, and his mother was extremely frustrated with the medical and educational systems. As their social worker, I noted that Evelyn was consistently sad, often crying and not able to articulate why she was tired. She appeared angry with José, yelling at him and telling us that he knew to take his medication and to tell her when he was not feeling well, but because "he was a bad kid and always getting into trouble" he would not do it.

Definition of the client

José is the identified patient. However, for José to receive the care that we recommend, we have to note household stressors that can distract the family, preventing them from focusing on José's medical needs. Thus, José remains at the center of the care plan with the understanding that at times I may focus on other family members or issues.

Goals

Our goal at the Center is to work with the family to address barriers to the child's medical care. Our assistance may come in the form of educational sessions with caregivers, community resources, forming a relationship with the school system to build consistency with medical management, or taking the time to troubleshoot problems to alleviate the family's burden. In this case, our goals were to better stabilize the family situation so that they could concentrate on José's care. I needed to hear from the family what they needed in order to focus on José's asthma. We built our care plan with José at the center to achieve comprehensive management.

Developing objectives and contracting

José's primary care physician and I met often to strategize about how to address this dysfunctional and dangerous situation. When I spoke to Evelyn, she listed the following barriers: (1) "My son, Carlos, is on and off the streets and might be using drugs. At the very least, he's dealing. It's making me crazy," (2) "José won't take his medicine," (3) "My ex-husband sees the kids and he never remembers José's medicine," (4) "I don't like José's school. They're always calling me and complaining about José. There's nothing that I can do. I don't know what they want from me," (5) "I'm tired and frustrated. I don't want to deal with this mess anymore." Evelyn's responses provided me with our framework. We developed an intervention to assist with stabilizing the outlying factors affecting Evelyn's ability to help José both medically and educationally. For the moment, my focus shifted from José to his mother.

Children come with guardians, and in order to intervene with children, I must consider and assist the adults who make decisions for them.

Meeting place and use of time

Most meetings took place within our clinic during José's follow-up or sick visits. To best support the family, I had to be flexible. During clinic visits, my time with the family depended on the physician's structuring of José's visit. I could meet with the family before or after the physician had completed the exam. This also depended on whether the family had time to meet with me after José's appointment. At times, Evelyn and I made appointments to speak privately. Also, I attended several school meetings and supported the family by phone.

Strategies and interventions

I began by clarifying with Evelyn that our program's help with other issues in the family was to help with José's less than optimal asthma management. Through coordinating services, I could ease some of the stress in the family. We discussed Evelyn's concerns about Carlos at length and considered how his lifestyle affects the rest of the family. We discussed how José and Sara perceive Carlos (their older brother). Through long discussions about how terrified Evelyn was about Carlos's future, she was able to connect that her feelings about this tenuous situation were similar to her younger children's feelings about Carlos. Evelyn said that she could see that they were scared and sad even though she was trying so hard to protect them from Carlos's lifestyle and struggles. Evelyn further explained that being overwhelmed by Carlos's problems left her with little energy to help her younger children. While identifying behavior and patterns does not eliminate them, Evelyn could begin to see that events and actions were linked and causal rather than completely out of her control and merely a series of tragic coincidences. Through discussions over the course of months, Evelyn began to take action with her eldest son and determined that his behavior caused his life to be at great risk. Evelyn made one of the most difficult decisions for a mother to make and agreed to collaborate with the police in assisting them in prosecuting her son, resulting in his incarceration with the goal of saving his life.

During this time, Evelyn seemed calmer and it appeared to me that making this decision was not solely about protecting her son, but about regaining control as the matriarch of the family. Evelyn came into our clinic and I assisted her with the phone call to her son's parole officer reporting Carlos's whereabouts and schedule. While his arrest and subsequent court hearings caused great anguish and stressed the family, Evelyn said she felt more at ease knowing that her eldest son would be safer now.

During the months of the above intervention, we also worked to reinforce asthma education, realizing that both Evelyn and José would need to take ownership of managing José's asthma. Initially, I thought that Evelyn had assumed the role of mother and José, the child. I began to notice, however, that Evelyn's expectations were that José was developmentally capable of fully managing his medical needs. While José should begin taking greater ownership of his asthma management at this stage of his life, it was inappropriate for an 11-year-old to take full responsibility. Additionally, José's learning disability further affected his capacity to understand the complexity of health, medication, and outcomes.

The physician, nurse, and I coordinated our approach by making sure that we gave the following consistent message to the family: we must work with José to teach him about asthma, but it remains an adult's responsibility to manage and redirect him as he gains comfort in taking on this role. We reinforced this message during every medical appointment and follow-up phone call with the goal of Evelyn's accepting that she held agency in this situation.

We worked with Evelyn to define what José's role should be with his asthma and directed her to verbalize her asthma plan. Should he always remember all medications? What happens if he forgets his medication? Is there a rewards system to encourage and reinforce this behavior? Should he report every sign and symptom without prompts from her? If he does report that he is not feeling well, what would she then do? Does she know what the next steps are? Coaxing this information from Evelyn helped her process these concepts. Most importantly, I had the full support of the pediatrician and nurse, so that we all reinforced these topics with the family. Both Evelyn and José had to verbalize their knowledge of asthma, medical management plan, and frustrations.

To focus on Evelyn's hope that José would manage his own preventive medication, I met with both Evelyn and José separately and together to develop realistic expectations for José's role in his health care. Evelyn wanted José to take all of his preventive medication and be responsible for it, including noticing when medication was running low and remembering every dose. José reported that he took his medication, but just "sometimes forgot." Developmentally, José was unable to fully connect cause and effect. While I worked on his understanding that the medicine was to improve his quality of life and lessen his symptoms, it was important to implement a concrete, age, and developmentally appropriate intervention.

I worked with José to figure out how to include taking medication into his daily routine. We began by looking at his daily schedule, reviewing his daily routine regardless of going to school or his mood. From here, José took control and formed his own plan. He needed to explain his plan to Evelyn and implement it with her assistance, signifying that both he and his mother controlled their individual roles in this plan. José determined that if he were to remember his asthma medication, he would need to keep it on the sink in the bathroom. He recognized that it could never be put away because then he would not remember it. He also realized that, to keep him on target, he needed a sign that he made to be kept on the bathroom wall. José took charge and explained his plan to his mother with the physician and me present. We reviewed the plan as a team and realized that this would ensure consistency with medication 5 days out of the week, but José may still struggle on weekends with his father. I spoke with Evelyn and José about what they could do to promote consistency with medications when José visited his father who seemed not to agree with a focused medical management plan for asthma and often put up barriers to care. If José, however, took his preventive medication regularly during the school week and as consistently as possible on the weekend with Evelyn's reminders, he would still be reducing his chances of symptoms. See Figure 27.1 for an ecomap of José's social situation.

Use of resources outside of the helping relationship

I referred the family to an asthma educational outreach program that provides families with asthma education via phone and is able to troubleshoot frequently asked questions through the anonymity of the telephone. The program reviews asthma triggers within the child's home, such as wall-to-wall carpeting, curtains, rodents and insects, pets, cleaning agents, and dust and paint chips. It also offers safety tips for storage of medications and tracking usage, and resources and ideas on how to eliminate these risk factors from their child's lifestyle and environment (Coughey et al., 2010), While we had provided much of this information

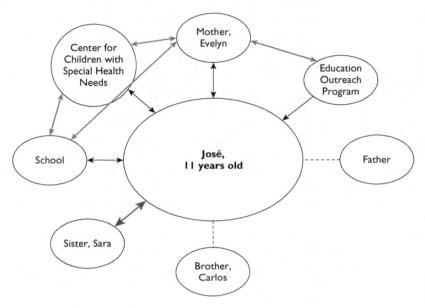

Figure 27.1 Ecomap for José

to the family in our office, it was greatly reinforced by this outreach program that the family deemed non-intrusive because all advice was delivered by telephone. I had decided that the more that Evelyn heard the facts in varying formats, the more she would retain further information on asthma, its impact, and its prevention. In addition to assisting José, this information would benefit anyone in the family struggling with asthma.

We then focused on José's elementary school. Despite José's placement in special education, he was doing very poorly and reports were showing that he was often in the nurse's office complaining of his asthma. At times, his asthma caused him to miss recess and physical education. When I called the school nurse and the teacher, they described José's asthma as a crutch; he would report that his chest was tightening resulting in an automatic visit to the nurse. When tracked, this behavior seemed to happen often during his academic subjects. The school further reported that while José's symptoms were often very real, he had a high level of anxiety around his asthma. José often began reporting his symptoms and if he was not given a nebulizer treatment urgently, he would become increasingly anxious. This further exacerbated his asthma until, regardless of the way they began, his symptoms would escalate.

The school had tried behavior modification by attempting to work with José to diminish his fears, lessen his anxiety, and teach him to compose himself so that his asthma symptoms would stabilize as opposed to spiking with increased anxiety. The challenge with behavior modification and any health concern with a child is that one should always err on the side of caution. It would, therefore, be increasingly difficult to discern what was true asthma and what was anxiety or an "excuse" to avoid participation for José. Such an intervention would need a meeting of all parties involved, including José.

I spoke with the school, the family, and my team to coordinate a meeting. We had two successful meetings at the school. I attended both and our nurse care coordinator attended one meeting as well on behalf of our medical team. The teachers, nurse, guidance counselor, principal, mother, child, and I met within the school to review everyone's concerns. José was present and we made sure that we spoke in an age-appropriate manner, but that he answered questions and provided us with feedback. The main concern was that José's asthma exacerbations were frequent, and the school wondered if some of his symptoms were more behavioral rather than true symptoms of asthma. The school would, in turn, frequently call Evelyn, frustrating her because it seemed to her to be another problem that she could not fix.

Interestingly, meeting with the school yielded insights into José's academic abilities and challenges. When José struggled, instead of asking for help, he misbehaved. As a team interested in José's success, we were able to reframe the meeting from being about how José "overreacted and mismanaged his asthma" to one concerning the additional strategies the school could use to assist José in better comprehending the most difficult subjects and, potentially, increasing his comfort while at school. The school recognized that this family took these issues seriously enough to work closely with their medical team in advocating for José's needs.

Also, articulating this child's medical and educational failures helped us all to see how closely the issues were intertwined. How could José concentrate if he was anxious about having an asthma attack? How could José learn if he was constantly in the nurse's office? Was José's anxiety about certain academics a trigger to shortness of breath and nerves that appeared as if they were symptoms of asthma? Was much of what would calm José down closely linked with receiving individualized attention from the school nurse? As a team, we were all struck with how health, behavior, academic performance, and family dynamics were so clearly linked.

Not easily broken, these cycles require consistent and finely tuned intervention. Because José spent a large portion of his time in school, the school was an ideal and necessary place to intervene. Much of our success came from our nurse's providing further asthma education for the teachers and the school's making accommodations in José's IEP to provide additional supports for his most challenging subjects. For the first time, José participated in school meetings so that he could see that everyone, including his mother, was communicating and making a plan with him rather than for him.

The school team reported that they noted increased anxiety in José whenever he showed any signs of asthma. While asthma and anxiety are closely linked, The American Lung Association notes that: "a common misbelief is that children with asthma have a major psychological problem that has caused the asthma. . . . Emotional stress itself (anxiety, frustration, anger) can trigger asthma, but the asthmatic condition precedes the emotional stress. . . . Many children with asthma suffer from severe anxiety during an episode as a result of suffocation produced by asthma. The anxiety and panic can then produce rapid breathing or hyperventilation, which further triggers the asthma" (American Lung Association, 2008, n.p.). According to the school's reports, José's anxiety affected his behavior. Potentially, many of the behavioral problems that the school reported could be stabilized if José felt better. Possibly, José would concentrate better in school if he were not anxious about his symptoms flaring up and if he were regularly taking his medication. Maybe José would feel more positively about school if he could consistently participate in all activities.

Throughout the process, Evelyn continued to struggle, but her struggles were less than when she worried about Carlos or was frustrated that the school did not take her seriously.

Now we had open communication between family, school, and medical team. Once we were able to stabilize Evelyn's concerns, we began to speak about what therapeutic assistance Evelyn needed for herself. Furthermore, I had gained her trust due to the success of the other interventions and knew that we could progress in our work for her children and the family as a whole.

Stance of the social worker

Reflecting on this case, I note the importance of a multi-systems approach. Finding the barriers to obtaining medical care, identifying the strengths of the family and the individual, and then coordinating care among all of the stakeholders empowered the family to manage the illness and supported successful outcomes. The focus shifts from the professionals' view of the family functioning, focusing instead on a family's managing its child's needs with the help of the medical team and the school. The parent deals with the key players in the child's life, the child is encouraged to share information about his symptoms, the adults will react accordingly, and we trust the child to be a part of the team. My goal for any case is that the family continues on this trajectory until they are requesting specific assistance from our team and coordinating meetings between the professionals independently. Eventually, as the child matures, he is the one dictating his care and needs to us. The family should become the central player in the care plan. Professionals will not always be consistent figures in the child's life. Physicians leave, nurses change positions, children graduate, and social workers may or may not continue to be involved. It would be a great service to adults if, throughout their youth, we had encouraged them to take on developmentally appropriate responsibilities for their care so that they could successfully manage their medical conditions throughout their lives.

Reassessment and evaluation

Much of this intervention depended on systems outside of the family: the medical team, the school, and the community asthma education program. At times, my role was primarily as a coordinator and communicator between parties. I worked with a physician who supported my interventions with this family and who would dedicate time and energy to educating them. Additionally, I depended on the physician and nurse to reinforce the importance of medical management, providing positive feedback to the family when they were appropriately managing care and redirecting the family when they faltered. The school also became an active part of this series of interventions. The school amended José's educational plan, met with José directly to create a plan to eliminate his asthma triggers, and conducted an open dialogue with mother and child creating a working, functional relationship.

In reassessing José's case and the series of interventions, it seems that if any goals were to be met, I had to be flexible, continually reconfiguring objectives and the means of obtaining them in order to meet the needs of the family. I could not strictly follow my agenda. One of the most positive aspects of this case was the cooperation between systems. The school's interest and dedication to José was remarkable. The school's nurse, principal, and teachers diligently created a comprehensive plan. They were able to support José through his struggles with his medical management without promoting dysfunctional behavior. In fact, the school discovered academic needs that may have been erroneously ascribed to behavior related to José's asthma. I have not formally spoken with the family about how fewer emergency room visits and better controlled asthma have impacted their lives. In the future, it would be valuable to meet directly with the family in order to review progress. It also seems that over time, individual and family therapy may greatly benefit this family due to past trauma, improving their current dynamic especially with fractured care between mother's home and father's home, and supporting chronic illness management.

Transfer, termination, and case conclusion

José's case will remain ongoing. Our center sees patients until they are 21 years old, and we will continue to reshape José's care plan based on his needs. This family continues to struggle. Their medical management, while improved, remains inconsistent. The foundation for good medical management and multi-systems communications has been built so that when there are inconsistencies of care, we have something to which we can return. Aspects of their lives have stabilized, but their foundation can be easily rocked, and Evelyn has not developed strong coping skills to weather change or new challenges.

José has had far fewer sick visits, emergency room visits, and has had no hospitalizations in the past year for his asthma. He continues to struggle with asthma, but not to the same extent. Evelyn now coordinates school meetings when she has concerns. She also took on the responsibility of inviting our medical team to participate in the meetings with the school. While José still struggles in school and admits to not always taking his medication, the reduced rate of overall hospital visits around asthma indicates that the family has improved their management of his chronic health condition at home, and he has missed fewer school days.

Differential discussion

While there have been successes and setbacks with José's case, the key element seems to be working across systems while empowering the caregiver and the child to take on this responsibility themselves. However, if the medical team or the school system were unwilling to take part in these discussions, José may have never received the necessary coordination to stabilize his asthma. José's case further illustrates the challenges of managing chronic illness at any point, but especially when there are difficult social issues that bar the caregiver from providing care. It seems that, in the minds of the family, José's asthma was not the utmost concern, and its management consistently fell second.

I wonder what would have happened in José's care if the medical team had reached out to the school earlier or if social services had become involved previously. While the family did have resources in the past, it seems that allowing for a long time period to manage and reconstruct this intervention was necessary to any success. Much depended on the family's connection with the medical office and a level of trust that led to disclosure of the barriers to managing José's asthma. Fortunately for this case, I was not given a time period or a deadline, but rather permitted to do ongoing work with the family. However, not all primary care offices are designed to be medical homes such as this one and many do not have social workers. Specific to our community, in recent years the Philadelphia School District has endured sweeping budget cuts that have reduced staff, especially school nurses. It has, therefore, become increasingly challenging to coordinate chronic care needs at school or have resources for creative interventions with children despite the reported high numbers of children diagnosed with asthma and missing school days because of it.

Discussion questions

1   Creating an environment in which an illness can be managed outside the hospital is a goal for families and social workers who are addressing chronic illness. It is a good example of thinking on the client level and the population level at the same time. How might thinking on both of those levels at once affect practice decisions, interventions or even outcomes?
2   This case study is as much about social as medical intervention. Is this realistic? How can social workers in health care keep the authority and autonomy to work in these ways?
3   José's mother was encouraged by the team to help the police to find her son. Do you agree that that was part of the team's responsibility? Relate that action to the National Association of Social Workers' work in social justice.

References

American Academy of Pediatrics (2015). The National Center of Medical Home Implementation for Children with Special Needs. Retrieved from www.medicalhomeinfo.org.

American Lung Association (2008). Retrieved from www.lung.org/

American Lung Association (September, 2012). *Trends in asthma morbidity and mortality*. Retrieved from www.lungusa.org

American Lung Association (2015). Retrieved from www.lung.org/

Bryant-Stephens, T., West, C., Dirl, C., Banks, T., Briggs, V., & Rosenthal, M. (2012). Asthma prevalence in Philadelphia: Description of two community-based methodologies to assess asthma prevalence in an inner-city population. *Journal of Asthma, 49*(6), 581–585. doi: 10.3109/02770903.2012.690476

CDC (Centers for Disease Control and Prevention) (2015). National Center for Chronic Disease Prevention and Health Promotion. Healthy Youth! Health Topics: Asthma. Retrieved from www.cdc.gov/healthyyouth/asthma/index.htm

Clark, N. M. (2012). Community-based approaches to controlling childhood asthma. *Annual Review of Public Health, 33*, 193–208. doi: 10.1146/annurev-publhealth-031811-124532

Coughey, K., Klein, G., West, C., Diamond, J. J., Santana, A., McCarville, E., & Rosenthal, M. P. (2010). The child asthma link line: A coalition-initiated, telephone-based, care coordination intervention for childhood asthma. *Journal of Asthma, 47*(3), 303–309. doi: 10.3109/02770900903580835

Findley, S., Rosenthal, M., Bryant-Stephens, T., Damitz, M., Lara, M., Mansfield, C., & Viswanathan, M. (2011). Community-based care coordination practical applications for childhood asthma. *Health Promotion Practice, 12*(6 suppl 1), 52S–62S. doi: 10.1177/1524839911404231

Imami, L., Tobin, E. T., Kane, H. S., Saleh, D. J., Lupro, T. H., & Slatcher, R. B. (2014). Effects of socioeconomic status on maternal and child positive behaviors in daily life among youth with asthma. *Journal of Pediatric Psychology, 40*(1), 55–65. doi: 10.1093/jpepsy/jsu066

Philadelphia Allies Against Asthma (2015). Linking families to untapped resources. Retrieved from www.pediatricasthma.org/community_coalitions/philadelphia

Spiegel, J., Love, A., Wood, R., Griffith, M., Taylor, K.R., Williams, G., & Redd, S. C. (2006). The inner-city asthma intervention tool kit: best practices and lessons learned. *Annals of Allergy, Asthma, and Immunology, 97*, 36–39. doi: 10.1016/S1081-1206(10)60778-8

Terre, L. (2011). Psychosocial factors in pediatric asthma. *American Journal of Lifestyle Medicine, 5*(1), 40–43. doi: 10.1177/1559827610377397

Ur-Rehman Malik, H., Kumar, K. & Frieri, M. (June, 2012). Minimal difference in the prevalence of asthma in the urban and rural environment. *Clinical Medicine Insights: Pediatrics, 6*, 33–39. doi: 10.4137/CMPed.S9539

Vital Signs (2011). Asthma prevalence, disease characteristics, and self-management education: United States, 2001–2009. (2011). *Morbidity Mortality Weekly Report, 60*(17), 547–552.

Chapter 28

Camp Achieve

A week-long overnight camp for children and teens with epilepsy

Sue Livingston, Emily Beil Duffy, Marikate Taylor, and Toba Schwaber Kerson

Context

The Epilepsy Foundation of Eastern Pennsylvania (EFEPA, www.efepa.org) is an affiliate of the national Epilepsy Foundation (Epilepsy Foundation of America, www.epilepsy.com). Founded in 1972 by local families and a neurologist who recognized a need for information and support beyond medical aspects of the disorder, the EFEPA serves approximately 14,000 people annually. Our mission is to stop seizures and SUDEP (sudden unexplained death in epilepsy), find a cure for epilepsy, and overcome the challenges created by epilepsy through efforts including education, advocacy, and research to accelerate turning ideas into therapies. We wish to create a community where people affected by epilepsy can experience the respect, support, and care they deserve to live fuller lives, and we envision the day when the stigmas associated with our community are permanently erased (Fiest, Birbeck, Jacoby, & Jette, 2014). One of the ways in which we provide education, support, and advocacy is through Camp Achieve, a camping experience that is meant to build self-esteem, confidence, independence, and friendships (Walker & Pearman, 2009). Camp Achieve is for children and teens ages 8–17 with a primary diagnosis of epilepsy, and it is a tremendously positive social experience for our campers.

Epilepsy and stigma

Despite great scientific advances, the word "epilepsy" bears a massive stigma that is driven by misconceptions and myths such as: epilepsy is contagious, people with epilepsy can see into the future, are possessed by the devil, or are of low intelligence (England, Austin, Beck, Escoffery, & Hesdorffer, 2014; Fernandes, Snape, Beran, & Jacoby, 2011; Kerson, 2010). Children and families can be affected more by social and psychological stigma than by the illness (Szaflarski, 2014). Embarrassment often keeps people suffering in silence. Children say that they feel different from their peers and are afraid of being teased about having seizures (Kerson, 2012).

Children's perceptions of epilepsy are heavily influenced by family, school, neurologist, and community (Brigo et al., 2015; Engel, 2013; Kerson & Kerson, 2008; Kobau, Dilorio, Thompson, Bamps, & St. Louis, 2015). Perception directly affects their quality of life. Families who refuse to discuss epilepsy, seizures, or medications with their children or do not use proper medical terminology perpetuate stigma and negatively affect their child's perception of their disorder (Kerne & Chapieski, 2015). Children are taught to be fearful, embarrassed, and not to ask questions. Imagine a young child whose parents tell him not to disclose his epilepsy to anyone but who then has a seizure in public. That child is now not only embarrassed and confused, but afraid and worried that he has done something wrong, something the parent has said not to do. This is a tremendous burden to put on children. We have found the Camp Achieve experience can improve children's attitudes towards their disorder, perceptions about epilepsy, and overall life quality.

Technology: epilepsy, seizures, and medication

Often called a seizure disorder, epilepsy is a collective term for a group of disorders affecting one in twenty-six people in their lifetime. It is caused by abnormal brain cell electrical activity and characterized by at least two epileptic seizures that are unprovoked by any immediately identifiable cause (International League Against Epilepsy, 2015). Seizures occur when brief, strong surges of electrical activity affect part or all of the brain. Usually, but not always, epilepsy involves convulsive movements of the body; sometimes it involves hyperactivity or only momentary inattention or staring.

Currently, of more than 25 antiepileptic drugs (AED) available, most are effective for only one seizure type. Finding the right combination(s) of medication and the dosage with the least side effects can be slow and frustrating for the patient, family, and health care provider. The seizure type determines which AED to try; then the effectiveness and severity of side effects are considered. For example, some medications will work best for a specific seizure type but actually worsen other types or cause unbearable side effects. Side effects commonly alter cognitive, emotional, and behavioral functioning. Finding "control" is defined as no seizures and no side effects. To achieve the right balance and dosage requires numerous medical tests as well as the experience and observational abilities of the neurologist (Shorvon, Guerrini, Cook, & Lhatoo, 2012).

Other treatment options include: surgery, vagus nerve stimulator (VNS), responsive neurostimulation (RNS), or a ketogenic diet (Klinkenberg, Majoie, Rijkers, Leenen, & Aldenkamp, 2012; Kossoff, 2008). For campers on the ketogenic diet, camp staff will work with parents and the camp kitchen to provide appropriate individual meals for the week. Most often, the diet is used in combination with AEDs; sometimes AEDs are completely eliminated. Some campers have undergone surgery, an option that may be used when several medications have failed to control seizures. The plasticity of the brain during childhood development and maturation may limit the postoperative cognitive side effects. The decision to pursue surgery is very personal, and people must weigh the possibility of being seizure free against the risks of surgery (de Tisi et al., 2011).

Camp Achieve must be prepared for epilepsy-related emergencies, and as a result campers are required to provide rescue medications even if their seizures have been controlled. One such emergency demanding immediate attention is when a camper is in status epilepticus, a period of time when a seizure is prolonged longer than 5 minutes without recovery or when seizures are repeated in clusters (short seizures that continue one after another). In the case of an emergency, the camper's designated counselor will contact the medical staff via walkie-talkie and ensure that the child is in a safe space while awaiting treatment. A few years ago, in order to respond quickly and effectively to camper needs, Camp Achieve gave the medical staff iPads containing every camper's medical and personal information. In this way, medical professionals are prepared immediately to individualize treatment.

Organization

Most children with chronic disorders such as epilepsy are not accepted at traditional summer camps because they need medical supervision that is not provided or there is not enough supervision for activities. In 1997, the EFEPA launched a 3-day Preteen and Teen Weekend

Retreat that preteens, ages 8–12, attended with one parent, and teens (aged 13–17) attended by themselves. Several years later, due to increased demand and the efficacy of the program, the Foundation transformed the retreat into Camp Achieve, a week-long overnight experience. In 2014, we hosted the largest camp to date with 54 campers 22 of whom were new to the experience.

The camp is managed by Camp Achieve's Medical Review Committee (CAMRC), a medical advisor (pediatric neurologist), five nurses, EFEPA executive director, camp medical coordinator, and camp coordinator. All volunteers (medical professionals, counselors, and junior counselors) must pass criminal and child abuse background checks, an FBI clearance, and be granted approval by the camp committee. Counselors are also required to submit a formal application. New applicants may be interviewed to determine their appropriateness for the program. Six to eight medical volunteers are always on the campgrounds, available 24 hours a day by walkie-talkie and cell phone. We have found it most effective to maintain a 2:1 counselor to camper ratio. All volunteers, both medical and non-medical, receive seizure first-aid training and epilepsy education. Historically, approximately half of the volunteer counselors have epilepsy. There are two to four counselors in each cabin of 8–10 campers, with one lead counselor taking responsibility for reporting any cabin issues to the camp coordinator. Counselors, EFEPA staff, and medical professionals communicate by walkie-talkie 24 hours a day and use them to radio for medical assistance. Caregivers are given staff cell phone numbers to check in as needed throughout the week. Campers are not allowed cell phones at camp. Counselors can use their phones away from campers if needed.

The EFEPA raises money for camp through private donations, pharmaceutical donations, and other grants. The Foundation charges a minimal registration fee of US$350 per camper; however, a camper is never turned away due to financial constraints. About 35% of campers receive financial assistance. We rely on a network of volunteers (counselors, medical professionals, and a social worker) who donate their time and expertise. Recently, we launched a new way for interested parties to support camp through an online "Wish-List" of supplies that individuals could purchase and donate. Figure 28.1 shows an organigraph of Camp Achieve.

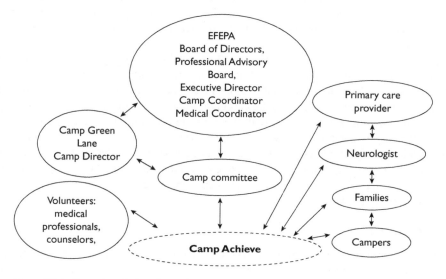

Figure 28.1 Organigraph for Camp Achieve

Decisions about practice

Definition and description of the typical camper

The campers are our primary clients and their caregivers, secondary clients (Shore, Perkins, & Austin, 2008). Campers include children and teens, ages 8–17 with a primary diagnosis of epilepsy who have the ability to complete activities of daily living (ADL) independently. This specific definition was made to maximize safety and the potential for a positive camp experience; we include it on Camp Achieve brochures, and it is addressed with all caregivers during the initial phone call. Many people with epilepsy also have co-morbid disorders affecting their functional ability. We have learned over the years that we cannot accommodate campers who are unable to complete ADLs independently or have another primary diagnosis, as evidenced by our having to send them home before completion of camp due to safety concerns.

The camp application is online. Once prospective campers' applications are completed by their caregivers, each camper's neurologist completes a form confirming that epilepsy is the primary diagnosis, assessing the child's appropriateness for Camp Achieve and capacity to complete all ADLs independently. Forms provide detailed seizure history, seizure type, triggers, other medical diagnoses, and a general medical background to ensure that each individual is medically, behaviorally, and physically able to attend camp. The camp committee then approves or denies admission. Several weeks before camp, the Foundation hosts a meeting so that caregivers can state their expectations and raise questions with the medical director, coordinator, executive director, and a member of the medical committee. In this way, new caregivers gain support from those with experience. Since campers face stigma and fear that has often resulted in social isolation, we strive to be as inclusive as possible, and we ask campers who have aged out to return as volunteer junior counselors when appropriate.

Caregivers are, in part, gatekeepers to their children's attendance. The idea of camp may be new to caregivers, and they are often reluctant to send their children. Many campers have never attended a summer camp or even spent the night away from home due to their seizure activity. In the past, caregivers attended camp with their children, but this ultimately inhibited campers' growth. Now, we believe that caregivers who allow their child to attend camp foster children's independence, curiosity, and feelings of psychological and physical safety. Sending children to Camp Achieve means that caregivers trust the Foundation to care for their children for an entire week.

In order to encourage more independence, we began a Facebook page just for caregivers. During camp, a staff member posts an end-of-day update including photos and an activity summary. Thus, caregivers feel involved at a distance. Open year round, our page supports continued conversation and strengthens the caregiver network. At the end of camp, in keeping with our maintaining a relationship with the entire family and expanding the impact of the camp experience beyond a single week, we host a caregiver "Coffee and Conversation." There, the executive director reviews the week and describes how caregivers can help their children continue to develop the skills learned at camp. This educational talk empowers caregivers and fosters a positive attitude towards epilepsy in caregivers and their children. It is also a time for family network building.

Goals and objectives

Our goal is to increase youths' ability to live well with epilepsy. Among our objectives are safety, supporting autonomy, and providing positive recreational and educational activities that result in a memorable, meaningful experience for the campers. Campers participate in positive and enjoyable recreational activities that promote social skills, problem solving, mutual encouragement, and a sense of accomplishment. Volunteers foster relationships and appropriate levels of autonomy, two necessary ingredients for healthy self-identity (Moola, Faulkner, White, & Kirsh, 2014). Prior to this experience, many campers are excluded from activities because of parental fear, social rejection, and concerns surrounding safety and perceived limitations associated with epilepsy. At camp, all freely participate in social and recreational activities. For example, one of the first recreational activities that campers try is wall climbing; they cheer each other on as each one climbs to the top of the wall. Last summer, Katie, who has cerebral palsy and whose left side is her helping side, climbed to the top of the wall with the whole camp cheering. And when Chuck, who was afraid to go down the water slide, saw Jeff doing it, he risked it as well, and it made his day. As campers begin to feel secure and comfortable, they learn how to give and receive support and build social skills. Additionally, each afternoon, cabin mates gather to discuss the day's activities, frustrations, excitement, joys, and fears in a safe and supportive environment. Counselors facilitate the conversation and provide meaningful feedback that helps campers process their emotions. Finally, Camp Achieve encourages mentorship and a sense of community as they mix cabin mates for each activity into "rings." Through the rings, rather than restrict each activity by age group, younger campers are assisted and guided by older campers, who learn to be leaders and role models for their younger friends.

The campers experience a new level of independence and build confidence in other ways as well. For many, this is the first time away from home, cleaning up after themselves (or not), dressing themselves, taking their medication without a caregiver's reminder, or even choosing their own food. This autonomy creates increased self-efficacy which directly influences the development of positive health habits and behaviors.

Daily educational activities are held to help campers to fight stigma, dispel myths, and feel empowered by their epilepsy – not fear it. Many campers know very little about epilepsy and how it relates to them. Addressing these kinds of issues puts the individual in charge, not the fear and negative anticipation of the next seizure. We know that children desire information on how epilepsy will affect them in the future, as well as strategies to manage seizures and ways to talk with others who have seizures. Past topics include: dating, drugs/alcohol, and driving, How to talk to your doctor, How to manage bullying in school, Understanding special education . . . What are your rights? What are all these medications? and Who are famous people with epilepsy? Camp Achieve medical staff also educate campers in daily casual encounters, freely answering questions about anything that might come up. We also invite guest speakers who have epilepsy or another disorder to encourage and motivate the campers. Speakers have included "Ms. Wheel Chair America," "Mighty Mike" Simmel who has epilepsy and plays for the Harlem Wizards, and Dirk Johnson, a professional football player whose sister has epilepsy. Access to real-life mentors and those thriving with epilepsy instills hope and inspiration.

Short-term memory is often affected by seizure activity so we try to create ways for campers to hold onto memories. Photos and videos are taken throughout camp and are posted online. Each camper is given a tee shirt, backpack full of gifts, and certificate of achievement to serve as positive, tangible reminders of camp. We also provide all participants with a contact list to encourage campers and families to socialize throughout the school year. Each winter we hold a reunion for campers, families, and volunteers.

Contracts

Camp Achieve depends on effective and explicit contracts between EFEPA and the camp director, caregivers, campers, volunteers, and neurologists. Contracts are written with the intent of maximizing the safety of our campers and providing information that is essential to the camp experience, and are revised annually to include critical, up-to-date information.

The EFEPA annually contracts with a traditional camp for use of its facilities, and that contract delineates financial obligations, insurance, and safety requirements. We negotiate issues related to the daily schedule including meal times, menus, reserved cabins, provision of lifeguards, athletic equipment, art supplies, and rainy day activities.

All volunteers must provide detailed information about themselves and pass criminal and child abuse background checks. All sign a letter agreeing to EFEPA guidelines. The information also helps us to pair volunteer counselors and junior counselors, assign cabin groups, and match activities to skill sets.

Meeting place

We decided to use this specific camp because it is convenient for our constituencies, meets safety specifications, and because the camp administration has worked with other special health care needs populations including youth with diabetes, asthma, and hemophilia. This traditional camp provides activity options and adequate medical facilities: a cafeteria, a pool with two slides, arts and crafts, miniature golf, athletic fields and courts, archery, wall climbing, a hockey rink, a ropes course, and several outdoor auditoriums. The camp and its buildings are accessible for the differently abled, cabins do not have bunk-beds and are in close proximity to each other, and the infirmary contains locked areas for medications.

Use of time

The camp and campers' school schedules determine the dates on which Camp Achieve will be held each year. This traditional overnight camp cannot accommodate us until after the completion of their regular camp season, and most of our campers attend summer school through mid-July. Therefore, camp is always scheduled at mid-August. The length of camp, five nights and six days, is determined by our concern for campers' well-being and budgetary challenges. Many campers have never spent time away from home, and families can be very apprehensive. Unfortunately, decreased sleep, excitement, and sun, natural parts of camp, can be seizure triggers.

Strategies and interventions

Most campers have never witnessed another person having a seizure, met another person with epilepsy, or slept away from home without a caregiver. In fact, results from the 2014 Camp Achieve program indicate that 69% of campers reported never having seen a seizure before (despite having epilepsy), and if they had seen one before, it made them afraid. The overall strategy of camp is to provide therapeutic recreational activities, purposeful interventions, and appropriate medical supervision.

Arriving one day before the campers, volunteers attend an orientation that focuses on epilepsy education, seizure first-aid, ice-breakers (bonding activities), a tour of the facility, group and cabin assignments, and an overview of guidelines and expectations. Orientation sets the tone for the week, and gives us an opportunity to thank the volunteers for their time. Our goal is for everyone to feel appreciated, excited, and prepared for the week. We finish the day with a "pizza party" as a token of our gratitude and a chance for volunteers to get to know one another.

Upon arrival, campers go immediately through registration, which can take several hours. Registration arrival time is staggered by last name in order to alleviate stress and allow caregivers to speak with camp staff. The most time-intensive process is medical registration. Campers have arrived with duffle bags full of medication for just one week and all medications must arrive in the original prescription bottles. Together, the volunteer medical professionals and caregivers organize the medications in individualized pill organizers. During registration, volunteers run an organized activity for campers to join and assist families in feeling comfortable when leaving their child.

Following registration, everyone gathers for camper orientation, which serves not only to familiarize the campers with their new surroundings, but also to create a sense of community. Camp guidelines are reviewed, group assignments are read, ice-breakers are played, and an educational video detailing what it looks like when someone has a seizure, various seizure types, and seizure first-aid, is shown to all campers. The video is a non-threatening way for campers to learn about seizures and to prepare them for what they will inevitably witness throughout the week.

The remainder of the week is purposefully designed. Each morning, after breakfast, the Camp Coordinator makes announcements including a special "word of the day" which is designed to remind campers about important camp concepts such as participation, community, and inclusion. Also, each day includes rest and free time, thus promoting camper interaction that is not facilitated by adults. Counselors encourage campers to participate in all activities to the best of their abilities. Through positive modeling, campers begin to encourage and motivate one another. As camp progresses, group cohesion forms, relationship skills and comfort levels increase, and the campers come to understand that they are no longer alone. Recreational activities promote a sense of normalcy and mastery. One specific example is yoga because studies have shown a positive relationship between seizure control and practicing yoga (Streeter, Gerbarg, Saper, Ciraulo, & Brown, 2012). Epilepsy disrupts the balance between the body and mind and yoga is a learned skill that can guide campers towards regaining control and balance. Yoga alleviates stress, induces relaxation, promotes a better understanding of the body, and enhances mental focus. The campers thoroughly enjoy it.

Also, campers use multiple media to create art based upon their experience with epilepsy, and may even draw a picture of themselves having a seizure; they are given an opportunity to share about their drawings. We have submitted campers' creations, with their permission, to Ortho-McNeil's publication, *Creative Expressions* and used others for a variety of EFEPA's publications. For this season, we plan to have an art therapist join the arts and crafts program. One of the week's highlights is the Talent Show. Most campers participate in some way, and every camper is cheered with great enthusiasm regardless of performance or talent.

Music is important, too. For several years, Jason who is now 18 and a counselor has made that his special purview leading gospel and other kinds of singing for everyone. Last summer, Jason, who had never had a seizure at camp, had a grand mal seizure. Recovering, he wanted to go home, but after resting for a short while in our infirmary, he said "I'm not here to go home just because I had a seizure." He stayed and enjoyed the rest of camp. He is a loving and compassionate fellow, and we are so glad he stayed.

Stance of the social worker

The role of the social worker is to assist counselors and staff in communications with each other and the campers and to help them also to understand campers' situations, struggles, and challenges. In months prior to camp, the social worker assists the staff with any issues that may arise with applicants. The social worker meets the counselors at their orientation, offering suggestions on topics for discussions as well as how to create a comfortable atmosphere for these discussions. She also visits the cabins at Cabin Conversation time for casual, impromptu talks with campers and counselors.

Use of outside resources

Outside resources are essential. In 2014, a local epilepsy center provided a useful workshop on bullying for the campers. Collaborative relationships with pharmaceutical companies, local pediatric neurology groups, and other epilepsy foundations help us better meet the needs of our campers and families. These relationships provide us with up-to-date medical knowledge, new funding streams, access to volunteers, as well as innovative strategies and interventions. We also create collaborative relationships with local schools and pediatric neurology groups in an effort to increase awareness about opportunities to attend camp or serve as a camp volunteer. We encourage neurologists' provision of care that goes beyond the traditional medical model to focus on educating children about their disorder and providing emotional support to the family. We would like neurologists to prescribe camp attendance to patients and families as one aspect of improving families' psychosocial functioning.

EFEPA's Board of Directors and Professional Advisory Board (PAB) serve as resources for funding and operational support. The PAB assists with fundraising to ensure the fiscal health of the organization. Board members are asked to volunteer as counselors, and in this way, they have the opportunity to meet campers and better understand their unique strengths and challenges. All Board members are invited to the annual cookout. The neurologists and lawyers who make up PAB assist with the creation and revision of medical forms within the camper packet, help develop medication routines, ensure that safety requirements are adequate and up-to-date, and are available to consult as needed on a variety of medical-related issues before and during camp. The medical advisor on the camp committee is selected from PAB.

Reassessment and evaluation

At the end of the week, campers and volunteers complete a survey that assesses their experience and lets them know that we value their opinions. These surveys collect feedback about the activities, guest speakers, educational sessions, quality of meals, orientation, and recommended changes/suggestions for next year. Campers' surveys are kept very simple due the varying levels of literacy. Campers rate activities on a scale of 1–4 and answer a series of yes or no questions. We encourage everyone to provide verbal feedback as well. Additionally, we ask counselors to provide feedback about camper's and junior counselor's level of "fit" and "appropriateness" at camp.

We also ask caregivers for verbal feedback about their experiences, beginning with their first contact with our organization all the way through to picking their child up at camp. We strive to remain flexible and open to all feedback in an effort to improve camp and better meet our goal to empower campers, their families, and caregivers to live well with epilepsy. It is also critical that we report to our various funders regarding our success in meeting identified goals and objectives. This process helps us to synthesize information and, ultimately, identify the necessary changes and areas for improvement for the following year. Finally, the camp committee meets shortly after camp ends to evaluate and assess camp in its entirety.

Termination and case conclusion

On the final day we hold a closing ceremony. Everyone gathers and the camp's coordinator and executive director highlight the fun, memorable, and positive experiences throughout the week. Each camper is called up to receive a certificate of achievement and a picture is taken to capture the moment. We distribute a master list of everyone's contact information and encourage campers to stay in touch, and remind them of the fall reunion for former and potential campers.

Differential discussion

Society has taught us to fear epilepsy and centuries of misunderstandings have deeply embedded the roots of stigma. Children with epilepsy still feel as though they are the only one in the world having seizures and hold tremendous fear about disclosing their disorder or having a seizure in public. This negative self-perception directly affects their health behaviors and quality of life. When kids walk into camp it is as though they have entered a new world, a safe one, a familiar one. Sometimes you can see them take a deep breath and smile as if it is their first *real* smile. They belong here; they are free to make friends and be themselves. After attending camp, we hope children and families can reframe their fear of disclosure or having a seizure in public as an opportunity to teach others about seizure first-aid and further uproot social stigmas. We hope they feel empowered, informed, and have an improved attitude towards their condition. This will improve their health behaviors (e.g., adherence to medication) and provide them with a sense of individual and family mastery.

Yearly we face funding constraints, difficulty obtaining volunteer medical providers, and other challenges, but despite these setbacks we are committed to providing our youth opportunities to participate in all life experiences. We believe summer camp positively affects their life trajectories and those of their families, schools, and communities. The yearly return of campers and counselors tells us that we are making a difference. The growth of campers into junior counselors and then into counselors speaks volumes about the long-term value of camp and the special place it holds for participants.

Discussion questions

1   If your work is focused on a certain social or diagnostic category, do you think that your constituents could benefit from such a camp? How would you go about creating it?
2   Are there ways in which you could adapt some of the extraordinarily positive dimensions of Camp Achieve to your own workplace?
3   What would you suggest to make Camp Achieve more financially secure?

References

Brigo, F., Igwe, S. C., Ausserer, H., Tezzon, F., Nardone, R., & Ottem, W. M. (2015). Epilepsy-related stigma in European people with epilepsy: Correlations with health system performance and overall quality of life. *Epilepsy & Behavior,* 18–21. doi: 10.1016/j.yebeh.2014.11.015

de Tisi, J., Bell, G. S., Peacock, J. L., McEvoy, A. W., Harkness, W. F., Sander, J. W., & Duncan, J. S. (2011). The long-term outcome of adult epilepsy surgery, patterns of seizure remission, and relapse: a cohort study. *The Lancet, 378*(9800), 1388–1395. doi: 10.1016/S0140-6736(11)60890-8

Engel, J. Jr. (2013). Social management. *Seizures and epilepsy* (2nd edn., pp. 644–664). New York: Oxford University Press.

England, M. J., Austin, J. K., Beck, V., Escoffery, C., & Hesdorffer, D. C. (2014). Erasing epilepsy stigma: Eight key messages. *Health Promotion Practice, 15,* 313–318. doi: 10.1177/1524839914523779

Epilepsy Foundation of America (2015). Retrieved from www.epilepsy.com

Fernandes, P. T., Snape, D. A., Beran, R. G., & Jacoby, A. (2011). Epilepsy stigma: What do we know and where next? *Epilepsy & Behavior, 22*(1), 55–62. doi: 10.1016/j.yebeh.2011.02.2014

Fiest, K. M., Birbeck, G. L., Jacoby, A., & Jette, N. (2014). Stigma & epilepsy. *Current Neurology and Neuroscience Reports, 14,* 444–454.

International League Against Epilepsy (2015). Retrieved from www.ilae.org

Kerne, V. & Chapieski, L. (2015). Adaptive functioning in pediatric epilepsy: Contributions of seizure related variables and parental anxiety. *Epilepsy & Behavior, 43,* 48–52. doi: 10.1016/j.yebeh.2014.11.030

Kerson, T. S. (2010). Epilepsy and media. In J. Pinikahana & C. Walker (Eds.), *Social epileptology: Understanding the social aspects of epilepsy.* New York: Nova Science Publishers.

Kerson, T. S. (2012). Epilepsy postings on YouTube: Exercising individuals' and organizations' right to appear. *Social Work in Health Care, 51*(10), 927–943. doi: 10.1080/00981389.2012.712634

Kerson, T. S. & Kerson, L. A. (2008). Truly enthralling: Epileptiform events in film and on television – Why they persist and what we can do about them. *Social Work in Health Care, 47*(3), 320–337. doi: 10.1080/00981380802174069

Klinkenberg, S., Majoie, H. J., van, der Heijden, M. M., Rijkers, K., Leenen, L., & Aldenkamp, A. P. (2012). Vagus nerve stimulation has a positive effect on mood in patients with refractory epilepsy. *Clinical Neurology and Neurosurgery, 114*(4), 336–40. doi: 10.1016/j.clineur0.2011.11.016

Kobau, R., Dilorio, C. K., Thompson, N. J., Bamps, Y. A., & St. Louis, E. P. (2015). Epilepsy, comorbidities and consequences: Implications for understanding and combating stigma. In E.K. St. Louis, D. M. Ficker, & T. J. O'Brien (Eds.), *Epilepsy and the interictal state: Comorbidities and Quality of Life* (pp. 15–25). Oxford, UK: John Wiley & Sons.

Kossoff, E. H. (2008). Three dietary therapies for epilepsy. In K. Chapman & J. M. Rho (Eds.), *Pediatric epilepsy case studies: From infancy and childhood through adolescence* (pp. 29–34). London: CRC Press.

Moola, F. J., Faulkner, G. E. J., White, L., & Kirsh, J. A. (2014). The psychological and social impact of camp for children with chronic illnesses: a systematic review update. *Child: Care, health and development, 40*(5), 615–631. doi: 10.1111/cch.12114

Shore, C. P., Perkins, S. M. & Austin, J. K. (2008). The seizures and epilepsy education (SEE) program for families of children with epilepsy: A preliminary study. *Epilepsy & Behavior, 23,* 157–164. doi: 10.1016/j.yebeh.2007.10.001

Shorvon, S., Guerrini, R., Cook, M., & Lhatoo, S. (2012). *Oxford textbook of epilepsy and epileptic seizures.* Oxford: Oxford University Press.

Streeter, C. C., Gerbarg, P. L., Saper, R. B., Ciraulo, D. A., & Brown, R. P. (2012). Effects of yoga on the autonomic nervous system, gamma-aminobutyric-acid, and allostasis in epilepsy, depression, and post-traumatic stress disorder. *Medical Hypotheses, 78*(5), 571–579. doi: 10.1016/j.mehy.2012.01.021

Szaflarski, M. (2014). Social determinants of health in epilepsy. *Epilepsy & Behavior, 41,* 283–289. doi: 10.1016/j.yebeh.2014.06.013

Walker, D.A. & Pearman, D. (2009). Therapeutic recreation camps: An effective intervention for children and young people. *Archives of Disease in Childhood, 94*(5), 401–406. doi: 10.1136/adc.2008.145631

Chapter 29

Following her lead

A measured approach to working with homeless adults

Annick Barker

Context

Founded in 1985, Health Care for the Homeless (HCH) works to prevent and end homelessness for vulnerable individuals and families by providing quality, integrated health care, and promoting access to affordable housing and sustainable incomes. HCH operates multi-disciplinary outpatient health care clinics in Baltimore City and County and funds similar programs in three other counties in Maryland. The Baltimore City clinic, where this case study originates, employs 170 staff and serves 9,000 people annually. Our program is one of over 200 federal HCH projects around the country. The organization strives to meet the highest standards of care and is accredited by the Joint Commission for ambulatory care and behavioral health, and it is also a Patient-Centered Medical Home.

Policy

Homelessness and adults with disabilities

Homelessness is a complex problem exacerbated by the diminishing value of median incomes, the increase in housing costs, and the shortage of comprehensive health services, problematic trends that have persisted over the last 40–50 years (HCH Clinicians' Network, 2005). These trends have devastating impacts on the poorest residents of many cities, as they do in Baltimore City. From 2011 to 2013, 24.5% of Baltimore's residents lived below the poverty level. Almost half of residents living in rental units spent more than 35% of their household income on rent (Maryland Department of Planning, 2014). In 2013, the Baltimore Mayor's Office of Homeless Services estimated that 2,638 individuals lived in shelters or on the streets on a typical night (Mayor's Office of Human Services, 2013).

People with physical and mental health disabilities are disproportionately burdened by these trends. The 8.3 million non-elderly people with disabilities who rely exclusively on Supplemental Security Income (SSI) are among the poorest in the United States. In 2012, the average monthly SSI payment for a single individual was US$721, almost 30% below the 2012 federal poverty level of US$11,170 (Technical Assistance Collaborative, 2013). As a result, SSI recipients face significant barriers finding housing in the private market. The National Low Income Housing Coalition reports that there is not a single jurisdiction in the United States where a disabled person who relies exclusively on SSI can afford an efficiency apartment in the private rental market (National Low Income Housing Coalition, 2014). In Baltimore City, the fair market rate in 2013 for a basic efficiency (US$846/mo) was about four times more than what the client described here could reasonably afford (US$213/mo) with the income she received from SSI (US$710/mo) (National Low Income Housing Coalition, 2014). The disparity between what is affordable for people receiving SSI incomes and the fair market rent in Baltimore persists to this day.

The role of supportive housing and Housing First initiatives

In response to these disparities, federal and local governments have increasingly invested in permanent supportive housing (PSH) programs. These programs provide subsidized housing and case management to vulnerable and chronically homeless adults and families. Since 2007, the City of Baltimore increased the number of PSH units by 60% (from 3,568 to 5,702 units). For adults without children, like Ms. Harper in this case, the number of supportive housing units increased by just over 100% (from 1,660 to 3,388 units) (U.S. Department of Housing and Urban Development, 2014). This number falls short of the supply needed to fully house low income disabled adults living in Baltimore, but it is movement in the right direction.

Historically, agencies serving homeless people have relied on continuum of care approaches to assisting severely mentally ill homeless adults. The continuum of care model provides outreach and engagement to homeless people, followed by treatment and transitional housing, and finally placement in permanent supported independent housing. The goal of such initiatives is to help applicants become "housing ready," helping them stabilize their psychiatric symptoms and achieve abstinence from street drugs and alcohol before securing permanent housing.

Over the last 10 years, observers and service providers have noted that this "housing ready" approach often leaves the most impaired and chronically homeless individuals without housing because it requires people to make significant behavioral changes while still confronting the burdens and trauma of homelessness (Stefancic & Tsemberis, 2007). In contrast, "Housing First" initiatives invert the approach, offering vulnerable people permanent housing right away and working with them intensively – at their own pace – to help them maintain their housing and improve their health outcomes.

SSI and the Representative Payee program

For many people with active symptoms of a serious mental illness (SMI), it is difficult to meet the basic demands of employment without significant support. For this reason, many people with SMI rely on income from the SSI program to meet their needs. In 2007, 40% of SSI recipients had mental health diagnoses other than mental retardation (Social Security Administration, 2007). Once awarded SSI benefits, people with SMI often struggle to manage their finances. More than a third of SSI beneficiaries participate in the Social Security Administration's Representative Payee program, whereby a third party administers the beneficiary's monthly SSI funds (SSA, 2007). Although the Social Security Administration (SSA) prefers to assign family members or friends as Representative Payee, regional offices report difficulty identifying appropriate Representative Payees for at-risk beneficiaries (Social Security Advisory Board, 2010). In such instances, SSA may assign human services agencies such as Health Care for Homeless to carry out the Representative Payee role.

Technology of medications

For people with schizophrenia, adherence to anti-psychotic medication regimens is a persistent challenge. The rate of medication non-adherence among patients with schizophrenia is approximately 50% (Glazer & Byerly, 2008). Treatment of SMI has improved, however, with the advent of new medications and methods of administration. Second-generation atypical anti-psychotic medications reduce the symptoms of schizophrenia without some of the troublesome side effects of older anti-psychotic medications. In 2003, a long-acting injectable form of risperidone, an atypical anti-psychotic, was introduced as an alternative to daily oral risperidone. Second-generation anti-psychotics have produced modest increases in adherence rates, and administration through long-acting injection has had a positive impact on efficacy as well (Keith, 2009). Motivational techniques, therapeutic alliance, and engagement of other clinicians and family members in a patient's treatment are equally, if not more, tied to both improved medication adherence and treatment outcomes (Farooq & Naeem, 2014). Not surprisingly, access to stable housing also significantly improves medication adherence rates (Gilmer et al., 2004).

Organization

Health Care for the Homeless is a Federally Qualified Health Center (FQHC) that provides outpatient medical, pediatric, dental, mental health, addictions, case management, and outreach services. Multi-disciplinary case conferences, shared electronic medical records, and co-located offices promote coordination of client care and client referrals among providers. As a recently certified Patient-Centered Medical Home (PCMH), HCH strives to maximize client access and integration of care.

HCH endorses a harm reduction philosophy of care among all providers. Staff members are taught to focus on the quality of their relationships with clients, to recognize that clients may not be ready to change behavior right away, and to understand that change often happens in small steps and that success should be measured accordingly. This incremental, person-centered approach is consistent with the recommendations of those who have studied models of care for people who are chronically homeless (HCH Clinicians' Network, 2014). It also parallels recovery-oriented approaches to mental health treatment in which consumers are given primary control and choice regarding the course of their care (SAMHSA, 2014).

Description of typical clients

In order to be considered homeless and eligible for HCH services, clients must be living on the streets; staying in emergency shelters, missions, single-room occupancy facilities, abandoned buildings or vehicles; or doubling up with a series of friends and/or extended family members (HRSA, 1999). Upon securing permanent housing, clients can receive HCH services for up to a year after they have become stably and permanently housed.

Decisions about practice

Description of case and client

When we first met in the early 2000s, Ms. Harper was a 40-year-old White woman with a history of paranoid schizophrenia. Ms. Harper was identified as a prospective client when an

HCH outreach worker encountered her living on the streets of downtown Baltimore. At the time, Ms. Harper was seen walking around downtown with a heavy dark coat draped over her head, obscuring most of her face and upper body. She appeared frightened and moved away when others approached. For 2 years, outreach workers attempted to make contact with her, offering tangible items such as snacks and toiletries. Eventually, Ms. Harper came into the clinic building in response to an intake worker's invitation and the offer of a shower. The intake worker introduced me to Ms. Harper in my role of Therapist Case Manager.

At our first meeting, Ms. Harper told me she had been staying in a local women's shelter but had been asked to leave because "the other women said I was doing things to them." After venting her frustration, Ms. Harper asked me for help with identification, alternative shelter, and income. I made phone calls to shelters and helped Ms. Harper obtain a photo ID card from the Maryland Transportation Authority (MTA). With no shelter beds available, I gave Ms. Harper two tokens so she could ride local buses, a form of shelter for many homeless people lacking alternatives. I explained that accessing housing would take time, but might be expedited if she maintained contact with HCH.

A few days later, Ms. Harper called me from a local hospital psychiatric unit to tell me she had been involuntarily admitted. I encouraged her to walk in to see me after her discharge. After a week, she was discharged with anti-psychotic medications to an emergency shelter and returned to HCH to see me. I asked her what help she needed and she again needed identification, food, clothing, toiletries, shelter, and bus tokens. We began working on getting her access to these. With her permission, I also contacted the state Disability Entitlement Advocacy Program (DEAP) to begin the application process for Medical Assistance, Food Stamps, and Social Security disability benefits. Ms. Harper complained of side effects from the medications prescribed by the hospital. I referred her to an HCH psychiatrist who conducted a brief evaluation the same day and provided her with samples of a different medication.

During our first month together, Ms. Harper's symptoms included flat affect, paranoid thoughts, hypervigilance, disorganization, and dysthymia. She denied auditory or visual hallucinations, but frequently appeared to respond to internal stimuli, laughing inappropriately and whispering to herself. During one of our encounters, she became very agitated. After initially resisting my requests that she lower her voice so we could talk, she quieted and became tearful and despondent. I encouraged her to use our meetings as a safe place to address her fears and other feelings.

Soon thereafter, Ms. Harper was again involuntarily admitted to a hospital psychiatric unit and discharged with anti-psychotic medication and a referral to a local shelter. She returned to HCH, saying she wanted to continue her psychiatric care with us. I scheduled another appointment with the staff psychiatrist and helped Ms. Harper contact a women's day-time shelter. Soon after, Ms. Harper disappeared for four months. I later learned that Ms. Harper had traveled to another state where her family of origin lives and was psychiatrically hospitalized there. Upon her return to Baltimore, she was once again homeless, frequently agitated, and had difficulty staying in the clinic building for longer than a few minutes. I arranged a psychiatric appointment and told her that she had been awarded Medical Assistance and Food Stamps. I also informed her that Safe Haven, a low-demand shelter for homeless adults with SMI, had a bed available. Ms. Harper declined Safe Haven, saying it was located too far away.

Ms. Harper returned the next day. She was too agitated to stay long enough to meet with the psychiatrist. She wanted some hot coffee, a change of clothes and toiletries, her mail (we had agreed she could use HCH's address), and to get her Medical Assistance card. The ensuing months were marked by rare and brief encounters with Ms. Harper. When she came into the clinic, I focused on her goals, checking her mail, and providing her with clothing. She was also approved for SSI 2 years after her initial application. I accompanied her to the local SSA office and we were told that Ms. Harper would require a Representative Payee to administer her SSI funds. Ms. Harper designated HCH as her Representative Payee and HCH assigned me to fill this role.

This was a turning point in our relationship. Although her psychotic symptoms persisted, Ms. Harper's visits to HCH became more frequent and regular. During that time, I proposed a variety of housing and case management programs for people with SMI. Each time an opportunity arose, however, Ms. Harper declined it. She was not interested in group home settings and rejected programs that required a significant portion of her SSI check toward rent. She also rejected programs that required transferring care from HCH. Staff at shelters where she had stayed before would not readmit her until her psychotic symptoms were more controlled. As a result, Ms. Harper remained on the street for much of the winter. She spent her days in the HCH waiting room, using the client bathroom to attend to her hygiene.

Eventually, Ms. Harper agreed to meet with a staff psychiatrist. She was initially guarded and declined medication, asserting that she had received an injection of Haldol that would last 15 years. I scheduled another appointment; with my prompting, Ms. Harper kept the appointment and agreed to try an anti-psychotic. The psychiatrist and I enlisted HCH's nursing staff to administer Ms. Harper's medication daily.

Ms. Harper's visits to the adherence nurses were sporadic and required frequent reminders from me. I used her struggle to secure shelter as an opportunity to discuss medication adherence, which at the time was required by most shelters and supportive housing programs. The psychiatrist also simplified Ms. Harper's medication regimen. Ms. Harper began to keep her appointments with me and other providers more consistently and became notably calmer. During one encounter, she grew angry with me but then stopped herself, stating "I don't need to speak that loud." She demonstrated increased insight, making statements such as "Will you see if (the shelter) will let me in if there is an attitude adjustment (on my part)?" and strategized about how to handle potential conflicts with fellow shelter residents. She expressed an optimism that had been absent before.

Ms. Harper continued to struggle with psychotic symptoms such as disorganized thoughts and auditory hallucinations. She was once again hospitalized after a heated argument during which she threatened to harm another client in the HCH waiting room. Upon discharge, Ms. Harper returned to HCH, lucid, calm, and goal-oriented. I found a low-cost rental room and she agreed to take it. She finally had permanent housing.

Securing housing and achieving the correct medication regimen constituted another turning point for Ms. Harper. After moving into the rental room, she had no further psychiatric hospitalizations, became less guarded and was able to have more relaxed, spontaneous interactions with others. Her thoughts were more organized and her memory improved. Her appearance and hygiene improved and she purchased new clothing.

Perhaps most notable was Ms. Harper's growing tolerance of conflict and better insight into her illness. That September, she traveled out of state to see her family for the weekend. Upon her return, she said, "My father wanted me to stay longer, but I had to come back to get my medicine." She had many successful visits to her family over the next couple of years.

After several months of being housed, Ms. Harper began reporting trouble with her landlady who made inappropriate requests such as asking Ms. Harper to buy alcohol and clean for her. The electricity was shut off several times because the landlady did not pay the utility bill. Despite our efforts to address these problems, they persisted and Ms. Harper eventually decided to move out and stay in emergency shelters until she could find better housing. Again, I contacted Safe Haven, the shelter for people with mental illness, and this time Ms. Harper agreed to move there. From Safe Haven, Ms. Harper eventually moved to a transitional housing program where she shared a house with three other women with SMI. After living there for over a year, Ms. Harper's 2-year-old application for the local Housing Authority's subsidized housing program was finally accepted. Three years after our initial contact, Ms. Harper at long last moved into her own efficiency apartment. She has since transferred her mental health care and medical treatment to a mainstream community health clinic and attends an adult day program.

See Figure 29.1 for Ms. Harper's ecomap before our work began and then Figure 29.2 for her ecomap after our 3 years of work together.

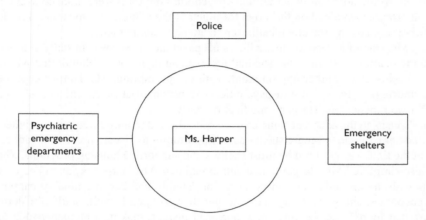

Figure 29.1 Ecomap of Ms. Harper's social network before intervention

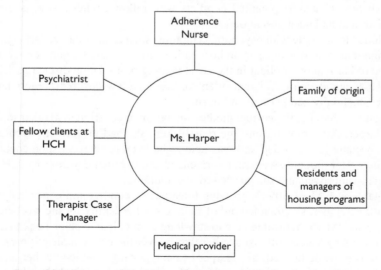

Figure 29.2 Ecomap of Ms. Harper's social network after intervention

Goals

Ms. Harper's primary goal was permanent independent housing. While that goal never changed, it evolved. Initially, she was only interested in the emergency shelters that had already barred her or in rental rooms in the private market. She was minimally interested in psychiatric care and too disorganized and paranoid to adhere to a medication regimen for long. When Ms. Harper finally engaged in psychiatric treatment, she began to understand that the type of housing she sought was unavailable, unaffordable, and/or inadequate. She was then able to modify her goal and consider other housing options.

I worked with Ms. Harper to have her identify her own goals and determine the pace and character of our relationship. To this end, I helped to secure housing from the very beginning even though I knew we were unlikely to be successful. We worked toward goals she identified that were more immediately achievable, such as income, identification, and, when she was ready, psychiatric care. This approach honored Ms. Harper's overarching goal of maintaining independence and allowed me to take the time needed to earn her trust. Recent research supports this approach, suggesting that giving clients choices and opportunities to collaborate with providers leads to improved mental health outcomes (Stanhope, Barrenger, Salzer, & Marcus, 2013).

Contract and objectives

It is challenging to discuss treatment planning with a client with SMI who does not yet consider herself to be in treatment. For Ms. Harper, a more clinically oriented approach to treatment planning would have undermined the relationship rather than enhanced it. Instead, we focused on securing shelter, obtaining a mailing address, and getting access to income, clothing, and food. As Ms. Harper became more comfortable with me, we talked about other objectives, such as applying for supportive housing programs and engaging in psychiatric treatment to reduce her psychiatric symptoms.

Our initial contracts were verbal and short term as Ms. Harper had difficulty tolerating a more formal approach. We renegotiated our contract at every session; themes included housing, income, help communicating with the outside world (through access to mail and the telephone), and access to tangible necessities (like toiletries and clothing). Eventually, Ms. Harper participated in a more formal contracting process regarding her goals for treatment as well as our Representative Payee relationship. We developed monthly budgets together and agreed on appointment schedules at the end of each month. Periodically, we wrote out a formal treatment plan outlining goals for the next six months.

Meeting place

Initially, HCH outreach workers approached Ms. Harper on the street. When Ms. Harper started seeing me, she sometimes tolerated brief visits in my office. Other times, I met with her briefly outside or on the first floor near the building entrance. She was uncomfortable with the large, crowded waiting room, and often waited for me outside across the street from the clinic.

Ms. Harper gradually stayed in the building longer and began using the clinic waiting room as a kind of day shelter, spending much of the morning there before going to lunch at a local soup kitchen. Eventually, Ms. Harper was comfortable both in the clinic and in my office for extended periods of time. She was well known to staff and developed friendships with other HCH clients.

Use of time

The frequency and duration of our sessions varied. Initially, I met with Ms. Harper whenever she came to the clinic as she rarely kept appointments. My goal was to build our relationship by interacting with Ms. Harper at least briefly, even if it was just to check mail and give her snacks and toiletries.

Once Ms. Harper began receiving SSI and I became her Representative Payee, her visits were more frequent, lengthier, and scheduled. Prior to receiving SSI, Ms. Harper visited HCH two to three times a month; after she received SSI, she visited an average of 11 times per month. As she secured stable housing and gained more control of her SSI funds, we reduced the frequency of her visits. Eventually her care at HCH consisted of daily visits with a medication adherence nurse and bi-monthly visits with me.

Strategies and interventions

Just as effective case managers nurture a therapeutic alliance with their clients (Chinman, Rosenheck, & Lam, 2000; Howgego, Yellowlees, Owen, Meldrum, & Dark, 2003), mental health practitioners recognize that attending to a client's immediate practical needs, such as shelter, is a priority (Kirsh & Tate, 2006). At the time of my work with Ms. Harper, HCH used a model of care which combined these two functions into the single role of "Therapist Case Manager." Therapist Case Managers at HCH were empowered to tailor their interventions to the needs and capacities of each client. While HCH has subsequently created a separate case manager role to help address the significant needs of our homeless clients, mental health therapists at HCH continue to prioritize the goals of clients as well as the quality of our relationships with them.

That said, providing SSI Representative Payee services for clients such as Ms. Harper presents both risks and opportunities for mental health therapists at HCH. On one hand, research suggests that for severely mentally ill SSI beneficiaries with no reliable family members, agencies and clinical professionals are the best equipped to carry out the Representative Payee role (National Research Council, 2007). People with SMI who participate in agency-based Representative Payee programs may spend fewer days in the hospital than before participation and make greater use of psychiatric services (Luchins, Roberts, & Hanrahan, 2003).

Nevertheless, engaging clinicians as Representative Payees raises the ethical question of whether managing a client's finances constitutes a dual relationship (Marson, Savage, & Phillips, 2006). When clients perceive clinicians using the payee role as leverage to compel treatment compliance, the therapeutic alliance can suffer (Angell, Martinez, Mahoney, & Corrigan, 2007). Yet studies also suggest that such relationships become more satisfactory to clients over time as the relationships are negotiated and clinicians maintain a client-centered and non-coercive stance (Rosen, Bailey, Dombrowski, Ablondi, & Rosenheck, 2005). In our case, I was careful never to make access to Ms. Harper's funds contingent on appointment or medication adherence. I used the Representative Payee relationship as a therapeutic tool, involving Ms. Harper in decisions about her SSI benefits, promoting financial autonomy, and attending to the conflicts that arose in the context of our Representative Payee–beneficiary relationship.

Stance of social worker

My initial stance was one of acceptance and responsiveness, designed to reduce barriers to Ms. Harper's engagement with HCH as a clinic and me as a provider. In addition to being flexible about the timing and location of encounters, I focused on being responsive to Ms. Harper's requests, respectful of her privacy, and holding back my thoughts and opinions unless she asked me for them. I avoided declarative statements that sounded judgmental and gave her time to express anger.

Once I was designated SSI Representative Payee, my stance became more active. I proposed applying to supportive housing programs and we talked about the role of mental health treatment in gaining access to these programs. She declined these suggestions; I reviewed them periodically in case she changed her mind. This was a challenging period for me because Ms. Harper could not find housing or receive psychiatric treatment as long as she declined both. If HCH and I had given up too early, we would have missed an opportunity for Ms. Harper to come to her own decision to engage in psychiatric treatment and find housing.

In the last stage of our relationship, I moved into a maintenance role. I made sure that Ms. Harper's rent was paid, that she had reliable access to her funds and medication, and that she was aware of upcoming appointments. Ms. Harper would ask me to advocate for her or use me as a sounding board when she was upset about housemates or other personal matters. She remained largely reserved about her personal affairs. Although I did not press her to disclose more information than she volunteered, I also felt freer to make suggestions as our relationship was stronger than it had been initially.

Transfer or termination

HCH provides services to homeless individuals for up to a year after they become permanently housed. Ms. Harper and I began talking about the need to transition to another clinic around the time she moved to a transitional shelter. I informed her that once she secured stable independent housing, we would look for other sources of mental and physical health care and case management. We also agreed to gradually increase her responsibility for managing her SSI funds with the goal of ending HCH's Representative Payee role. Transition is often a difficult time for clients who, like Ms. Harper, have been coming to HCH for a long time. Just as engagement in services takes time, termination is a process that takes time as well. Ms. Harper telephones me periodically to let me know how she is doing. As of our last phone conversation, she was doing well and was still living in the same efficiency apartment.

Differential discussion

Today, Ms. Harper is doing remarkably well. She now has safe and permanent housing, friendships, and has close contact with her family. One of the most striking aspects of Ms. Harper's experience, however, is how long it took for her to obtain shelter, even after making contact with HCH and other service providers. As noted earlier, chronically mentally ill individuals often have difficulty complying with the requirements of supportive housing or shelter programs.

Over the last 15 years, "Housing First" has emerged as an alternative model that offers individuals housing regardless of their sobriety, psychiatric state, or interest in treatment (U.S. Department of Housing and Urban Development, 2007). Medical care, mental health services, and substance abuse treatment are offered to clients, but access to housing is not contingent on their adherence to treatment. Early evaluations of Housing First programs suggest that they are more successful at helping chronically homeless individuals secure and maintain permanent housing than continuum of care ("Housing Ready") and other models of assistance (Groton, 2013). The Housing First approach has been identified as a core strategy by the U.S. Interagency Council on Homelessness (2010) and is a centerpiece of Baltimore City's Ten Year Plan to End Homelessness (Baltimore Homeless Services, 2008).

In 2007, around the time Ms. Harper finally moved into a public housing unit, HCH received a federal SAMHSA grant to implement a Housing First program in Baltimore City. The program has since housed and provided intensive services to over 100 chronically homeless people whose life stories parallel Ms. Harper's in many ways. HCH also now participates in the SSI/SSDI Outreach, Access, and Recovery (SOAR) program, a federal initiative to expedite and improve access to Social Security disability benefits for homeless individuals diagnosed with a mental illness and/or co-occurring disorders. In 2014, 87% of applicants assisted by the SOAR program were awarded SSI or SSDI in an average of 71 days. Both the Housing First and the SOAR programs have increased our clients' ability to meet their goals of permanent housing, personal independence, and recovery from mental illness.

Discussion questions

1 What societal and life experiences likely contributed to Ms. Harper's homelessness?
2 How might have Ms. Harper's experience been different if Health Care for the Homeless had engaged her in a Housing First program? What benefits and challenges would this approach have presented?
3 Should mental health clinicians provide Representative Payee services for their clients? What factors should clinicians take into account when deciding whether or not to provide this service?

References

Angell, B., Martinez, N., Mahoney, C., & Corrigan, P. (2007). Payeeship, financial leverage, and the client-provider relationship. *Psychiatric Services, 58*(3), 365–372. doi: 10.1176/ps.2007.58.3.365

Baltimore Homeless Services (2008). *The journey home: Baltimore City's ten year plan to end homelessness.* Retrieved from www.baltimorecity.gov/mayor/downloads/0108%2010%20Year%20Plan.pdf

Chinman, M., Rosenheck, R., & Lam, J. (2000). The case management relationship and outcomes of homeless persons with serious mental illness. *Psychiatric Services, 51*(9), 1142–1147. doi: 10.1176/appi.ps.51.9.1142

Farooq, S. & Naeem, F. (2014). Tackling nonadherence in psychiatric disorders: Current opinion. *Neuropsychiatric Disease and Treatment, 10,* 1069–1077.

Gilmer, T., Dolder, C. Lacros, P., Folsom, D., Lindamer, L., Garcia, P., & Jeste, V. (2004). Adherence to treatment with antipsychotic medication and health care costs among Medicaid beneficiaries with schizophrenia. *American Journal of Psychiatry, 161,* 692–699.

Glazer, W. M. & Byerly, M. J. (2008). Tactics and technology to manage nonadherence in patients with schizophrenia. *Current Psychiatry Reports, 10*(4), 359–369.

Groton, D. (2013). Are Housing First programs effective? A research note. *Journal of Sociology & Social Welfare, 40*(1), 51–63.

HCH Clinicians' Network (2005). Closing the door to homelessness: How clinicians can help. *Healing Hands, 9*(5). Retrieved from www.nhchc.org

HCH Clinicians' Network (2014). Partnering with people for life-saving change. *Healing Hands* 18(3). Retrieved from www.nhchc.org

HRSA (Health Resources and Services Administration) (1999). *Program assistance letter 1999–12*: *Principles of practice – A clinical resource guide for Health Care for the Homeless programs.* Retrieved from http://bphc.hrsa.gov/policy/pa19912.htm

Howgego, I., Yellowlees, P., Owen, C., Meldrum, L., & Dark, F. (2003). The therapeutic alliance: The key to effective patient outcome? A descriptive review of the evidence in community mental health case management. *Australian and New Zealand Journal of Psychiatry, 37*(2), 169–183. doi: 10.1046/j.1440-1614.2003.01131.x/abstract

Keith, S. (2009). Use of long-acting risperidone in psychiatric disorders: Focus on efficacy, safety and cost-effectiveness. *Expert Review of Neurotherapeutics, 9*(1), 9–31.

Kirsh, B. & Tate, E. (2006). Developing a comprehensive understanding of the working alliance in community mental health. *Qualitative Health Research, 16*(8), 1054–1074. doi: 10.1177/104973230 6292100

Luchins, D. J., Roberts, D. L., & Hanrahan, P. (2003). Representative payeeship and mental illness: A review. *Administration and Policy in Mental Health and Mental Health Services Research, 30*(4), 341–353. doi: 10.1176/appi.ps.57.2.197

Maryland Department of Planning (2014). *Demographic, socioeconomic, housing and journey to work data for Maryland's incorporated and unincorporated areas & jurisdictions. American Community Survey 2011–2013 three-year estimates.* Retrieved from www.mdp.state.md.us/msdc/American_ Community_Survey/2011-2013/ACS_2011-2013_SummaryProfile.pdf

Marson, D. C., Savage, R., & Phillips, J. (2006). Financial capacity in persons with schizophrenia and serious mental illness: Clinical and research ethics aspects. *Schizophrenia Bulletin, 32*(1), 81–91.

Mayor's Office of Human Services, Homeless Services Program (2013). *2013 homeless point in time count report.* Retrieved from http://humanservices.baltimorecity.gov/HomelessServices/ DocumentsandResources.asp

National Low Income Housing Coalition (2014). *Out of reach 2014.* Retrieved from http://nlihc.org/oor/2014/

National Research Council (2007). *Improving the Representative Payee program*: *Serving beneficiaries and minimizing misuse.* Washington, DC: The National Academies Press.

Rosen, M. I., Bailey, M., Dombrowski, E, Ablondi, K., & Rosenheck, R. A. (2005). A comparison of satisfaction with clinician, family members/friends and attorneys as payees. *Community Mental Health Journal, 41*(3), 291–306.

SAMHSA (Substance Abuse and Mental Health Services Administration) (2014). *Recovery and recovery support.* Retrieved from www.samhsa.gov/recovery

Social Security Advisory Board (2010). *Disability programs in the 21st century*: *The Representative Payee program.* SSAB Issue Brief Series Vol. 2, No. 1. Washington, DC: Social Security Advisory Board. Retrieved from www.ssab.gov/Documents/Rep_Payee_Program.pdf

SSA (Social Security Administration) (2007). *SSI Annual Statistical Report.* Retrieved from www. socialsecurity.gov/policy/docs/statcomps/ssi_asr/

Stefancic, A. & Tsemberis, S. (2007). Housing first for long-term shelter dwellers with psychiatric disabilities in a suburban county: A four-year study of housing access and retention. *Journal of Primary Prevention, 28*(3–4), 265–279.

Stanhope, V., Barrenger, S. L., Salzer, M. S., & Marcus, S. C. (2013). Examining the relationship between choice, therapeutic alliance and outcomes in mental health services. *Journal of Personal Medicine, 3*(3), 191–202. doi: 10.3390/jpm3030191

Technical Assistance Collaborative (2013). *Priced out in 2013*: *The housing crisis for people with disabilities.* Retrieved from www.tacinc.org/media/33368/PricedOut2012.pdf

U.S. Department of Housing and Urban Development (2007). *The applicability of housing first models to homeless persons with serious mental illness.* Retrieved from www.huduser.org/portal/publica tions/hsgfirst.pdf

U.S. Department of Housing and Urban Development (2014). *The 2014 Annual Homeless Assessment Report to Congress.* Retrieved from https://www.hudexchange.info/resource/4074/2014-ahar-part-1-pit-estimates-of-homelessness/

U.S. Interagency Council on Homelessness (2010). *Opening doors*: *Federal strategic plan to prevent and end homelessness*. Washington, DC: USICH. Retrieved from http://usich.gov/resources/uploads/asset_library/Opening%20Doors%202010%20FINAL%20FSP%20Prevent%20End%20Homeless.pdf

Resource

For more information about working with homeless adults, see National Health Care for the Homeless Council: HCH 101 webinar, https://www.nhchc.org/training-techical-assistance/online-courses/hch-101/

Chapter 30

Pediatric public health

Educating professionals and communities about children's health and environmental exposures

Bambi Fisher

Context

The Pediatric Environmental Health Specialty Unit (PEHSU) at Mount Sinai is part of a network of 12 centers established since 1998 to educate health care providers, policymakers, and the public about environmental risks to children's health. Several disastrous events in the 1990s demonstrated community professionals' lack of knowledge about children's exposures to toxic environmental substances. In two such events, children were exposed to mercury and pesticides, and in each case, health providers failed to recognize the toxic exposure as the cause of their illnesses. PEHSUs were created in response to those events to help develop expertise among community providers and to provide trustworthy knowledge in the intervening time. The PEHSU mission is to educate health professionals and others about issues related to children's health and the environment, particularly the effect of chronic, low-level exposures to air and water pollution, lead, mercury, mold, and low doses of pesticides.

In an article published in 2005, Lanphear, Vorhees, and Bellinger called upon the United States to require industry to submit to toxin testing regulations similar to the European Union's "Registration, Evaluation and Authorization of Chemicals (REACH)" program because even low-level chemical exposures have been scientifically linked to spontaneous abortion, developmental delays, and pediatric illness and disorder. Systematic reviews show strong evidence linking organophosphate exposures (pre- and post-natally) to attention deficits and other neurodevelopmental negative outcomes in pre-school and early childhood (González-Alzaga et al., 2014). Specific components of air pollution have been found to be associated with children's poorer school performance in Louisiana. Air pollution is thought to affect poor and minority populations more intensely because such populations tend to live in more heavily polluted areas (Scharber, Lucier, London, Rosofsky, & Shandra, 2013). Nevertheless, politicians have been slow to implement REACH or similar legislation due, in part, to concerns that the costs of clean-up would be detrimental to industry.

The PEHSU work is based on the knowledge that children are not little adults and that they are especially vulnerable to hazards in the environment. Exposures that occur during the nine months of pregnancy and in the earliest months of life are among the greatest concerns. Five fundamental differences between children and adults exist. First, infants' normal growth demands for food, water, and air are disproportionate to adults', therefore toxins become more concentrated in infants' bodies due to the greater pound for pound exposure that infants and children get from the food and water they ingest and the air they breathe. Similarly, children's short stature and ground level activities (crawling, playing) expose them to toxins that are heavier and which become concentrated lower in the air/environment. Babies and children have age-appropriate hand-to-mouth behavior that puts them at risk for consumption of toxins in dust, soil, and ground surfaces. A third vulnerability is that children's metabolic pathways are immature, especially in the first months after birth; they are less able than adults to break down and excrete toxic compounds. Due to children's rapid growth and development, the time of early development creates windows of exquisite vulnerability. The developmental processes in the young are very complex and easily disrupted by toxic exposures. Finally, because children have more years ahead than adults, they have more time to develop chronic diseases that may be initiated by these early toxic exposures (Children's Environment Health Center, 2015)

Policy

The overarching goal of the PEHSU is to protect children from environmental threats. The United States Environmental Protection Agency (EPA) provides funds to ATSDR, the Agency for Toxic Substances and Disease Registry, which in turn lays out the therapeutic goals and specifications which the PEHSU follows in order to receive funding. PEHSU practices are therefore influenced and dictated by the specifications and the limitations of available funds. Initially, the national PEHSUs were funded to improve the environmental health of children by enhancing educational and consultative services to individuals, clinicians, health professionals, and the community. PEHSUs rely on evidence-based and unbiased information from a network of experts in environmental health (Centers for Disease Control, 2015). More recently, funders have requested that the focus be more heavily on the education of, and consultation with, health professionals; they want to focus less on individual patient encounters or calls. This is due to shrinking funding and attempts to put the already limited resources of this program into areas where the outcome will be the greatest.

Technology

To satisfy the requirements of the PEHSU grant, for the next 5 years we will collect data, document our work, and gather feedback to demonstrate that program goals are being met. Data will include tracking the number of presentations developed and delivered, informational documents created, articles or book chapters disseminated, and health and community educational sessions delivered. Surveys will be distributed to collect data to assess target audiences' increased knowledge and behavioral changes as a result of PEHSU activities.

The PEHSU utilizes various types of technology to gather data and assess whether program goals are being met. One presentation the PEHSU gives to health and community providers is how to make the best use of technology in understanding and making decisions about children's environmental health. We work to increase and improve providers' use of internet technology and social media, as these popular technological options are known to reach large audiences and could prove to be an effective method of conveying important information.

Technology also influences the referrals received by the PEHSU nationally. Worried parents often are concerned about their children's environmental exposures. We have a toll-free number and an easily referenced website; calls are received frequently from parents who search the internet and question us about the next steps to take in assessing environmental toxins to which they believe their children have been exposed. Support and carefully researched consultation is provided via telephone and email. On occasion, we may meet with a family to assist them in managing medical interventions and to minimize unnecessary stress due to worries about exposures.

Organization

Environmental health in a hospital setting draws professionals from a variety of disciplines, all sincerely interested in working together for the common goal of improving children's health. The PEHSU team is exemplary in its inclusiveness and interdisciplinary work. Each disciplinary perspective is respected and the team includes physicians, social workers, industrial hygienists, researchers, and students. The Mount Sinai PEHSU has a fluid definition of social work's role and the social work voice is valued for the biopsychosocial perspective the profession brings to each case, issue, outreach, or presentation discussed.

In 2000, as the Mount Sinai PEHSU was developed, a pediatrician advocated for social work involvement with the unit because social work could add the translational and psychosocially informed perspective to effectively convey complex knowledge to diverse groups. Shortly after this, the World Trade Center 9/11 tragedy occurred in New York City. As pediatricians and social workers worked closely responding to this unprecedented disaster, the need for collaborative work within the PEHSU became even clearer. The Mount Sinai PEHSU stepped in and social workers joined pediatricians speaking with traumatized parents and school officials as they planned for children's return to schools, educating them about the potential psychological effects on children. The PEHSU developed and disseminated several fact sheets pertaining to air quality and environmental issues affecting children in downtown New York City (Mount Sinai Pediatric Environmental Health Specialty Unit, 2002). The PEHSU was respected and sought after during this crisis for its trusted, unbiased, and evidence-based information.

Social work enhances the work of the PEHSU due to our knowledge base and person-in-environment perspective. Our training about how to effectively communicate with varied populations is beneficial. Much of the PEHSU work centers on translating the complex language of environmental issues into understandable concepts for a wide range of audiences. My social work perspective helps shape how to best present complicated material so audiences will listen and comprehend. My social work role helps to interpret dense scientific information in a way that people can understand. Further, we help convey the information in a way that health professionals and consumers can integrate into their work and their lives more easily.

Description of typical clients/situations

The Mount Sinai PEHSU serves New York, New Jersey, Puerto Rico, and the Virgin Islands. Clients are typically self-referred and range from individual callers using our toll-free phone line, to schools and communities who are concerned about broader environmental exposures. Below, an individual case is described, yet most of our cases are communities. Our primary focus is to educate health providers in the geographical area about how children's health can be impacted by such exposures.

Example of typical client and intervention

Clients in the PEHSU may be individual families or communities struggling with a possible environmental exposure in the home, school, day care, or play area. One such community exposure occurred in Suffolk County, Long Island. Several families contacted the PEHSU due to illegal dumping of contaminated soil in a playground near a populated cul-de-sac of homes (Bolger, 2014). In this situation, parents were individually provided guidance, based on their child(ren)'s possible exposure. Evidence-based advice was given about how to understand the risks and benefits of proceeding with testing and advocacy. The "client" we were working with in this case expanded to include the local pediatrician who served many of the affected families, the Suffolk County Department of Health, and the community at large. Few pediatricians or other health providers are formally trained to diagnose, treat, prevent, or advise on environmental problems in children. The PEHSU team can help close this gap in knowledge, providing case-by-case consultation with health providers and community-based organizations. Social work works hand in hand with the PEHSU team to carefully craft the messages that are given to communities where an environmental concern exists.

The Suffolk County community dumping case above illustrates the comprehensive way the PEHSU intervenes when a potential environmental threat to children may exist. Fact sheets for health care providers and the general public were developed as quickly as possible to aid in clinical decision-making and provide further resources. These fact sheets were developed using message maps, tools for conveying concise, accurate information (Melcrum, 2015). Message maps use evidence-based, lay-person-friendly health messages that draw from existing local, regional, and national resources to convey information about the community's exposure (Figure 30.1 and 30.2). These message maps guide health care providers

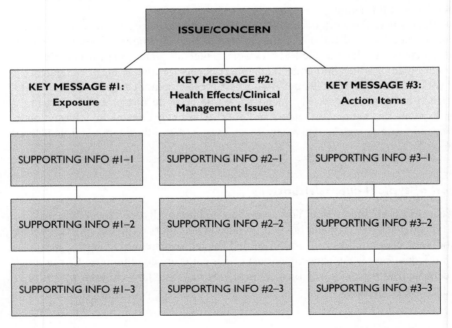

Figure 30.1 What is a message map? Message maps are a framework in which messages – particularly for complex environmental situations – can be organized and help to ease the communication with patients or the media. Typically the first key message explains the exposure of concern, the second key message explains the potential health effects or clinical management issues, and the third key message provides action items for physicians and families

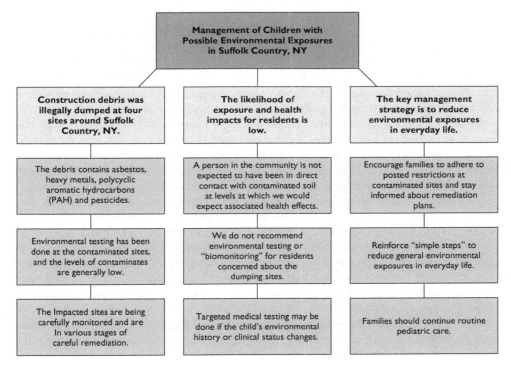

Figure 30.2 Example of a message map for Suffolk County exposures

in communicating risk, organizing messages, and assuring that information is relayed in a clear, consistent, and simple way. In-person trainings are used to educate health care providers about how to conduct an environmental health history, provide risk communication, and advocate for proper protection of children, while helping families to identify future steps. We work to increase the capacity and knowledge of health care providers locally so that they can manage exposures and be more effective partners to families. We use telephone consultations and follow up to maintain communication with health care providers, families, and community group members, allowing us to answer any additional questions.

In all services and interventions, environmental health information is carefully and painstakingly dissected and reassembled in a way that is accurate and fact based, but not alarmist. Our aim is to provide the most helpful information and guidance to health care providers who are working day to day with the concerned community. We want them to be fully informed so that they can comfort and guide families concerned about their children's health.

Decisions about practice

Definition of the client (individual case)

The clients and the problems addressed in the pediatric environmental arena vary. We recently worked with a family whose home had exceedingly high levels of tetrachloroethylene (PCE).

Tetrachloroethylene and trichloroethylene are used as solvents for cleaning metal and in dry cleaning; exposure at high levels can have serious health effects (see Agency for Toxic Substances & Disease Registry, 2014a, 2014b). This case was handled by a pediatric environmental fellow who used our multi-disciplinary team recommendations to assist the family in understanding the dangers of their environmental exposure and in advocating for change. The family has lived in their home for 19 years and only recently learned that their home was built on contaminated land. The father contacted our PEHSU with concerns about the possible health effects of long-term exposure to PCE in his indoor air (resulting from nearly two decades of soil and groundwater contamination on his property). It seemed reasonable to assume the home had been affected. During the family's 19 years of residency, the mother had been pregnant with each of their two children and the children had lived in the home for their entire childhood. Both children have health problems and one child has developmental issues that the father assumes may be a result of their exposures. Aside from the possible physical health effects associated with this family's chronic PCE exposure, the situation was an ongoing source of significant distress for the family once the contamination was discovered. The parents are understandably concerned about their children's health and the chronic exposure to PCE. Our PEHSU team recognizes that stress itself is linked to many mental health and physical health problems, as well as quality-of-life issues. The father has exhibited high levels of stress due to his sense that every breath his children have taken in the home has damaged their health; the family members feel dread whenever they return home because they know the air is contaminated.

The PEHSU researched the impact of PCE specific to this family's circumstances; we gave them information that is accurate and concerned, but not alarmist. In addition to the scientific data about toxic exposures that drives the work of the PEHSU, the team also intervenes to ameliorate the stress associated with the exposure. Experiencing chronic stress can have a lasting, negative effect on key systems in the body (Sandel & Wright, 2006). Therefore, PEHSU advocated with state agencies on behalf of this family, primarily with the New Jersey Department of Health and the New Jersey Department of Environmental Protection, to support the best action plan: in light of the toxic exposure and the high level of stress entailed, we asked them to assist the family to relocate.

Goals, objectives, and contracting

Goals and objectives differ based on whether the client is a family or a community and whether the target of intervention is educating local health care providers or remediating the pollutant or toxic exposure. Environmental justice is the larger goal embraced by the team and that informs the advocacy and objectives of the program. The PEHSU team was committed to providing information and support to this distressed family. The toxic home environment with its extensive soil and groundwater contamination was created by an industry formerly situated on the property. The industry no longer exists and is, therefore, not financially or legally responsible for any environmental hazard it may have left behind. Yet this family had nearly two decades of exposure and our hope was to help them relocate to reduce both ongoing exposures and stress. The larger policy message this case highlights is the importance of oversight about where homes and schools are built. The hazards of chemical and other exposures are slowly being recognized and legislation is being changed to reflect understandings about housing and school safety.

Example of a social justice goal in a community case

In 2006, the PEHSU helped to address a vapor intrusion problem in a day care center in New Jersey (see Public Health Services Branch, 2006, pp. 5–7). The daycare was housed in a building used earlier to manufacture mercury-containing thermometers. Elevated mercury levels were found in the indoor air and surface wipe samples. The building was closed and day care activities were canceled. Over the next months, the PEHSU helped parents and staff get a better understanding of how much elemental mercury exposure had taken place. The PEHSU's work, together with other state and local agencies, led to landmark legislation in January of 2007 requiring all child-care centers and educational facilities to get certification that the indoor environment is safe from contaminants (Public Health Services Branch, 2006). The larger goal of environmental justice requires different objectives for individual versus community cases. In each case, the goals and objectives are framed by the importance of addressing children's environmental health needs at micro, mezzo, and macro levels of practice.

Meeting place

Much of the PEHSU's work is done over the phone or in training sessions with community health providers and interested parties. In the individual (PCE) case, work with the family was done primarily over the phone and included helping them to get accurate information and to think about how to access help from the Department of Environmental Protection and the Department of Health. Our work is often done around our conference table as we gather accurate, non-alarmist scientific data about the exposures, identify the key messages that people need to ease communication, and help advocate for best outcomes and health follow-up for the children.

Stance of the social worker

Introducing social workers to the concepts of environmental health can open new doors for social work roles in health care settings. Mount Sinai's PEHSU funding for social work is limited, but we still play a vital role on the team. Each week, a 1–2 hour interdisciplinary PEHSU team meeting takes place. The agenda includes sharing individual case calls from the week, discussion of presentations, outreach and advocacy events taking place, and funding updates, as needed. Social work contributes to all these areas and my input is valued.

My stance is one of trying to put myself in the shoes of the people who must receive these scientifically complex messages that have emotional implications. I help the team consider ways of accurately conveying the information while recognizing the emotional reactions those messages may inspire. The intervention is like that of a translator or interpreter; I work to promote compassionate, informative communication.

In pediatric health care there is mounting evidence that there is an association between the environment and children's health. Pediatric social workers who are in direct contact with children, families, and the community can play a key role in identifying children at risk, recognizing environmental health concerns in all populations, and maximizing reliable information shared with parents. Pediatricians often have time limitations in clinic or office visits and social workers are well positioned to assess environmental risks by considering environmental histories.

Use of outside resources

Social workers need to increase their knowledge base in pediatric environmental health. We need to gain comfort and build expertise in asking questions about the environment and identifying best resources. Social work is well placed in pediatrics to be helpful and effective in environmental health. A pediatric environmental health history assesses places where children interact and spend time: home, school, playground, day care, or even the grandparent's residence. In other words, any place children live, grow, play, and learn. When social workers are educated about what goes into an environmental history, they can incorporate this focus into existing social work assessments in pediatric settings and that can allow social workers to add to this specialty field.

Basic and concise questions make up a pediatric environmental history and these fit well within social work biopsychosocial assessments. Questions as basic as the age of the child and his or her local situation (home, school, day care) combine with questions about whether the child lives in a low-income or marginalized community where children and families may live in less than adequate housing, and the answers can inform health providers about potential risky exposures. These families may be under extreme stress and living with hazardous environmental circumstances that they may not have identified. These screening questions about environmental health are easily accessed at http://who.int/ceh/capacity/Paediatric_Environmental_History.pdf. As social work roles in medical settings expand to include home visits and consultation with teachers and communities, social work is a natural discipline to embrace environmental health assessments. In this way, social work fulfills its mission to advocate for social justice and promote the well-being of all individuals. It allows us to manage and prevent potential threats to children's health. Social work offers a critical additional service to patients and families by providing another expert source to turn to for evidence-based information. Too often families are confronted with sensational headlines about environmental threats to children's health that range from plasticizers in food packaging, to arsenic in rice, to flame retardants in home furnishings. There can also be periodic events in communities like Superstorm Sandy or a building explosion (as happened in East Harlem and in the East Village in New York City). At times like these, families may experience increased anxiety, raised by the abundance of sensational information available on the internet; health professionals with accurate, non-alarmist environmental information and guidance can prove priceless.

Case conclusion

Unfortunately, at this time, the family in this case is still living in the house, despite our efforts to advocate for relocation. The Department of Environmental Protection and the Department of Public Health collaborated to install a remediation system that purportedly has cleaned the toxins from the home's environment and rendered the home safe. The family remains anxious about whether they and their children are truly safe, but they have few resources to enable moving out of the home without additional assistance. When individuals are affected rather than whole communities, it is harder to mobilize media and legislative actions to assist individual families. Nevertheless, there is still hope; a bill introduced in New Jersey will allow for funds to relocate families in this situation if it is passed.

Differential discussion

Informed social workers can help manage family's emotional reactions to information so that they can hear accurate information and consider problem-solving strategies to promote their children's health. Targeted environmental questions can be asked about housing to supplement what is already part of the social work intake assessment. Areas of focus might include specifics regarding the type of dwelling (private house, apartment, etc.) and how old the housing construction is, due especially, but not entirely, to lead paint issues. Asking about smoking at home, recent painting or renovations, and indoor pesticide use sheds additional light on possible childhood exposures. As pediatric social workers are assessing and learning about the behavioral practices of children in the areas they serve, "red flags" might be raised. For example, it is important to ask additional questions about where a child goes to day care or school, and if a child's hobbies include paints and solvents, glues, pesticides, or chemicals. We also need to sensitively ask about any alternative medicines, and/or cultural or religious practices that might involve products from other countries as there may be harmful products from abroad used in such practices. Discovery of hazards will help develop appropriate intervention and treatment plans. We must also explore parents' work-related habits and hazards as part of the social work assessment, especially if they work in factory or other environments where they are exposed to potential toxins. Valuable environmental information may be unearthed. Specifics about where the parent works, what materials they are exposed to at work, and habits they have upon return to home can ascertain what exposures are occurring. With this information, we can encourage parents to engage in handwashing and changing out of work clothes and shoes before entering the home and interacting with children in order to reduce children's exposure to workplace residues.

On a larger scale, social workers are trained to understand the macro/community level and are thereby well positioned to refer families to resources and advocacy groups related to environmental advocacy. The state of the art in environmental health is still evolving, meaning that situations are often uncertain. Social workers are often more comfortable in this gray zone than other professionals and can assist families in developing comfort zones and strategies for coping until the knowledge base evolves. We have the expertise to advocate for policies to protect the environment and children's health. It is a role we can embrace.

It is feasible for social work to more fully integrate environmental histories and environmental health practice by overcoming several barriers. Social work graduate schools and training or internship programs need to incorporate environmental health into the curriculum. Social workers in home visiting programs and those performing lengthy preventive admission assessments could incorporate environmentally focused assessments and interventions. Adding environmental health questions into existing clinical forms would make social work's pediatric assessments more complete and substantive and allow our referrals to be more holistic. With social work spearheading work in pediatric environmental health, the profession would be able to stress the value and importance of environmental health to patients and families and promote environmental awareness in schools and communities. This would strengthen the families we serve and allow the profession to take on a wider educational role.

The new relationship between the American Academy of Pediatrics, the American College of Medical Toxicologists, and the national PEHSU network can substantially enhance the program's outreach and effectiveness, and reinforce its linkages with a wide range of health care professionals, government agencies, and community-based organizations. However, given limited funds, it is essential that the PEHSU identify other environmental champions to help move its valuable work forward. This is where pediatric and perinatal social workers can step in and be in the right place at the right time. Given the social work profession's close involvement with patients, families, communities, and multi-disciplinary health care teams, we are well situated to partner with current experts to increase the health system's capacity to provide pediatric environmental health services.

The lessons learned from the social work role in the Mount Sinai PEHSU are in some ways unique to this program and in other ways able to be more universally applied to the social work role in health care settings. This work has taught me the importance of taking on new roles within existing job descriptions, without initially receiving designated compensation for the new work. New roles may require self-education through searching professional literature and obtaining mentorship regarding pediatric environmental health. Promoting attention to these issues in graduate and continuing education also needs to happen. Given the complexity of environmental science and patient/family/community general health literacy, social work can serve an important function in decoding and messaging (translating and interpreting) information for the people they work with. This expanded social work role fits with social work principles and with the profession's larger agenda of social and environmental justice, both locally and globally. The time is right: these factors – the need for more professional environmental health education, parents' desire for more environmental health information, and the high cost of pediatric environmental health problems – indicate a need and an area where social work can have an impact. Social work can join the growing number of pediatricians, nurses, public health specialists, and researchers who are part of much needed leadership in children's environmental health.

Discussion questions

1   What obstacles might keep you from incorporating environmental health history questions into your current biopsychosocial assessments? How can you overcome those obstacles?
2   Have you noticed common environmental health problems in the populations with whom you have worked? How does a public health lens of considering environmental exposures help you to think about these circumstances differently?
3   During your graduate education, were you ever exposed to questions about how the physical and biological environment affects the clients you serve? Why do you think social work education is strong on training for psychosocial assessment and weaker on training for biopsychosocial and environmental assessment?

References

Agency for Toxic Substances & Disease Registry (2014a). Tetrachloroethylene (PERC) Fact Sheet. Retrieved from www.atsdr.cdc.gov/PHS/PHS.asp?id=263&tid=48
Agency for Toxic Substances & Disease Registry (2014b). Trichloroethylene (PCH) Fact Sheet. Retrieved from www.atsdr.cdc.gov/toxfaqs/tf.asp?id=172&tid=30
Bolger, T. (2014, May 30). More carcinogens found in park amid growing Islip dumping probe. *Long Island Press*. Retrieved from www.longislandpress.com/2014/05/30/more-carcinogens-found-in-park-amid-growing-islip-toxic-dumping-probe/
Centers for Disease Control (2015). Retrieved from www.cdc.gov/features/pehsu/
Children's Environment Health Center (2015). *Patient care*. Retrieved from www.mount sinai.org/static_files/MSMC/Files/Patient%20Care/Children/Childrens%20Environmental%20 Health%20Center/NYS-Children-Environment.pdf
González-Alzaga, B., Lacasaña, M., Aguilar-Garduño, C., Rodríguez-Barranco, M., Ballester, F., Rebagliato, M., & Hernández, A. (2014). A systematic review of neurodevelopmental effects of prenatal and postnatal organophosphate pesticide exposure. *Toxicology Letters, 230* (Environmental contaminants and target organ toxicities), 104–121. doi: 10.1016/j.toxlet.2013.11.019

Lanphear, B. P., Vorhees, C. V., & Bellinger, D. C. (2005). Protecting children from environmental toxins. *PLOS Medicine, 2*(3), 203–208. doi: 10.1371/journal.pmed.0020061

Melcrum (2015). Developing a message map. Retrieved from https://www.melcrum.com/research/engage-employees-strategy-and-change/developing-message-map

Mount Sinai Pediatric Environmental Health Specialty Unit (2002). *WTC particulate matter fact sheet.* Retrieved from http://icahn.mssm.edu/static_files/MSSM/Files/Research/Programs/Pediatric%20Environmental%20Health%20Specialty%20Unit/pm-faqs3.pdf

Public Health Services Branch, NJ Division of Epidemiology, Environmental and Occupational Health (2006). *Annual report.* Retrieved from www.state.nj.us/health/eoh/cehsweb/documents/cehs06.pdf

Sandel, M. & Wright, R. J. (2006). When home is where the stress is: expanding the dimensions of housing that influence asthma morbidity. *Archives of Disease in Childhood, 91*(11), 942. doi: 10.1136/adc.2006.098376

Scharber, H., Lucier, C., London, B., Rosofsky, A., & Shandra, J. (2013). The consequences of exposure to developmental, neurological, and respiratory toxins for school performance: A closer look at environmental ascription in East Baton Rouge, Louisiana. *Population & Environment, 35*(2), 205. doi: 10.1007/s11111-013-0185-9

Resources

Agency for Toxic Substances and Disease Registry, www.atsdr.cdc.gov/about/

Association of Occupational and Environmental Clinics, www.aoec.org/

Centers for Disease Control, www.cdc.gov/

EPA. Evaluating exposures to toxic air pollutants: A citizen's guide, www.epa.gov/ttnatw01/3_90_023.html

World Health Organization Pediatric Environmental Health Assessment, http://who.int/ceh/capacity/Paediatric_Environmental_History.pdf

Internationally related public health

Chapter 31

Community-based health and social services for Bhutanese refugees

Jessica Euna Lee and Parangkush Subedi

Context

The Office of the United Nations High Commissioner for Refugees (UNHCR) defines a refugee as someone who has been forced to flee his or her country because of persecution, war, or violence for reasons of race, religion, nationality, political opinion, or membership in a particular social group (UNHCR, 2015). Since the 1970s, the United States has received over 3 million refugees (U.S. Refugee Act of 1980, 2012). These diverse individuals have established new homes and lives across all 50 states; up to 70,000 refugees have arrived annually to the United States for the last 5 years (U.S. Department of State, 2015a). The main countries of nationality include Iraq, Burma, Bhutan, and Somalia. After the initial resettlement period funded by the Office of Refugee Resettlement (ORR), refugees are quickly expected to assimilate to life in the United States and become self-sufficient. This is very challenging as they face a myriad of resettlement obstacles; it can be even more daunting for refugees with particular vulnerabilities and high medical needs. This chapter will focus on a community-based organization founded by Bhutanese refugees in one U.S. city.

The United States has been the prime destination for Bhutanese refugees and approximately 78,000 refugees have resettled in 40 states (U.S. Department of State, 2015a). The Bhutanese American Organization-Philadelphia (BAOP) provides post-resettlement health services and peer-support programs to the community. BAOP grew out of the community's recognition of the need for mutual assistance in order to build bridges with existing health and social service providers; to develop programs that will decrease social isolation; as well as to provide community-based English language classes that are accessible to vulnerable community members.

Policy

The U.S. Refugee Act of 1980 adopted the UNHCR's definition of refugees, and presently the ORR directs the dissemination of benefits for refugees resettled in the United States (U.S. Refugee Act of 1980). Refugees arriving in the United States are granted refugee status by the U.S. Department of Homeland Security prior to arrival and are placed under the sponsorship of a resettlement agency participating in the Department of State's Reception & Placement Program (U.S. Department of State, 2015b). During the first 90 days from arrival, resettlement agencies provide newly arrived refugees with initial support and case management funded by ORR (Figure 31.1).

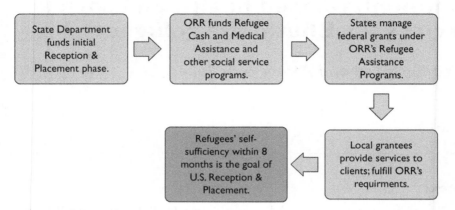

Figure 31.1 Overview of U.S. refugee resettlement process.

Source: Adapted from the Office of Refugee Resettlement (2014)

About 800 refugees arrive in Philadelphia each year. Their resettlement and health services are coordinated by members of the Philadelphia Refugee Health Collaborative (PRHC), which comprises three resettlement agencies and eight medical institutions (PRHC, 2013). According to federal protocol, refugees must obtain a domestic health screening (immunizations and screening for tuberculosis, infectious diseases, parasites, and posttraumatic stress disorder) as well as an orientation to the U.S. health care system within 30 days of arrival (ORR, 2014). State health departments or state refugee coordinators may facilitate this medical screening process, but this does not occur in Pennsylvania. Therefore, the PRHC plays an integral role in coordinating initial health screenings and follow-up screenings for newly arrived refugees (PRHC, 2013). All refugees receive federally funded Refugee Medical Assistance (RMA) for their first eight months in the United States. After the eight-month period of RMA, refugees are required to obtain health insurance on their own. Prior to the Affordable Care Act, the majority of refugee adults in Pennsylvania did not qualify for Medicare and so became uninsured upon termination of RMA. The Affordable Care Act now enables all refugees to have ongoing health insurance at variable costs. As most ORR-funded benefits for refugees are time-limited, agencies and health care providers do not have the capacity to meet clients' long-term needs. Thus, community-based support is invaluable to clients' resettlement experiences.

Organization

The BAOP is a nonprofit community-based organization (501c3) launched a little more than 2 years ago. Bhutanese community members in Philadelphia conceived of and initiated BAOP. Its mission is to empower Bhutanese refugee families and to support them in integrating into a new environment and maintaining healthy living practices. It provides short-term and long-term services to Bhutanese refugees while fostering a community-building and placemaking mission. BAOP has become a problem-solving center for refugee families who face challenges navigating systems and adjusting to life in the United States. BAOP values teamwork and is staffed and run by Bhutanese refugee community members who share the resettlement experience and are able to assist newly arriving people in acclimating to life in Philadelphia. Stakeholders with English fluency and competency to build networks within and out of the Bhutanese community have become community leaders. These individuals uphold the bylaws of the organization, build capacity, and lead the organization. BAOP leaders are mindful of power dynamics and diversity as they work with fellow community members, as there are differences in English language skills, education, income, age, gender, and able-bodiedness. Volunteers, comprising stakeholders as well as partners outside of the Bhutanese community, provide various services to address the needs of refugee clients. BAOP collaborates with many partners outside of the community. These include members of the PRHC, local universities, city agencies, and nonprofit organizations. BAOP has interdisciplinary programs and functions that are established according to the community's needs and interests. Programs focus on health care, English language, culture, and general social services. Since BAOP's inception, Bhutanese community members identified health care access as a major concern. It is within this context that BAOP community members partnered with local health care providers to develop the Health Focal Points (HFP) project that currently provides community-based health support to Bhutanese refugees in Philadelphia (Subedi et al., 2014). BAOP believes that clients' satisfaction and independence are the priorities of the organization's work. BAOP continues to broaden its outreach to the community and to build capacity among local service providers and organizations.

Technology

BAOP staff members facilitate clients' access to and understanding of technology, though technology is not a central feature of BAOP's work with clients. Bhutanese refugees arrived from refugee camps in Nepal where many people lived in thatched-roof huts with no electricity. Therefore, community members' encounters with technology prior to arrival were limited. Bhutanese refugees describe the transition from camp life in Nepal to life in the United States as a culture shock, and technology is a contributing factor. Health care in the

Table 31.1 Overview of Bhutanese American Organization-Philadelphia's programs

Health program	English language classes	Cultural programs	General social services
• HFP project provides health care navigation, care management, and walk-in hours • Series of health fairs and free clinics organized in collaboration with local health care providers • Staffed by volunteer community members • Experts from local agencies and medical institutions provide supervision and consultation	• English and literacy classes are provided • Staffed by community leaders with expertise in teaching English as a second language as well as volunteers • Education experts provide consultation and support	• Festival and holiday celebrations are organized • Regular social gatherings organized, some in collaboration with local organizations • BAOP hosts sewing programs in collaboration with local groups • In collaboation with SEWA-International, yoga classes are held	• Provides peer support and community-building for Bhutanese refugees • Community members assist non-English speakers with language interpretation • Drop-in hours held to assist clients in navigated systems such as: job applications, college applications, funeral processes, etc.

United States relies heavily on hospital systems and medical technology. Thus, BAOP case managers often assist clients in understanding medical procedures and technologies that they may encounter.

Description of typical clients and situations

The BAOP welcomes all Bhutanese community members living in the Greater Philadelphia region. Community members, resettlement agency staff members, health care providers, social workers, and educators often refer newly arrived refugees to BAOP for community-based post-resettlement support. BAOP serves "self-identified clients," who seek help from the organization for specific needs. The clients served by BAOP are Nepali-speaking Bhutanese individuals referred to as *Lhotshampas* (Hutt, 2003). In the late 1980s, the Bhutanese government began its "One Nation One People" program, which marginalized *Lhotshampa* peoples (Hutt, 2005). By the early 1990s, *Lhotshampas* were compelled to flee the country, and they landed in Nepal for safety and security (Sinha, 2003).

The majority of these refugees are Hindu; smaller percentages are Christian, Buddhist, or other religions. Refugees lived in UNHCR-funded camps in Nepal for nearly two decades until third-country resettlement became an option in late 2007 (Basu, 2009). UNHCR and the International Organization for Migration (IOM) coordinate refugees' resettlement to third countries. Pennsylvania is one of the top receiving states for Bhutanese refugees, with approximately 8,700 Bhutanese refugees arriving from 2008 to 2014 (Pennsylvania Refugee Resettlement, 2015). The PRHC reports that 20% of refugees arriving in Philadelphia have high medical needs (Lee & Stair, 2013). Health research indicates that Bhutanese refugees exhibit disproportionately high rates of suicide, mental disorders, micronutrient deficiency, and latent tuberculosis (CDC, 2012; Schinina, Sharma, Gorbacheva, & Mishra, 2011).

According to researchers, refugees' resettlement challenges and vulnerability result not only from individual or population-specific characteristics, but also from structural issues and services that they encounter during resettlement (Shrestha, 2011). The post-resettlement period, after the first 90 days of arrival, is a critical time of transition and vulnerability for newly arrived refugees. They are still acclimating to their new home and interfacing with various systems, but may no longer be receiving regular case management or ORR-funded support. Refugees in Philadelphia report great appreciation for the case management provided by their resettlement agency, while also stating that they desired a longer period of services (Lee & Stair, 2013). Navigating the U.S. health care system, particularly in managing the immunization process for immigration, understanding health insurance, and scheduling appointments, is a major challenge for refugees and adds to their stresses during resettlement (SEARAC, 2011).

As newly arrived community members, Bhutanese refugees are struggling to remain stable and self-sufficient. Because the first Bhutanese refugees only began arriving in 2008, there are no long-established Nepali–Bhutanese communities in the United States to receive and educate new immigrants. Thus, community members have limited awareness of mainstream social services, which may or may not be linguistically or logistically accessible to them. Acculturation is a difficult process and age, too, affects the experience. BAOP notes that problems with connecting to services and adapting to life in the United States appear to be the most acute among elderly and non- or semi-literate community members, as well as individuals with mental illness. Family units are typical clients of BAOP, as most Bhutanese refugees in Philadelphia are resettled in families and reside in large households. Nepali–Bhutanese culture highly values family and places less value on individualism, relative to the U.S. norm. Families who are unable to overcome challenges during resettlement or health-related problems approach BAOP for support.

Decisions about practice

Definition of the client

BAOP's clients are Bhutanese refugees residing in the Greater Philadelphia area. Two client examples will be discussed here to illustrate BAOP's health and social service impact. BAOP's clients are generally families; problems that an individual faces are contextualized within the family system. The Ansari family and the Dorji family were resettled in Philadelphia by local resettlement agencies. Both families arrived from a refugee camp in Nepal. Like most Bhutanese families, their lack of English proficiency and understanding of U.S. systems have been barriers to these families' adjustment. The families received cultural orientations in Nepal prior to departure; however, this did not prepare them for life in the United States. In addition, members of the Ansari and Dorji families have significant medical needs; thus, managing the families' health care and navigating the hospital and welfare systems have been significant problems for both families. BAOP provided health services and social support to these client families. Their resettlement process, which is generalizable to many Bhutanese refugees in the United States, is illustrated in the timeline shown in Figure 31.2.

The Ansaris are a family of seven. Karma, a 42-year-old man, and his wife Sonam, a 39-year-old woman, have five school-going children between the ages of 19 and 10: Reena, Junu, Kumar, Raju, and Sanjay. Karma Ansari suffers from paralysis and Sonam has a speech disability. They live in a rented apartment in an area that is far away from most of the other community members. The Ansari family relies totally on public assistance, as neither Mr. nor Mrs. Ansari is able to work. The family has had to interact a great deal with the welfare office as well as hospital systems in Philadelphia. Because of the parents' medical conditions and their lack of English proficiency, the Ansari family struggled with navigating appointments and relied heavily on relatives and church members for escorts to appointments and language

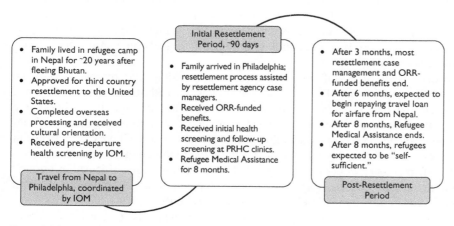

Figure 31.2 Resettlement timeline for Ansari and Dorji families

interpretation. The family's relatives became their de-facto case managers. Community members referred the Ansari family to BAOP via telephone and communicated the family's health and social needs to BAOP leaders. Their initial interactions with BAOP were during walk-in hours at the BAOP community center, as well as during a visit to a BAOP community leader's home. Managing medical needs and navigating health appointments were the main short-term problems identified by the family. BAOP volunteers helped the Ansari family to meet these needs, while also fostering a sense of community.

Husband and wife, Tashi and Puja Dorji, and their five children are the second case example. They live in an apartment complex where large numbers of other Bhutanese community members reside. Mr. Dorji, a 60-year-old man, and one of his elder daughters, Deepa, aged 27, are the sole earners for the household. Mrs. Puja Dorji, aged 55, and two daughters, Gita, aged 30, and Kali, aged 24, have high medical needs and are physically too weak to work. The sons Sumesh, aged 22, and Tilak, aged 19, attend high school. Mr. Dorji was overwhelmed with the pressure to financially support the family, pay their bills, and manage the care of his three ill family members. Regretting the decision to resettle in Philadelphia, he was frustrated by not being able to navigate U.S. systems independently due to language barriers. The Dorjis were referred to BAOP by neighbors and resettlement agency staff for post-resettlement support. The family identified health care navigation for Mrs. Dorji, Gita, and Kali as problems to be addressed by BAOP's Health Focal Point program, as well as supports for Mr. Dorji to better manage his household's bills and related matters. HPF volunteers provide medical case management for the Dorji family and the family regularly utilizes BAOP's walk-in hours for other social services.

Goals, objectives, and contracting

After doing an initial assessment of the family's presenting problems, BAOP staff work with clients to set goals and plan a course of action to address their needs. Clients of BAOP seeking health services generally come with time-limited needs and the Health Focal Points project's goals are mainly to resolve acute health navigation needs. The short-term goals for the Ansari and Dorji family included increasing the family's awareness of system navigation, assisting them in managing the family's medical appointments and care, and empowering them to mobilize their resources in adjusting to life in the United States. Clients actively participate in the goal-setting process. If outside resources are required, other agencies and institutions, such as health care providers, may also be part of the goal-setting process. Since BAOP is a community organization, goals may shift after clients' short-term needs are met.

The broader vision of BAOP includes community-building and placemaking; thus, clients' involvement with BAOP may evolve over time. In addition to short-term goals, long-term goals may be set for clients' sustainable adjustment to life in Philadelphia. These long-term goals often include English language learning, community engagement, citizenship attainment, and upward economic mobility in the United States. Clients may engage in English classes or community activities to pursue these long-term goals. For the Ansari family, BAOP staff members worked toward preventing the family's social isolation through community engagement. For the Dorjis, Mr. Dorji set the long-term goal of gaining English fluency and he eventually enrolled in English classes at BAOP.

Formal contracts are not written with clients; however, client goals and services are documented by BAOP staff members. Health Focal Points was formalized as a program during the past 2 years and is currently an organized case management program. Case files are kept in a safe locker, which only HFP staff members, who are trained in Health Insurance Portability and Accountability Act of 1996 (HIPAA) Privacy Rule, can access. HIPAA regulations provide protections for identifiable health information held by covered entities (U.S. Department of Health and Human Services, 1996), which includes health information for BAOP clients, who receive treatment at PRHC refugee clinics.

Meeting place

The majority of meetings and HFP case management sessions occur in the BAOP community center. The first BAOP community center was a two-story townhome-style building, located close to the homes of many Bhutanese community members. In recent months, BAOP moved to a building just a few blocks away from the original community center. Health clinics and workshops organized by BAOP and local health care providers are held at the community center. Due to the various programs and classes held in the center, it is a dynamic and vibrant space. Members of the Ansari and Dorji families visit BAOP to schedule medical visits, make appointment at welfare offices, meet with HFP volunteers, and to access other services. Mr. Dorji visits the BAOP community center at least once a week during walk-in hours and to meet with community leaders. The new BAOP community center is larger than the first building and has more rooms, which better accommodate programs and classes. For members who live far away from the BAOP community center, meetings may take place offsite, such as at community leaders' homes or at churches. As Karma Ansari is paralyzed and the family lives far away from the center, HFP volunteers meet with him and his family at their home or at BAOP community leaders' homes. Volunteers may also escort clients to medical visits and other appointments if the clients require assistance navigating systems and language barriers.

Use of time

BAOP's Health Focal Points program is short term and addresses clients' acute health care navigation needs. The Ansari family and the Dorji family schedule appointments with their HFP case manager as needed, during which time the volunteer facilitates their health needs. Walk-in hours for the health program and general social services are scheduled daily between 9:00 am and 5:00 pm on weekdays at the Center. During walk-in hours, volunteers are available to assist clients with questions and to provide language interpretation. The BAOP community center hosts English classes, as well as cultural classes such as sewing and yoga classes. Because BAOP serves long-term community-building purposes, time is often dedicated to celebrating cultural holidays and holding community events. The BAOP center is open most weekends for informal gatherings, where community members meet to discuss current problems and concerns that the community may be facing. No prior appointment is needed to meet community leaders in their houses or at the center. In addition, BAOP provides a series of health fairs and free health clinic hours at the community center in collaboration with local medical institutions. Over the past 2 years, BAOP was able to obtain grant funding and developed ties with other refugee stakeholders and inter-agencies such as the school district, health care providers, post-resettlement agencies, and other community organizations. As a result, too, BAOP is now able to employ paid staff members, who provide organized HFP case management and support other services.

Strategies and interventions

BAOP's community-based health care navigation program grew out of a series of community meetings and surveys. Members of BAOP and local health institutions adapted an evidence-based community health worker model for the community (Subedi et al., 2014). Both the Ansari and Dorji family were enrolled in BAOP's HFP program in order to better navigate the health care system. HFP case managers act as facilitators for the client's health and social needs (Children's Hospital of Philadelphia Policy Lab, 2014; Subedi et al., 2014). Strategies include assisting families with navigating medical appointments, and public assistance appointments, helping them understand systems, enrolling kids in school, and finding a way for long-term adjustment to city life. Twenty-two Bhutanese community volunteers were trained on medical bill clearance, scheduling appointments in hospitals, enrolling in health insurance, taking public transportation, and applying for welfare (Subedi et al., 2014). These community volunteers work on a rotational basis at the Center. Because of the increasing number of clients and greater demands for more health system navigation services, BAOP hired a part-time staff member to support HFP clients in a sustainable manner. See Figure 31.3 for the Ansari family's genogram.

Karma Ansari and Sonam Ansari required assistance in managing their medical needs and their HFP case managers acted as facilitators. The case managers assist clients with their health navigation needs and also provide education and empowerment so that clients can learn to manage their own health care in the long term. Since Karma is paralyzed and the family does not live close to the Center, their HFP care team meets with them at their home or at community leaders' homes. The Dorji family requires assistance navigating medical appointments for the three family members. As the family members lack English proficiency, they often come to BAOP's walk-in hours for assistance with making appointments, making sense of bills and paperwork from health clinics. Finding jobs, adjusting to city life

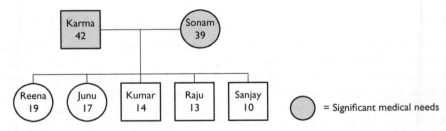

Figure 31.3 Ansari family genogram

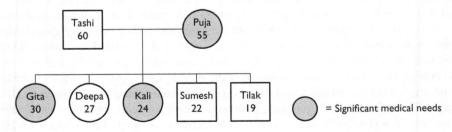

Figure 31.4 Genogram for Dorji family

and learning English are long-term needs for the Dorji family. See Figure 31.4 for the Dorji family's genogram.

Prior to the Affordable Care Act, some members of the Ansari and Dorji family were uninsured after RMA; therefore, the BAOP health clinic served as their primary health care site. BAOP is mindful of long-term resettlement needs and therefore may refer HFP clients to other programs. BAOP recognizes the heightened vulnerability of Bhutanese refugees who lack education levels and English language skills. Thus, members of the Ansari family and the Dorji family were referred to English classes at BAOP. Members of both families also participate in informal community gatherings and celebrations that increase their community engagement.

Stance of case management and BAOP staff members

BAOP's health services and care management are both short term and long term. Short-term care management includes HFP volunteers' assisting client families in navigating immediate health matters and gradually meeting their post-resettlement health goals. The long-term goal is refugees' adjustment to U.S. city life. Thus, long-term care management takes the form of continued peer interaction and adjustment to city life through English as a Second Language (ESL) and cultural classes as well as community gatherings. As its staff and volunteers are stakeholders, the organization fosters community and a sense of belonging. Until November 2014, BAOP had only unpaid staff volunteers, but ORR funding has allowed for hiring paid staff members. The BAOP staff and board are deeply committed to sharing their knowledge, time, and energy to assist fellow community members. BAOP's priorities and systems are governed by the needs of their clients, all members of the Bhutanese community.

Because BAOP leaders, staff, and the majority of volunteers are stakeholders, their boundaries with clients are complex. BAOP's relationship with clients depends on the type and scope of the problems the clients identify. For example, the role of the HFP case manager at BAOP is that of a facilitator; the role of BAOP education instructors is that of a teacher; and the role of walk-in hour volunteers is that of language interpreter and troubleshooter – all while being fellow community members, neighbors, and peers. Thus, boundaries between BAOP staff members and clients are much less formal than boundaries between non-community-based agency staff members and clients. Also, BAOP staff members and clients occupy numerous roles, sometimes simultaneously, which may change depending on the situation. As they are all stakeholders, BAOP staff members and clients are co-decision makers, initiators, advocates, and community members.

Use of resources outside of the helping relationship

BAOP partners with numerous organizations and health institutions and, therefore, has built a broad network of resources. Experts from outside the community who are affiliated with local universities and institutions supervise both the health and English language programs. BAOP has also focused on outreach to city agencies, such as the Mayor's Office of Immigrant and Multicultural Affairs. As BAOP staff and volunteers serve as facilitators of clients' health and social issues, anything requiring direct intervention from professionals such as social workers, doctors, or lawyers are immediately referred or forwarded to the respective resources. One major resource is the PRHC network. Resettlement agencies work hard to meet the needs of their clients; however, their capacity to provide post-resettlement services is limited. Thus, the BAOP is positioned to meet the significant need for post-resettlement support among the Bhutanese refugee community. PRHC and other organizations serving refugees and immigrants in Philadelphia recognize the value of BAOP and its mission. BAOP provides health clinics and workshops led by outside health service providers. Staff members of non-profit organizations and initiatives also often partner with BAOP in order to develop and coordinate programs. For instance, BAOP has collaborated with the Mural Arts Program and Nationalities Service Center's Growing Home Garden programs. Social workers employed by PRHC partners who practice in various capacities, such as resettlement case managers, hospital staff, and program coordinators, collaborate with BAOP when community-based support is required. Thus, social workers partner regularly with BAOP in order foster community-based peer support for sustainable adjustment and placemaking.

Transfer and termination

As BAOP is a community-driven organization, termination of services for clients is not formalized. Once clients' short-term goals are met, they may transition to longer term interactions with BAOP such as using BAOP's walk-in hours as needed, instead of scheduling appointments with an HFP case manager. Such was true for both the Ansari family and the Dorji family. Clients may also choose to participate in classes or community events, which have differing timelines. Clients' outcomes are not measured but their satisfaction and eventual self-reliance are taken into account as programs are reassessed and maintained.

Case conclusion

The Ansari family is making a very good adjustment to their new home. Mr. Ansari is building connections with community members and beginning to manage his health appointments independently. The family has found sustainable ways to schedule and get to medical appointments on their own. Mr. Ansari still utilizes BAOP's services episodically when he has specific questions and his older children now serve as volunteers at BAOP. The children are thriving in school and the family has begun to feel more acclimated. As they maintain relationships with BAOP community members, the family feels less isolated and has developed a sense of belonging. The Dorji family has transitioned away from HFP's case management, as their acute health navigation needs have been met. These days, Mr. Dorji visits the BAOP center approximately once a week during walk-in hours if he has specific questions or needs. He is well-connected with community members and feels that BAOP's volunteers are accessible and reliable when he is in need of their services. Puja, Gita, and Kali have learned how to manage their medical appointments and health care needs. Mr. Dorji is currently attending ESL classes taught at BAOP and developing long-term goals for his employment. Sumesh and Tilak serve as volunteers during BAOP's walk-in health services hours after school. The Dorji family now feels more optimistic about their future.

Differential discussion

Empowering community members through awareness, English classes, and workshops is BAOP's central mantra in order to enable Bhutanese community members to become self-reliant. Community members are taught to navigate systems and address their problems independently, while building a sense of community. Both the Ansari and Dorji families greatly benefited from work with BAOP's health volunteers, who provided health care navigation and language support. Members of both families have become active participants of BAOP. As in these two families, members of other families who utilized health services have also become BAOP volunteers. As the health and welfare needs of newly arriving refugee families were so great, BAOP has not been able to focus on the education and employment issues of the younger members of Bhutanese families. The focus is changing now, so that BAOP can assist Bhutanese youth in successfully finishing high school and accessing college. BAOP is continuing to seek and secure funding, such as the ORR's community grants, which will hopefully grow the organization and enable it to provide more comprehensive services and community-building initiatives to Bhutanese refugees.

Discussion questions

1   If there is a refugee or immigrant population in your area, what do you think the health needs might be for these communities? How would you assess these needs and how might you work with the community to intervene?

2   How do issues related to accessing health care intersect with other resettlement challenges that newly arriving refugee groups in your region may face? What implications may arise?

3   Policy allowing for medical assistance initially quickly gives way to needing to buy insurance through the ACA Health Marketplace, still much more expensive than many can afford. If you could write policy for refugees and immigrants, how would you weigh the needs of the community versus the needs of the larger community to keep health costs in check?

References

Basu, P. S. (2009). *The fleeing people in South Asia: Selections from Refugee Watch*. London: Anthem Press.

CDC (Centers for Disease Control and Prevention) (2012). An investigation into suicide among Bhutanese Refugees in the US 2009–2012. Stakeholders Report. Retrieved from www.refugeehealthta. org/files/2011/06/Bhutanese-Suicide-Stakeholder_Report_October_22_2012_Cleared_-For_ Dissemination.pdf

Children's Hospital of Philadelphia Policy Lab (2014). Building a healthcare navigation program with the Bhutanese refugees of Philadelphia. Retrieved from http://policylab.chop.edu/project/ building-healthcare-navigation-program-bhutanese-refugees-philadelphia

Hutt, M. (2003). *Unbecoming citizens: Culture, nationhood, and the flight of refugees from Bhutan*. New Delhi: Oxford University Press.

Hutt, M. (2005). The Bhutanese Refugees: Between verification, repatriation and royal realpolitik. *Peace and Democracy in South Asia, 1*(1). Retrieved from himalaya.socanth.cam.ac.uk/collections/ journals/pdsa/pdf/pdsa_01_01_05.pdf

Lee, J. & Stair, K. (2013). Health access and perceptions of newly arrived refugees in Philadelphia. Philadelphia Refugee Health Collaborative. Retrieved from philarefugeehealth.org/wp-content/ uploads/2014/08/PRHC-PA-DOH-Report-Sept-2013.pdf

ORR (Office of Refugee Resettlement) (2014). Refugee resettlement process. Retrieved from www. acf.hhs.gov/programs/orr

Pennsylvania Refugee Resettlement (2015). Demographics and arrival statistics. Retrieved from www. refugeesinpa.org/aboutus/demoandarrivalstats/index.htm

PRHC (Philadelphia Refugee Health Collaborative) (2013). Retrieved from http://philarefugeehealth.org/

Schinina, G., Sharma, S., Gorbacheva, O., & Mishra, A. K. (2011). Who am I? Assessment of psychosocial needs and suicide risk factors among Bhutanese refugees in Nepal and after the third country resettlement. International Organization for Migration. Retrieved from www.iom.int/files/live/sites/iom/files/What-We-Do/docs/Mental-Health-Assessment-Nepal_Final_11March.pdf

SEARAC (2011). *Needs assessment of refugee communities from Bhutan and Burma*. Conducted with the Intergenerational Center at Temple University. Retrieved from www.searac.org/new/searac-announces-new-report-needs-assessment-refugee-communities-bhutan-and-burma

Shrestha, C. (2011). Power and politics in resettlement: A case study of Bhutanese refugees in the USA. *New Issues in Refugee Research*, Research Paper No. 208; UNHCR Policy Development and Evaluation Service. Retrieved from www.unhcr.org/4dca7f129.html

Sinha, A. C. (2003). *Himalayan Kingdom Bhutan: Tradition, transition and transformation*. New Delhi: Indus Publishing Company.

Subedi, P., Kuikel, L., Paul, P., Shown, A., Kangovi, S., & Yun, K. (2014). The Bhutanese health focal points initiative: Lessons on starting a community-based healthcare navigation program. North American Refugee Health Care Conference (Presentation), Rochester, NY, June 2014.

UNHCR (United Nations High Commissioner for Refugees) (2015). Who we help: Refugees. Retrieved from www.unhcr.org/pages/49c3646c125.html

U.S. Department of Health and Human Services (1996). Health Insurance Portability and Accountability Act of 1996. Retrieved March 12, 2015 from www.hhs.gov/ocr/privacy/hipaa/administrative/statute/index.html

U.S. Department of State (2015a). Refugee admissions. Retrieved from www.state.gov/j/prm/ra/

U.S. Department of State (2015b). The reception and placement program. Retrieved from www.state.gov/j/prm/ra/receptionplacement/index.htm

U.S. Refugee Act of 1980 (2012). Retrieved from www.acf.hhs.gov/programs/orr/resource/the-refugee-act

Chapter 32

Research for health efforts in the West Bank, Palestine

Cindy Sousa

Context

Both social work and public health have the obligation to work across multiple levels to alleviate immediate symptoms of suffering while also working to locate and prevent the cause of the suffering. In line with this mandate, recently both fields have intensified their efforts to understand and address the fundamental ways that war and global conflict affect health. Inspired by this growing focus on global conflict, health, and social justice, I was compelled to explore the health effects of the ongoing conflict in Palestine, and to try to find ways to root the work in the principles of what Paul Farmer terms *pragmatic solidarity*: "the rapid deployment of our tools and resources to improve the health and well-being of those who suffer . . . violence" (Farmer, 2005, p. 221). I approached the effort with what I hoped to be a spirit of partnership and humility, knowing that outside researchers can often enter "the field" with colonialist or elitist approaches that alienate rather than assist. This chapter describes the resulting collaborative project that I undertook with one of the oldest and largest health care non-governmental organization (NGO) in Palestine, the Palestinian Medical Relief Society (PMRS). This case highlights how social work practitioners might develop partnerships in international public health settings to prevent and alleviate the health consequences of war. My work focused on two areas of practice: program development and advocacy efforts. These practice areas fulfill crucial roles within both social work and public health as these undertakings are entwined with our historical roots, ethical mandates, and multi-level frameworks for practice.

Description of setting

The West Bank, part of Palestine, is a region well known for its history of protracted conflict (for historical timeline of the conflict and an analysis of its relationship to health see Giacaman et al., 2009, and other articles in *The Lancet* series on health in Palestine). The West Bank is the site of persistent military occupation of civilian areas, which began in 1967 (Giacaman et al., 2009). Political conflicts and violence between Israel and Palestine (encompassing both the West Bank and Gaza) are ongoing.

Policy

In 1967, the Israeli Ministry of Defense took over the government-controlled portions of Palestine's health sector (previously controlled by the Egyptians in Gaza Strip and Jordanians in West Bank, with the presence of the UNRWA (UN Relief and Works Agency), private sector entities, and charities) until the Oslo Accords of 1993. In 1993, government control was officially transferred to the Palestinian Authority (PA). The PA inherited a system that was fundamentally ineffective, in large part due to the de-investment in the public sector under Israel's occupation. Examples of this include the facts that in 1967, more than 85% of health services in Palestine were delivered in the public sector; by 1991, under Israeli control, that number had shrunk to around 37% (World Bank, 1993). Between 1967 and 1993, there was also no increase in the number of beds in government hospitals (despite the population nearly doubling in the years 1970 and 1990), and government hospitals were only fully staffed an average of one or two days each week (World Bank, 1993). Health scholars charge this de-investment in the public sector was part of a larger Israeli policy of purposeful debilitation of a health system that would benefit and strengthen Palestinian infrastructure (Giacaman et al., 2009). Most problematic results are due to the fragmentation of health care within Palestine and the challenges this poses to coordination and planning. Health care is spread out over multiple sectors, including NGOs, programs and facilities, along with Ministry of Health clinics and hospitals; the UNRWA services; the military health system; and private clinics, doctors, and hospitals.

Nonetheless, health care provision might adequately meet the needs of the population if the occupation did not further cripple the delivery of health care through the requirements for permits and coordination to pass into areas both within the West Bank and between Israel and Palestine, along with the extensive series of checkpoints and roadblocks that are in place (Hamdan, Defever, & Abdeen, 2003). These physical impediments are such that, for example, in 2007, when this assessment began, the United Nations reported that more than one-third of the West Bank consisted of Israeli infrastructure, including checkpoints, road barriers, gates, and roadblocks (United Nations Office for the Coordination of Humanitarian Affairs (UN-OCHA) Occupied Palestinian Territories (oPt), 2007).

Organization

In light of the constant conflicts and strategies of de-development as well as the shifts in control and government structures, NGOs in Palestine have historically occupied an integral place in efforts for independence and the ability of the civil sector to organize itself. The empowerment of NGOs was both a strategic move to keep control of health infrastructure under Palestinian, rather than Israeli, control, and a way to utilize health as a way to promote community development and grassroots mobilization (Giacaman et al., 2009).

One of the oldest and largest Palestinian health care NGOs is the PMRS, established in 1979. Values of justice, equity, dignity, respect, inclusion, and centrality of marginalized people underlie PMRS. The agency also views health promotion as an important avenue for justice and development. These values inform the commitment of PMRS to a holistic advocacy-based approach that seeks to address the underlying determinants of the health of the Palestinian population rather than simply employing a biomedical model. PMRS operates a great many programs, including community-based rehabilitation, women's health, chronic disease, emergency, health education, and mental health. They also run a School of Community Health.

Description of the client situation

PMRS was well aware of the challenges they face. Several official international agencies have assessed the impacts of the conflict on health and the health care system. One of the most comprehensive reports was released by the Palestinian Health, Development, Information and Policy (HDIP) Institute, which assessed the effects of the closure policies, including the 8-metre high, 436-mile long concrete separation wall on which construction began in 2002. HDIP concluded that the path of the wall created or will create more than 25 enclaves that are effectively cut off from services, including seven communities that will have no access to any type of health care (HDIP, 2005). Other organizations, including the World Health Organization (WHO), Medecins du Monde, and various United Nations agencies, have also documented how, within the area of the West Bank itself, the wall and its associated divisions compromise access to regular preventive services, medication, pregnancy care, post-partum care, emergency care, and specialty services. Among the many impacts are the sheer loss of work time due to delays and incidents at checkpoints; for instance, between January 2007 and April 2008, medical personnel encountered 929 incidents at checkpoints, resulting in a loss of over 11,000 work-hours (UN-OCHA, 2008).

PMRS was also aware of the evidence about how the conflict affects Palestinian mental health, having heard from the many women they serve about the ways the conflict has created or contributed to anxiety, sadness, hopelessness, and increased anger and aggression within families. These reports from PMRS clients align with findings from the increasing body of scholarship about the mental health effects of conflict; the WHO concludes that one-third to one-half of those exposed to political violence will have some sort of mental health disorders due to the experience (WHO, 2001). While this was a known consequence of the situation of the organization, PMRS did have some questions related to mental health, including what the rates of exposure to political violence and the mental health consequences might be for their particular patient pool. PMRS also wanted to investigate the critical question of what types of protective factors their programs might build on to help promote resilience within their women's groups. To this end, in the assessment of mental health, I investigated exposure to political violence (past month and lifetime); various mental health consequences (including post-traumatic stress disorder (PTSD), distress, and an overall mental health measure); and many potential protective factors (proactive coping; self-reliance; reliance on political, family, and religious support; and political/civic engagement).

Decisions about practice

Definition of the client

PMRS provides leadership and operates an array of essential programs in a challenging environment. The conditions under which staff members work offer little time or human resources to embark on research or formal quality improvement. Thus, partnerships focused on research, advocacy, and program development are small but hopefully useful in helping to sustain the health of the organization and the people, families, and communities they serve. Yet, despite the practical advantages of partnerships such as the one fostered through this project, these types of relationships within social work and public health are full of relatively underexplored dynamics (Minkler, 2012; Stoecker, 1999). I fully intended that the partnership benefit PMRS, and I also hoped to emerge with data from which I might publish. Thus, I knew, as did PMRS, that I, like many others who regularly approach the agency (and indeed, like many who engage in research collaborations), stood to benefit far more than those with whom I collaborate. As the initiator of the project, I felt acutely aware of these types of tensions, and I conceived of the project with the goals of mutuality and collaboration.

Goals, objectives, and contracting

I knew well the often troubling relationships of outside volunteers and researchers, so my strategy was to lay out my qualifications and skills and to ask PMRS to dictate the focus of the partnership. When I approached Raniya,[1] my main contact (one of the lead administrators, who is trained as a social worker), I presented her with details of my skills and time frames. I asked her to consider projects that would most benefit the agency and its work. Under Raniya's suggestion, I began by meeting with lead administrators, along with many program directors and their staff. After visiting programs and having this series of exploratory meetings with program directors, staff, and volunteers, Raniya and I met to establish goals for the partnership. We decided that the overarching goal of my work would be to assess how the ongoing conflict in the region affects health and healthcare delivery; I would then apply findings to improve programs and advocate relevant policy modifications. This meant working on two primary tasks: (1) documenting and helping with advocacy regarding the challenges PMRS health care workers and administrators face due to the conflict; and (2) investigating the consequences of the conflict on women's mental health, subsequently using the results to assist PMRS' women's health and empowerment programs with developing and evaluating their services. Once the projects were agreed on, we completed a data sharing agreement. As I was the person who was leading the research arm of the project, I worked through the Human Subjects Division at my university (University of Washington), who approved all study procedures.

Strategies and interventions: overview

There were two distinct phases of the intervention: (1) the process of choosing the topics for exploration and methods by which to examine them; and (2) the process of disseminating findings and applying these to both practice and policy (see Figure 32.1). I will describe each phase below.

This project brought to light how, when one engages in solidarity work, commitments must be clearly articulated and consistently fulfilled. Like other populations who tend to be simultaneously over-studied and under-served, Palestinians experience research fatigue from the constant struggle against having their lives and contexts regarded simply as laboratories for data gathering, rather than locales where research helps in the struggle for social justice (Maira, 2013). In this context, I found that people, from study partners to participants, often met the research with considerable hesitancy. The most dramatic instance of this suspicion occurred early in one of our focus groups: when we told the women that we would be taping the dialogue (and asked them to omit names – both their own and others), one by one each of the women stood up and walked out.

Not all interactions were this dramatic, of course, but with striking regularity people asked how the findings of the assessment would better their lives. Most of the people I interviewed (and many of the patients who saw me observing), kindly asked (and in some cases, firmly demanded) that PMRS act on the findings by providing tangible projects and services. Because I was clearly a foreigner, many insisted I return home and tell people about what I was seeing. PMRS staff and volunteers were also clear that they viewed my work as not so much the programmatic research in Palestine, more, they wanted the findings liberally disseminated in the United States, where the issue is so poorly understood. It was clear they themselves already possessed an incredible amount of talent and also tenacity to persevere

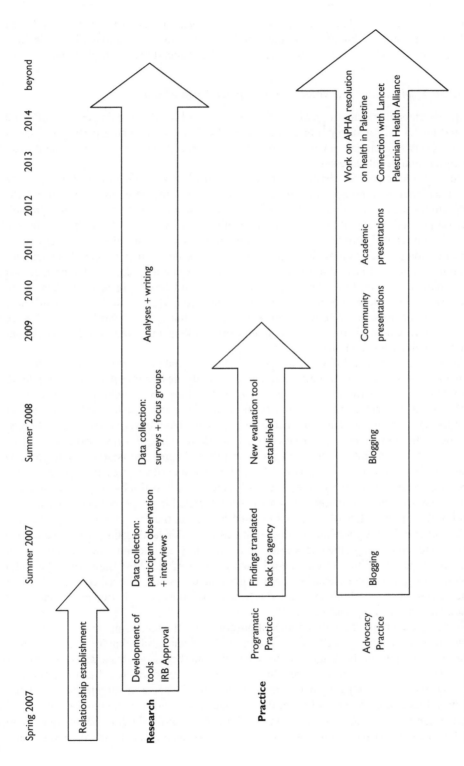

Figure 32.1 Timeline of project

even in the face of many challenges. Thus, the imperatives of this project were established not only with the agency, but also with the people with whom I strived to act in solidarity – imbuing the project with deep (and necessary) ethical and social justice implications.

Phase I: Data collection – activities, meeting places, use of time

When the partnership began, my main work was to assess how the ongoing conflict affected health and health care delivery. For this question, I collected data using participant observation, interviews, literature reviews, and analyses of secondary data from humanitarian, human rights, and health care agencies.

To conduct participant observation, I traveled with PMRS mobile clinics, traveled with medical personnel attempting to transfer a patient to a specialty care clinic, visited PMRS' standing clinics, traveled with and observed health care workers and administrators in their daily activities, and went with PMRS' mental health team to several of their sites to observe group and individual therapy sessions. Most observations of the mobile clinic teams consisted of full, long days – joining the team early in the morning as they prepared the vehicles and set out; eating breakfast with the team before they opened the clinic; watching them set up, serve patients, break down the clinic and pack up; and driving back with them in the vehicles. During my observation times, I conducted informal interviews with health care providers (e.g., doctors, lab technicians, nurses, and community health workers), ambulance drivers, health care administrators, and mental health workers. Interviews ranged from about 20 minutes to more than an hour.

In one case, I spent a full day with an incredible tour guide, Jaiyana, a woman who is a phenomenal leader in her community, and regularly dedicates hours upon hours to helping internationals with their research – all in the hopes that they do something useful with the findings. As she described the town, the conflict, and its effects on the well-being of her community, she generously shared her personal stories and reactions. For instance, as I noted in my blog, with obvious hurt in her voice, Jaiyana told us that Qalqiliya used to be a place where there was a great peace between Israelis and Palestinians, and Israelis would come to get their cars worked on or to buy plants. She told us that it used to be a city of peace. Yet it was also the first area to be targeted by the wall project. With justifiable anger, Jaiyana said it proves to her that the government of Israel is not interested in peace, but in confiscation of land and water. Jaiyana also told us about her family – about the very personal impact of the wall. Her father died this year, and his one wish was to see his land again before he died. He was not able to pass through the checkpoints to do this. Jaiyana told me how she had wanted desperately to get her mother to treatment in another part of the West Bank after she had a heart attack. Because of the closures, she was not able to do this. She asked me, "Can you imagine, sitting there watching someone die, when you know there is treatment that is not very far away, that you just can't get to?"

I also completed more than 50 participant observations at checkpoints in the West Bank, as a passenger in a taxi, ambulance, or mobile clinic. During checkpoint observations, I collected information on the length of the delay, the number of vehicles delayed, whether any of these vehicles were ambulances, how Israeli soldiers conducted the stops, and any special occurrences (i.e., apparent harassment, detentions, the apparent targeting of particular groups or individuals). The hours I spent doing these observations in the mobile clinics and ambulances gave me considerable time to talk with PMRS staff. Like Jaiyana, many of them shared with me the very real details about how the occupation affected their daily lives; many of them had to make considerably detailed plans to get to their workplace, and those who lived beyond checkpoints (of which there were many) often had to make contingency plans in case they could not get home after work.

During the following 2 years, I collected additional data for the separate project that investigated trauma, resilience, and health among Palestinian women using focus groups ($N = 32$) and surveys ($N = 122$). We conducted the focus groups and collected surveys at PMRS clinics. Data collected for the mental health project consisted of five focus groups, each lasting about an hour, and surveys that patients filled out in about 20–45 minutes. Upon my return to the United States, the remainder of the work needed to take place electronically. I used email to send various draft reports back and forth and to do some member-checking (asking participants to comment on my interpretations and whether they found my analysis valid). I also worked with my translators and assistants via Skype.

Phase II: Application of findings – activities, meetings places, use of time

The findings of this particular assessment echoed what PMRS staff has long known: the conflict has profound effects both on health care delivery and on the health status of civilians. In response to this, PMRS fashioned their work so as to develop and maximize creative, community-based strategies that can improve the health of communities despite the challenges they face. PMRS has always viewed health as a catalyst for community action. Their model exemplifies how complex health problems, such as those that war and conflict create and sustain, require solutions that simultaneously cut across multiple levels of intervention (individual, family, community).

Our findings illustrated how even creative, well-organized programming from strong local agencies cannot prevail over the health impacts of an ongoing conflict. Thus, this work highlighted the need to merge on-the-ground practice solutions with strong advocacy efforts. This task, in line with pragmatic solidarity (Farmer, 2005), was the main goal of the collaboration. The goal, shared by PMRS and me, was not to drastically alter their standing initiatives. Rather, there were two desired outcomes of the project: (1) for me to apply findings to policy advocacy activities, particularly within the United States and the international arena; and (2) for me to communicate findings back to PMRS program directors to assist them in evaluating, reporting on, and applying for additional funding for their programs.

On the policy advocacy side of this project, I worked to uphold some of the key essential functions of public health, including the tasks of building information, education, and empowerment for health and helping to mobilize partnerships and actions to promote health. As an international observer, I felt a particular responsibility to try to use findings to affect the political and social context within which these programs operated. I presented findings at both academic and non-academic conferences, published in peer-reviewed journals (Sousa, 2013; Sousa & Hagopian, 2011), and applied results to advocacy efforts within community settings and the American Public Health Association (APHA). Tasks within APHA included joining with others to present on the health effects of the conflict and helping to author a proposed resolution on health in Palestine. Our project explored the effects of the conflict on maternal and child health; mental health; the conditions in which Palestinians live (including poverty and unemployment); and health systems.

Regarding the implications for direct practice, I provided findings, along with developing evaluation tools and program reports, for the women's mental health and community development program. I had shadowed (observed, explored, and analyzed) the program during my time in the West Bank. I also provided findings to two programs that I worked with extensively for the first project on health care provision, the community health worker program, and the mobile clinic program, community-based initiatives that I highlighted in a peer-reviewed paper that was published as a result of this collaboration (Sousa & Hagopian, 2011).

I had originally envisioned this as a long-term partnership, and indeed it has become quite long term (see Figure 32.1). Each of the specific projects within the partnership took on longer timeframes than I had originally anticipated, as often happens in research in general and international research specifically. Indeed, partnerships, particularly those with aims for advocacy and program development, often take on a life of their own. While data were collected in 2007 and the initial article based on the findings was completed and published in 2011, advocacy efforts really took on an increased energy in 2012, 2013, and 2014, when I joined a team that was working on the issue within the APHA.

Stance of the social worker

This project demanded of me a renewed commitment to a stance that focused on respect and mutuality. While this has, of course, always been a priority within social work, the need for this stance became particularly acute in conflict zones. I particularly felt this in Palestine, where the ongoing conflict affects not only people's safety and freedom, but also infrastructure that supports research done by Palestinians. Here, I was acutely aware of the ethical risk that I would impose an outsider perspective, a legitimate critique of international research. Outside researchers in international contexts have been responsible for unsuitable decisions about all aspects of research; these uniformed research findings have then resulted in programmatic suggestions that are ill-fitting with the host culture and often ultimately short-lived (Weiss, Saraceno, Saxena, & van Ommeren, 2003).

To counter this dynamic, it was important that I consider my own positionality and outsider status (Stoecker, 1999). Unlike my research partners, I was free to come and go as I pleased. Travel around and in and out of the West Bank was relatively easy for me. My academic and professional training and endeavors were not interrupted by the restrictions many of my partners faced (checkpoints, financial constraints, school closures). Being honest and clear on these areas of access and privilege was central to this collaboration, as was attending to building long-term, close relationships and friendships to build the foundation for the project.

Challenging the lines between researcher and researched, I often asked both my official research partners and various respondents what they wished to happen with the results of the project. Answers ranged from interventions that PMRS could (and was) enact(ing) (more women's discussion groups, for instance) to interventions that depended on my responsible use of my outsider status (bringing this information to an international audience, educating people in the United States about the civilian costs of the conflict). In this way, the relationship between my partners and me reflected a consistent commitment on my part to honoring the principle of self-determination – always central to public health and social work, but imperative in a location such as Palestine.

Use of resources outside of the helping relationship

As noted, the primary objective here was to advance both practice and policy for PMRS; as such, connecting with outside resources was central. I shared findings with PMRS program leaders, funders, and current or potential PMRS volunteers, along with academics and community leaders in the United States working on the conflict (especially the health effects).

Particularly when the results of the project demanded efforts related to international education and advocacy around the health effects of the conflict, there was a need for outside resources. Ongoing involvement in both U.S.-based and international efforts has been essential to the effort. This work has included connecting with the Lancet Palestinian Health Alliance, launched in 2009 by the Lancet alongside the Institute of Community and Public Health based in Birzeit University, Palestine. This alliance supports research on health conditions by Palestinian public health scientists and leaders. The purpose of this initiative was to support networks between scientists in Palestine and scientists around the world. In the first report in the series, published in 2009, Richard Horton, Chief Editor of the Lancet noted that health could be the catalyst to promote peace and justice in the region, particularly for and with Palestinian people. This project also provided inspiration for continued work within the APHA, detailed above.

Transfer, termination, evaluation, and case conclusion

While the partnership remains, transfer from one contact person to another is frequent. Allowing time for relationships to build has been an important component of the work. In-person visits are central to building these; one challenge is certainly the time that has passed since my last trip. As yet, the work continues, and it likely will for some time, as one of the primary principles of this project was to create and maintain a lasting partnership. An enduring challenge is determining who is responsible for the relationship on behalf of the agency and how to make these connections last, particularly when in-person visits are not possible for long periods of time. Providing frequent updates is helpful, along with harnessing technology, including social media, to keep each other updated. We did not set up measurable outcomes for the project, but rather larger overarching goals about its uses (i.e., publications, professional, and scholarly presentations, written products for PMRS and its funders), all of which have been realized.

Differential discussion

Reflections on this case bring up several important pieces of learning. Despite my thorough theoretical and practical preparation on both a scholarly and a personal level, this case presented many surprises and challenges. This project made clear to me that engaging in international partnerships requires a great deal of time and energy, and justifiably so. It should not be entered into casually, or with the idea that one will drop in, collect data, leave to "do the work," and then move on. Gaining trust and entry in order to collect data, accurately representing findings, and diligently using them for the priorities outlined by those most affected by the problem at hand, all require not only sensitivity and humility, but also the kind of knowledge and relationships that only time can establish. Going into the project with more foresight around this reality would have enabled me to better navigate some of the logistical and relational challenges around international partnerships.

Other challenges also presented themselves, including issues around staff being suspicious of the project (as they thought we might be evaluating them, rather than their situations), issues about who represents the community and is allowed to speak and give consent on its behalf, and challenges around communication and follow-through: each of these challenges was heightened once the work had to take place via long distances. All of these, along with the usefulness and health of the collaboration itself, would have benefited if I had made a clearer arrangement at the outset. While the data-sharing agreement was quite a positive and important document, a Memorandum of Understanding (MOU) or some other written document might have further clarified some of the terms of the partnership. It should be noted that this, also, would be vulnerable to some of the challenges above, including who is authorized to commit to the scope of the work and partnership, and how accountability plays out across various arrangements of power. To be sure, this work benefits from some of the innovative and important work that health and social work scholars are doing around community-based research and around scholar–practice collaborations (see Minkler, 2012). These challenges notwithstanding, this case provided an example of the power of connecting internationally to promote knowledge and action across multiple levels of intervention.

Discussion questions

1   Political strife exists across the world. How does one make decisions about how research can help to ameliorate suffering as a result of such strife? What are one's duties politically?
2   War diminishes access to health care facilities while also creating more need for such facilities. How might you develop policy at an international level to recognize this reality and work to protect civilian populations?
3   An important ethical imperative of research is to respect and inform the researched population. Doing so can be challenging and often we must resort to informing the heads of programs or people in charge. How would you create and foster more direct connections between researchers and the communities they seek to research and assist?

Note

1 All names used in this chapter are changed to protect confidentiality.

References

Farmer, P. (2005). *Pathologies of power. Health, human rights and the new war on the poor*. Berkeley, CA: University of California Press.
Giacaman, R., Khatib, R., Shabaneh, L., Ramlawi, A., Sabri, B., Sabatinelli, G., Khawaja, M., & Laurance, T. (2009). Health status and health services in the occupied Palestinian territory. *The Lancet, 373*(9666), 837–849. doi: 10.1016/S0140-6736(09)60107-0
Hamdan, M., Defever, M., & Abdeen, Z. (2003). Organizing health care within political turmoil: the Palestinian case. *The International Journal of Health Planning and Management, 18*(1), 63–87.
HDIP (Health Development Information and Policy Institute). (2005). *Health and Segregation II: The impact of the Israeli separation wall on access to health care services*. Ramallah, Palestine: Health Development Information and Policy Institute (HDIP).
Maira, S. (2013). *Research ethics (report): A review of relevant research literature*. Birzeit, Palestine: Birzeit University. Retreived from: http://sites.birzeit.edu/research-ethics/images/doc/maira-enf.pdf
Minkler, M. (2012). *Community organizing and community building for health and welfare* (3rd edn.). Piscataway, NJ: Rutgers University Press.
Sousa, C. (2013). Political violence, health, and coping among Palestinian women in the West Bank. *American Journal of Orthopsychiatry, 83*(4), 505–519. doi: 10.1111/ajop.12048

Sousa, C. & Hagopian, A. (2011). Conflict, health care and professional perseverance: A qualitative study in the West Bank. *Global Public Health*, 1–14. doi: 10.1080/17441692.2011.574146

Stoecker, R. (1999). Are academics irrelevant? Roles for scholars in participatory research. *American Behavioral Scientist, 42*(5), 840–854. doi: 10.1177/00027649921954561

UN-OCHA (United Nations Office for the Coordination of Humanitarian Affairs). (2008). The Humanitarian Impact of the Barrier (West Bank, oPt). Retrieved from https://www.ochaopt.org/documents/barrier_report_july_2008.pdf

UN-OCHA Occupied Palestinian Territories (oPt) (2007). *The humanitarian impact on Palestinians of Israeli settlements and other infrastructure in the West Bank.* East Jerusalem: UN-OCHA OPT.

Weiss, M. G., Saraceno, B., Saxena, S., & van Ommeren, M. (2003). Mental health in the aftermath of disasters: Consensus and controversy. *The Journal of Nervous and Mental Disease, 191*(9), 611–615.

World Bank (1993). *Developing the Occupied Territories: An investment in peace*, vol. 6: *Human resources*. Washington, DC: The International Bank for Reconstruction and Development/The World Bank.

WHO (World Health Organization) (2001). *The world health report 2001 – Mental Health: New understanding, new hope*. Geneva: World Health Organization.

Resources

United Nations-Health, www.un.org/en/globalissues/health/
World Health Organzation, www.who.int/en/

Summary

Chapter 33

Conclusion

Judith L. M. McCoyd and Toba Schwaber Kerson

Use of the Practice in Context (PiC) framework

Applying the Practice in Context (PiC) framework allowed our contributors to share cases in a way that permits us to identify themes inherent in social work practice in health settings. It also let them reflect on often overlooked contextual aspects of practice decisions. We believe the PiC framework helps social workers identify explicitly the constraints and possibilities of context and recognize how it influences decisions. By seeing how these seasoned social workers made practice decisions in the cases they presented here, we may infer something akin to best practices in social work in health care.

Context – constituted in the PiC as policy, technology, and organization – frames the work but is not static. Policies constrain and enable, but they also evolve. Our authors show that when the social worker is creative, flexible, willing to make the extra effort, and is competent and respected within the team, advocacy can be effective, policies changed, and win–win situations created. From Schlup's extraordinary familiarity with adoption policies (Chapter 3) that allowed her to advocate and manage her client's adoption desires, to Miller and Addis's use of policy to advocate for their patient to receive a liver transplant (Chapter 15), to Brooks and McCoyd's suggestions for new policies regarding palliative care and hospice (Chapter 22), our authors engage policy in ways that respect its purpose and understand its malleability.

Technology developments affect each client's diagnoses, their functional abilities, and the course of their diseases or disabilities, and social workers must therefore understand each of those aspects of clients' lives. Helping clients cope with the use and results of technology is a major social work role, as is advocating for equitable access to technology. At the same time, technology may raise ethical dilemmas for social workers. Technological innovations may allow clients to live longer, but they guarantee neither fine life quality nor client interest in using the latest technology. Fetal surgery may allow babies to be born who would otherwise have suffered and possibly died, but this is not without great cost to the mother and her family, as Inglis, Hertzog, and Ousley (Chapter 4) illustrate. Similarly, neonatal nurseries can keep an infant's body alive, but cannot allow that child to have a fully engaged life when there are major cognitive deficits, leading to challenges for the parents (and their social workers), as Stewart so ably portrays (Chapter 5). Likewise, Wilkenfeld (Chapter 8) demonstrates the ethical issues involved in enlisting the patient/client's involvement in use of technologies and how even the most expensive technology fails if it is not used. Maus and Kerson (Chapter 20) also illustrate (along with Brooks and McCoyd) how technologies at the end of life have the potential to harm more than help and that comfort care with psychosocial support ("high touch" as Maus refers to it) can assure that social workers follow our duty to respect the dignity and worth of humans and work to enhance a client's well-being while also respecting the client's right to self-determination.

Overall, the case chapter authors take great pride in their organizations, the teams of which they are a part, and the work they do. The team at Children's Hospital of Philadelphia, (CHOP) (Chapter 6) are clear that they not only work together, but truly enjoy the time they spend together and the organization of which they are a part. Sometimes, the organizations that provide physical care cannot provide necessary, on-going psychosocial support and many of our authors have found collaborative ways to assist clients through modified private practices such as Healy's work with individuals pursuing gender-conforming medical care (Chapter 12), Werner-Lin and Merrill's work to support those with genetic diagnoses that add layers of uncertainty to life and family relationships (Chapter 9), or Harris and Durkin's work with individuals coping with dementia (Chapter 21). On the occasions where explicit policies or traditional practices of the organization conflict with clients' needs, social workers work to protect clients from the organization or its staff, as when Fenstermacher supports consultation with other medical providers (Chapter 7) or when Cunningham extends her boundaries beyond what organizational policies allow (Chapter 19). In the current stingy environment where psychosocial services are limited and economic supports are tight, social workers must be creative and more thoughtful than ever about advocacy and the interpretation of policy. These areas of context – policy, technology, and organization – continue to frame and circumscribe the work social workers do, while also challenging social workers to think broadly about how to influence each area as well.

In direct work with clients, social workers' practice decisions define the work and are grounded in hope. Ideally, they are tenacious and unrelenting, even when others have given up. Social workers lend the vision of a better future when clients are dispirited and hopeless, as when Sousa brings hope to Palestinians unable to access health care (Chapter 32) or when Hahn persistently supports the morale of a severely burned young man who needs to believe he can live successfully (Chapter 10). Social workers sometimes risk crossing professional lines (sometimes just flexing boundaries and other times challenging authority) to help clients reach goals (as Cunningham (Chapter 19), Findley (Chapter 17), and Barker (Chapter 29) all illustrate dramatically). We worry about becoming too close to patients and thus compromising their care (and we are professional enough to recognize the concern and attend to it). We are also boundary spanners, willing to assume tasks outside our professional purview in order to support the work in professional ways. Recent interprofessional education research indicates that professionals who "practice at the top of their license" are valued by patients and colleagues (Robert Wood Johnson Foundation, 2015); this means that in the service of a patient's well-being they expand their practice into areas where they are needed and capable of developing competence quickly. Across the board, social workers understand that we must support a client's motivation and sometimes get the client's family to buy in to the goals and objectives of the work. We also know that sometimes we need to do the same thing with our health care teams.

Social workers must remain flexible, altering our views about the definition of the client, where the work can happen, who can be included, what outside resources to use, and how to manage the time frame. Several of our contributors are involved with camps and other extended day services that have them go well beyond a typical social work role. (See Xenakis' work with young women with disabilities in Chapter 11; Ciporen's creative programming for children with diabetes in Chapter 26; Boyd and Kerson's involvement with children managing asthma in Chapter 27; and Livingston and her colleagues' willingness to attend a week-long camp for children with epilepsy in Chapter 28.) Team and interdisciplinary work has never been more important. Social workers understand the need to enlist the help of other professionals, organizations, friends, and family members in order to make things happen.

Case chapter authors universally demonstrated their professionalism and their humility in disclosing decisions about practice that, in retrospect, seem less than ideal and different from what they would do now. Cunningham (Chapter 19) and Fenstermacher (Chapter 7) are especially articulate about how they stretched their boundaries, and now see those practice decisions to have yielded mixed results that could have been better. This confirmed to us the place of the differential discussion at the end of every case; we see again the benefit when we take time to reflect upon and evaluate the practice decisions we made in each case and to consider what we might do differently in a similar situation. The "decisions of practice" section of the PiC is designed to guide such reflection, providing a structure to consider everything from the definition of the client through the interventions and outside resources one used and the ways time and meeting places influenced the work.

Themes of best practice

This edition of our casebook, like its predecessors, demonstrates that social workers in health care are compassionate and committed professionals able to assume new roles even as we remain committed to the values and ethics of the profession. We analyzed the themes that emerged from the cases in the four previous editions of this casebook (McCoyd & Kerson, 2013), and we found five themes that characterized the work of seasoned health social workers:

- Theme 1: The conscious use of self as a catalyst for patient/client progress.
- Theme 2: A willingness to engage in authentic relationships with patients/clients.
- Theme 3: Self-reflection and use of professional consultation to manage boundary issues from self-disclosure to over-involvement.
- Theme 4: The willingness to use the time and energy to advocate for patients/clients.
- Theme 5: A profound commitment to self-determination and autonomy, even when patients/clients make what seem like poor decisions.

These themes also appear throughout this latest edition of the *Social Work in Health Settings* casebook. Below, we discuss these perennial themes and then report new themes we see reflected in this edition.

Theme 1: The conscious use of self as a catalyst for patient/client progress

This refers to utilizing one's skills in deliberate, specific ways that match the needs of the context and the client. Every chapter in this casebook shows how the social worker tailored her or his work to meet the needs of the client/patient. From Fenstermacher's (Chapter 7), Cunningham's (Chapter 19), and Barker's (Chapter 29) extension of self into emotionally demanding and professionally risky circumstances through Werner-Lin and Merrill's (Chapter 9) and Scarvalone, Oktay, Scott, and Helzlsouer's (Chapter 13) movement into new roles in genetics that require learning new material, our contributors are willing to extend themselves, learn new things, and be flexible about their roles and ways to use themselves to catalyze positive change. Likewise, when Moulton (Chapter 14) realizes that a peer who has survived gynecological cancer may be better able than she to support women at the time of diagnosis, she arranges to train and support such volunteers to do so. Lee and Subedi (Chapter 31) recognize that community members can do powerful work with immigrants as they become accustomed to societal services and expectations in a new country. Using oneself as a catalyst to promote relationships (to be a liaison between groups) is another way we social workers consciously modify our roles and behaviors to promote positive change.

Although most obvious when life-threatening illness is present, palliative intervention (work to comfort and relieve suffering) is an inherent part of social work practice and thus is a core feature the conscious use of self. Social workers intervene to both comfort and cause reflection, sometimes moving the client and his or her supporters to an uncomfortable realization that (hopefully) precedes some significant degree of relief. Schlup (Chapter 3) helped Chris meet with the court to relinquish her triplets; Stewart (Chapter 5) helped Brooklyn's parents bring her home and eventually allow her to die comfortably; Ray and Condon (Chapter 16) helped veteran RF realize that her bronchiolitis would be chronic and that to avoid persistent impairment she needed to make healthy changes in lifestyle; and Fisher (Chapter 30) provided accurate, non-alarmist information in the face of pediatric exposures to substances that parents fear will damage or kill their children. In each of these cases (and many others) social workers use themselves in conscious ways to inform, gently confront, nudge, and on occasion urge people to recognize and adjust to dire circumstances. Recognition achieved and changes begun, the social worker can then assume more often the role of comforter as the patient/client grapples with circumstances in a realistic manner.

Theme 2: A willingness to engage in authentic relationships with patients/clients

This refers to the social worker's authenticity and genuine empathy, positive regard and interaction in the relationship with the client. Our contributors do not hold themselves apart from their clients, lording expertise and access to services over clients. To the contrary, they engage clients in relationships based on partnership and mutual respect. This is guided by social work's commitment to respect the dignity and worth of all human beings and to honor a client/patient's right to self-determination. Yet our contributors go beyond mere adherence to the NASW Code of Ethics. Within professional requirements to be appropriate and to disclose about themselves only what will help the client, they engage fully and authentically. They eschew "professional distance," employing humor in purposeful ways, for example (Fenstermacher, Chapter 7; Harris and Durkin, Chapter 21), and care about their clients beyond the circumscribed, medical reasons that brought them together originally. There is ample evidence that these qualities of positive regard, empathy, and authenticity can themselves induce positive change (Sudberry, 2002).

Theme 3: Self-reflection and use of professional consultation to manage boundary issues from self-disclosure to over-involvement

This involves the social worker's willingness to be open and vulnerable in the supervisory relationship, a pre-condition of using supervision to grow in one's professional role and modify oneself to consciously practice in a way that most effectively helps clients. This requires a healthy degree of humility. Fenstermacher (Chapter 7) and Cunningham (Chapter 19) are most articulate about the questions they have about their own practice and the ways they used peer supervision and reflection to consider having allowed their boundaries to drop enough that they had difficulties maintaining their professional roles. Still others name the influence of supervisors and colleagues (Birmingham et al., Chapter 6 and Barker, Chapter 29) as enabling them to do the emotionally consuming work they must do.

Theme 4: The willingness to use the time and energy to advocate for patients/clients

Advocacy can be directed at changing social and/or organizational policies, creating new programs for underserved clients, or providing liaison with additional resources: the tenacious social worker is creative, flexible, and willing to span boundaries to promote the best outcomes for the clients they serve. Even when their organizations do not value the advocacy role, good social workers know its importance. This grows from our professional commitment to social justice and our belief in the dignity and worth of all human beings (NASW Code of Ethics, 2008). Sometimes advocacy is on the micro level, as when Cunningham (Chapter 19) worked exceptionally hard to assure that Junior got treatment for his congestive heart failure even when the physician refused to admit him for treatment as punishment for non-compliance. The work of Miller and Addis (Chapter 15) in advocating with policymakers and their team to enable Mark's liver transplant, or Ray and Condon's (Chapter 16) work to promote understanding that RF's symptoms were not the result of psychosomatic illness are also examples of good case advocacy. These social workers extended themselves and their work to understand the policies that needed to be changed (or circumvented) on behalf of their clients. In this sense, they went beyond the boundaries of their organizations – in Sousa's case (Chapter 32) beyond the boundaries of her country – to advocate for similar clients in the future. This said, case advocacy, especially, has important ethical boundaries, the most important of which is respect for procedural justice. Ethical advocacy does not use special access to secure favorable treatment for one client at the expense of others similarly situated. Attempts to help clients "jump" a fairly determined queue for services or benefits run afoul of fairness (Lipsky, 1980) and require the social worker to advocate for better circumstances for all who are in similar circumstances.

Theme 5: A profound commitment to self-determination and autonomy, even when patients/clients make what seem like poor decisions

The commitment to client self-determination is part of the ethical foundational of social work, but is often difficult to maintain within settings where medical staff think the social worker's job is to convince patients to comply with the treatment plan. The challenge of supporting clients who may seem to act against their best interest is illustrated by Cunningham (Chapter 19), who supported Junior even when he was not compliant with medical care, and Brooks (Chapter 22), who despite her strong disagreement, continues to honor Lisa's decision to avoid hospice care. Burgos (Chapter 25) refrained from expressing disapproval when Ms. Garcia continued her relationship with abusive Juan, instead helping her consider the pros and cons of the relationship and its effects on Ms. Garcia and her children.

The social workers who contributed to this casebook revisit such decisions to be sure that clients are aware of their ramifications and that they, too, take opportunities to reconsider. But good social workers never punish clients for making poor decisions; they avoid paternalistically forcing rigid adherence to treatment. As DeBonis, Zerden, and Jones point out about smoking cessation (Chapter 18), room for relapse and failure permits important lessons to be learned about how to go forward.

New themes of Practice in Context

As illustrated above, this new edition of the book reflects the significant themes we identified in its predecessors. In addition, three others have emerged in this edition: assuring informed consent, "thinking globally, acting locally," and promoting self and team care to enable good client care.

Assuring informed consent

Social workers now seem more aware of how the concept of informed consent is integral to their work. One aspect of effecting informed consent is to assure understanding. No one questions the need for translators and interpreters when a patient speaks another language, and the world of health care has its own jargon and culture that patients must negotiate. Just like people learning a new language, patients may indicate understanding when it is in fact quite limited. According to the National Assessment of Adult Literacy, only 12% of U.S. adults have proficient health literacy (U.S. Department of Health and Human Services, 2015). Social workers must translate this information, helping parents understand a medical team's sense of medical futility (see Stewart, Chapter 5), homeless adults understand the stability necessary for medication regimens to be effective (see Barker, Chapter 29), and children understand the need for exercise and dietary restrictions (see Ciporen, Chapter 26). Fisher (Chapter 30) states the matter clearly: "Much of the PEHSU work centers on translating the complex language of environmental issues into understandable concepts for a wide range of audiences." Indeed, nearly every chapter has some instance of the social worker acting as translator between medical team members and the client constellation. In Moulton's chapter (Chapter 14) on women cancer survivors who volunteer with newly diagnosed women, translation from English to Spanish took place, along with "translation" of health literacy (as the volunteers and social worker assessed the patient's understanding of her medical condition), and between the patient and the medical provider (as the patient's physician was helped to see the limitations of the patient's understanding). Informed consent requires complete understanding of the potential benefits and challenges of treatment, and social workers have a major role in helping medical systems assure that full informed consent is gained prior to onset of treatment. This is a critical legal aspect of care that protects patients from manipulation and health care institutions from litigation.

Assuring informed consent also involves helping clients/patients process health information in view of their life circumstances and values. In this way, social workers assure that consent is informed not only about medical risks, but by the patient's awareness of how life changes, family dynamics, and other non-medical aspects of life must be considered in the risks/benefits calculation that underlies informed consent. This is particularly apparent in the chapters on genetics by Scarvalone, Oktay, Scott, and Helzlsouer (Chapter 13) and Werner-Lin and Merrill (Chapter 9), yet many contributors identify how social workers assure that patients are aware of the potential impacts of adherence or non-adherence to recommended medical treatments. The ethic of patient self-determination is predicated on the patient's full understanding of psychosocial barriers to care and adherence (e.g., fear/anxiety, substance involvement, family tensions, social stigma) and not just the medical implications of care. As Werner-Lin and Merrill point out:

> At-risk families wishing to decline all testing or screening for either themselves or their children pose a challenge to the genetic counselor or physician, as it is difficult to know if they are making informed decisions for reasons consistent with their personal values, if they have limited resources or information, or if decisions were based on misperceptions (p. 123).

Helping patients identify how their psychosocial context may affect planned medical treatment, and helping them manage psychosocial outcomes and navigate family dynamics related to medical care are all clearly within the social work role.

Think globally, act locally

The necessity to "think globally, act locally" is a theme that emerges most insistently but not exclusively from our contributors in public health. Pockett and Beddoe (2015) call for global sociological thinking in social work, noting that health disparities are growing worldwide and that our commitment to social justice requires social workers to intervene across micro, policy, research, and advocacy dimensions of practice. This approach is obvious in Lee and Subedi's work (Chapter 31) and Sousa's (Chapter 32), but also in Chapters 24–30, which focus on population-level interventions for particular groups. This theme is implicit in many other chapters as well, particularly Birmingham et al.'s (Chapter 6) work with HIV-positive children, children who, thanks to a combination of medical technology and public health efforts, are now seldom infected at birth. Many chapters discuss programs designed to help members of marginalized populations access quality care; indeed, Chapters 11–18 all demonstrate responses to larger population needs that our contributors managed on the micro level, yet each identified mezzo and macro interventions as well.

The PiC framework promotes such attention to the larger social context. On the transdisciplinary team, our distinct ethical call is to attend to social justice implications and to advocate for social justice. This requires that we take a broader view than a strictly medical one: we are to identify the places where poverty, oppression, and polarization of economic goods and services mean that populations and individuals are being short-changed. We are called to identity where, when, and how injustice occurs, to advocate for equity, and intervene to minimize negative impacts on our most vulnerable societal members. Our contributors show how this can be done in health settings.

Care for self/team to enable care of the client

A last theme whispers through our new contributors' work: to enable the best care for our clients we must assure self-care and care of our teams. Social workers have long made reference to the airline safety slogan that passengers must "put their own oxygen mask on before helping others." In Chapter 6, contributors from Children's Hospital of Philadelphia show that self-care promotes teamwork and prevents compassion fatigue when working with a traumatized and economically challenged population. Recognizing that the care team's morale matters, members plan lunches and special outings for the whole team. Hospice and palliative care social workers have long known that attention to self-care enables them to continue with such emotionally challenging and occasionally draining work (Vachon, 2011, 2015). Vachon (2015) recognizes the temptation to use substances, screen time, and isolation to escape the intensity of the work, and emphasizes that healthy ways of dealing with work stressors include exercise and physical activity, willingness to take time off, and meditative and reflective practices. She identifies the traits of "exquisite empathy" with good boundaries, resilience, and spirituality, as qualities that enable compassionate practice. She encourages social workers to attend to their "compassion satisfaction," the satisfaction we get from helping others. By monitoring and protecting compassion satisfaction, we can avoid compassion fatigue. Vachon does not see "venting" or otherwise focusing on the negative aspects of work or its frustrations as helpful. Instead, enjoying and returning the support of colleagues is constructive (Vachon, 2015).

Although our contributors only occasionally mention the need for self-care, it is clear they all know that authentic relationships require emotional energy, creativity, and work, requirements that make self-care imperative. Barker's experience (Chapter 29) is a nice example: the faith in purpose required to spend years reaching out to an individual with serious mental illness who is sometimes abusive and whose progress is slow and sporadic, depends on consistent self-care.

Angelo McClain, the CEO of NASW, recently observed:

> An organizational commitment to wellness not only empowers staff, but addresses important organizational goals, such as improving retention and increasing productivity. In fact, focusing on social worker wellness is a win-win-win situation, because social workers with lower levels of stress are more productive in their work with clients and more committed to the organization. (2015, July, p. 3)

As this suggests, strategies of self-care are important, but so is institutional support for it. Social workers who have supervisory and program development roles must work to ensure that their colleagues have opportunities to process the frustration that comes with working in resource-poor, unjust social worlds with angry, traumatized, ill, and frightened people. Health organizations should be sure that team members can support one another through challenging cases and times, perhaps in the manner of the lunches and outings enjoyed by the CHOP team. These efforts at self- and team-care support good morale and allow social workers to extend themselves for their clients, even when doing so is frustrating and requires significant energy over a long time.

Conclusion

In retrospect, each case chapter reaffirms the utility of the PiC framework. The context of social work in health care has three primary dimensions: policy, technology, and organization. Together these elements provide parameters for practice decisions that social workers and clients make to determine the structure of their work. The practice decisions are often seen as "givens," yet the PiC forces its users to consciously consider how they define who the client(s) is/are, how objectives and outcome measures are developed, what and how the contract is established, how meeting place and use of time affect the work, what strategies and interventions to employ, how to consciously use oneself to catalyze change (hence varying the stance of the social worker), how to mobilize outside resources, and how to reassess the effectiveness of each of these decisions throughout the case. In considering the case termination and using the differential discussion to consider each of these decisions, social workers are helped to reflect on lessons learned for that case that may carry over to other similar cases in the future. In sum, a large measure of the art of social work is the ability to structure the relationship between social worker and client in ways that maximally support the work. To do this, social workers must be able to understand, influence, and alter many dimensions of practice in context.

Social work in health care settings is undoubtedly changing as a result of economic pressures in health care. Health organizations are less willing to fund social work departments to do work they may not always recognize as critical to the well-being of patients. Judd and Sheffield (2010) found that discharge planning was the primary social work role in hospitals in the United States after "reengineering." They found little evidence that social workers were used to assess patients' understanding of their diagnoses or the process of adjusting to disease. Social workers were minimally involved in the institutions' processes of bioethical reflection, nor did they do systematic advocacy or intervene to minimize health disparities. Still, recent work in Australia affirms that even one-shot social work contacts can utilize such interventions as these contacts, lasting from a half hour to nearly an hour and a half, yield interventions including assessment (30%), case management and coordination (22%), counseling (11%), and advocacy (11%) (Plath & Gibbons, 2010). Our chapter authors give us hope that the "high touch" of social work interventions continue to comfort and assist patients. Even as Judd and Sheffield lament the loss of traditional social work roles and interventions in health care, we see good role models exemplified by the work of our case contributors. We trust that students reading this text will be guided by the PiC framework and the cases in this book to make practice decisions that support the best outcomes for clients/patients.

References

Judd, R. G. & Sheffield, S. (2010). Hospital social work: Contemporary roles and professional activities. *Social Work in Health Care, 49*(9), 856–871. doi: 10.1080/00981389.2010.499825

Lipsky, M. (1980). *Street level bureaucracy: Dilemmas of the individual in public service.* New York: Russell Sage Foundation.

McClain, A. (2015, July). Wellness requires a multifaceted approach. *NASW News, 60*(7), p. 3.

McCoyd, J. L. M. & Kerson, T. S. (2013). Teaching reflective social work practice in health care: Promoting best practices. *Journal of Social Work Education, 49*(4), 674–688. doi: org/10.1080/10 437797.2013.812892

NASW (National Association of Social Workers) (2008). Code of ethics. Washington, DC: NASW Press.

Plath, D. & Gibbons, J. (2010). Discoveries on a data-mining expedition: Single session social work in hospitals. *Social Work in Health Care, 49*(8), 703–717. doi: 10.1080/00981380903520525

Pockett, R. & Beddoe, L. (2015). *Social work in health care: An international perspective. International Social Work.* Published on-line before print, 0020872814562479, February 16, 2015. doi: 10.1177/0020872814562479

Robert Wood Johnson Foundation (2015). Lessons from the Field: Promising Interprofessional Collaboration Practices. Retrieved from www.rwjf.org/en/library/research/2015/03/lessons-from-the-field.html

Sudberry, J. (2002). Key features of therapeutic social work: The use of relationship. *Journal of Social Work Practice, 5,* 231–262.

U.S. Department of Health and Human Services. (2015). Quick guide to health literacy. Retrieved from www.health.gov/communication/literacy/quickguide/factsbasic.htm

Vachon, M. L. S. (2011). Four decades of selected research in hospice/palliative care: Have the stressors changed? In I. Renzenbrink (Ed.), *Caregiver stress and staff support in illness, dying, and bereavement* (pp. 1–19). New York: Oxford University Press.

Vachon, M. L. S. (2015). Care of the caregiver: Professionals and family members. In J. M. Stillion & T. Attig (Eds.), *Death, dying, and bereavement: Contemporary perspectives, institutions, and practices* (pp. 379–393). New York: Springer Publishing.

Index